CW00867585

Anesthesiology

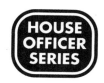

Anesthesiology

EDITORS

Arnold J. Berry, M.D.

Associate Professor of Anesthesiology
Department of Anesthesiology
Emory University Hospital
Atlanta, Georgia

Gundy B. Knos, M.D.

Department of Anesthesiology
The Emory Clinic
Atlanta, Georgia

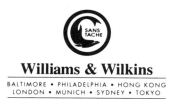

Williams & Wilkins

BALTIMORE • PHILADELPHIA • HONG KONG
LONDON • MUNICH • SYDNEY • TOKYO

A WAVERLY COMPANY

Editor: Charles W. Mitchell
Managing Editor: Linda S. Napora
Copy Editor: Anne K. Schwartz
Designer: Dan Pfisterer
Illustration Planner: Ray Lowman
Production Coordinator: Charles E. Zeller

Copyright © 1995
Williams & Wilkins
428 East Preston Street
Baltimore, Maryland 21202, USA

All rights reserved. This book is protected by copyright. No part of this book may be reproduced in any form or by any means, including photocopying, or utilized by any information storage and retrieval system without written permission from the copyright owner.

Accurate indications, adverse reactions, and dosage schedules for drugs are provided in this book, but it is possible that they may change. The reader is urged to review the package information data of the manufacturers of the medications mentioned.

Printed in the United States of America

Library of Congress Cataloging in Publication Data

Anesthesiology / Arnold J. Berry, Gundy B. Knos.
     p.   cm. — (House officer series)
  Includes index.
  ISBN 0-683-01018-2
  1. Anesthesiology. I. Berry, Arnold J. II. Knos, Gundy B.
III. Series.
  [DNLM: 1. Anesthesia. WO 200 A5728 1994]
RD81.A5423   1994
617.9′6—dc20
DNLM/DLC
for Library of Congress   94-7759
                                              CIP

95 96 97 98
1 2 3 4 5 6 7 8 9 10

Preface

Since Dr. Crawford Long administered the first ether anesthetic in 1842 in Jefferson, Georgia, a small community 60 miles northeast of Atlanta, anesthesiology has matured into a medical specialty with more than 30,000 physician practitioners. Our understanding of anesthetic pharmacology and the development of new technology has made anesthesia safer for patients and has made more invasive and complex surgical procedures possible. Paralleling the growth of the specialty, there has been a proliferation of textbooks and journals adding to and synthesizing information for students of anesthesiology.

In addition to these resources, we believe that it is necessary to have a concise, practical, clinically oriented text for students and residents. We are pleased that this book in the House Officer series was written and edited by individuals who are current or former faculty, fellows, or residents in the Department of Anesthesiology at Emory University School of Medicine. The authors have drawn upon their knowledge and experience to cover the most important areas of perioperative anesthetic management. It has been our pleasure as editors to work with our colleagues to put together a resource for students and residents learning about the practice of anesthesiology. We hope that this information will provide a basis for further study using the References or Suggested Readings included with most chapters.

We would like to thank the chapter authors and their secretaries who have worked to make this book possible. We also thank our secretaries, Louise Evans, Cathy Hefner, and Joy Ramsey, who have assisted us in the editorial process. Finally, we would like to acknowledge the help of the editorial and production staff at Williams & Wilkins for their assistance and encouragement on this project.

Arnold J. Berry, M.D.
Gundy B. Knos, M.D.

Contributors

Carolyn F. Bannister, M.D.
Assistant Professor of Anesthesiology, Emory University School of Medicine, Atlanta, Georgia

Arnold J. Berry, M.D.
Associate Professor of Anesthesiology, Emory University School of Medicine, Atlanta, Georgia

John T. Bonner, M.D.
Associate Professor of Anesthesiology, Assistant Professor of Surgery, Emory University School of Medicine, Chief of Anesthesia Services, Veterans Administration Medical Center, Atlanta, Georgia

Stuart Bramwell, M.D.
Assistant Professor of Anesthesiology, Assistant Professor of Gynecology and Obstetrics, Emory University School of Medicine Atlanta, Georgia

Barry W. Brasfield, M.D.
Private Practice, Johnson City, Tennessee

Grace W. Brown, M.D.
Department of Anesthesiology, Carolinas Hospital System, Florence, South Carolina

Mary V. Clemency, M.D.
Assistant Professor of Anesthesiology, Emory University School of Medicine, Clinical Director of Anesthesia, Grady Memorial Hospital, Atlanta, Georgia

Boleslaus A. Falinski, M.D.
Anesthesiologists Associated of Chattanooga, Attending Anesthesiologist, Memorial Hospital, Parkridge Medical Center, Chattanooga, Tennessee, North Park Hospital, Hickson, Tennessee, Hutchison Medical Center, Rossville, Georgia

Ghaleb A. Ghani, M.D.
Associate Professor of Anesthesiology, Emory University School of Medicine, Associate Clinical Director, Anesthesia for Surgical Specialties, Emory University Hospital, Atlanta, Georgia

James R. Hall, M.D.
Associate Professor of Anesthesiology, Emory University School of Medicine, Atlanta, Georgia

William D. Hammonds, M.D.
Associate Professor of Anesthesiology, Emory University School of Medicine, Atlanta, Georgia

Dean M. Harless, M.D.
Department of Anesthesiology, Grady Memorial Hospital, Atlanta, Georgia

Allen H. Hord, M.D., F.A.C.P.M.
Director for Division of Pain Medicine, Department of Anesthesiology, Emory University Hospital, Atlanta, Georgia

Ira J. Isaacson, M.D.
Associate Professor of Anesthesiology, Deputy Chairman of Clinical Services, Emory University School of Medicine, Associate Chief of Anesthesia Services, Emory University Hospital, Atlanta, Georgia

Debra Jones, M.D.
Department of Anesthesiology, Emory University School of Medicine, Atlanta, Georgia

Georgina Odom Kesterson, M.D.
Assistant Professor
Department of Anesthesiology, Emory University School of Medicine, Atlanta, Georgia

Gundy B. Knos, M.D.
Assistant Professor of Anesthesiology, Emory University School of Medicine, Atlanta, Georgia

Scott M. Kreger, M.D.
Assistant Professor of Anesthesiology, Emory University School of Medicine, Atlanta, Georgia

Diane L. Lefebvre, M.D.
Scottish Rite Children's Hospital, Atlanta, Georgia

Thomas J. Mancuso, M.D.
Assistant Professor of Anesthesiology, Assistant Professor of Pediatrics, Emory University School of Medicine, Atlanta, Georgia

Deborah A. McClain, M.D.
Assistant Professor of Anesthesiology, Emory University School of Medicine, Atlanta, Georgia

Ann Marie McKenzie, M.D.
Assistant Professor of Anesthesiology, Emory University School of Medicine, Atlanta, Georgia

John G. Morrow III, M.D.
Assistant Professor of Anesthesiology, Emory University School of Medicine, Atlanta, Georgia

Amy Mortensen, M.D.
Staff Anesthesiologist, National Naval Medical Center, Assistant Professor of Anesthesiology, Uniformed Services University of the Health Sciences, Bethesda, Maryland

Albert H. Santora, M.D.
Associate Professor of Anesthesiology, Emory University School of Medicine, Atlanta, Georgia

Michael Schneider, M.D.
DeKalb Anesthesia, Decatur, Georgia

Yung-Fong Sung, M.D.
Associate Professor of Anesthesiology, Emory University School of Medicine, Chief of Anesthesia Services, Ambulatory Surgery Center, The Emory Clinic, Atlanta, Georgia

Brian L. Thomas, M.D.
Assistant Professor, Department of Anesthesiology, Emory University Hospital, Atlanta, Georgia

Steven R. Tosone, M.D.
Assistant Professor of Anesthesiology, Emory University School of Medicine, Chief of Anesthesia Services, Henrietta Egleston Hospital at Emory University, Atlanta, Georgia

Karen R. Trulson, M.D.
Assistant Professor of Anesthesiology, Emory University School of Medicine, Atlanta, Georgia

Steven Weissman, M.D.
Attending Anesthesiologist, University Community Hospital, Tampa, Florida

Cheryl Westmoreland, M.D.
Assistant Professor of Anesthesiology, Emory University School of Medicine, Atlanta, Georgia

David M. Wimberly, M.D.
Associate Professor of Anesthesiology, Deputy Chairman of Clinical Services, Emory University School of Medicine, Associate Chief of Anesthesia Services, Emory University Hospital, Atlanta, Georgia

Contents

Chapter 1

Preoperative Evaluation

All physicians involved in the care of patients—internists referring the patients, surgeons operating on them, and anesthesiologists providing anesthesia and life support during the intraoperative and early postoperative period—share the common goals of producing the best possible surgical outcome and minimizing risks to the patients' survival and well-being.

Evidence indicates that perioperative management affects referring the patients, surgeons operating on them, and anesthesiologists providing anesthesia and life support during the intraoperative and early postoperative period—share the common goals of producing the best possible surgical outcome and minimizing risks to the patients' survival and well-being.

Evidence indicates that perioperative management affects outcome for better or worse, and central to achieving the best possible outcome is a thorough preoperative evaluation intended to *(a)* identify the health problems that place the patient at increased risk, *(b)* resolve or control the disease(s) as well as possible, and *(c)* define a management plan that minimizes preoperative, intraoperative, and especially postoperative risks. Communication and cooperation among the patient, internist, surgeon, and anesthesiologist are the keys to success in the quest for the best possible outcome for the patient.

A complete preoperative evaluation consists of a systems-oriented history and physical, including a surgical and anesthetic history, drug and allergy histories, any necessary laboratory and diagnostic tests, and formulation of an anesthetic plan (including preoperative medication), with informed consent obtained from the patient. Additional consultation with other specialists may or may not be necessary.

HISTORY

In each of the following systems addressed by the history, introductory comments are followed by a list of important conditions and their significance or anesthetic implication.

Cardiovascular

Much of the morbidity and mortality associated with anesthesia is cardiac in origin.

• Hypertension	May herald intraoperative blood pressure instability; risk factor for atherosclerotic coronary artery disease (ASCAD)
• Angina pectoris (or anginal equivalent)	Known risk factor for ASCAD; in some studies, itself a predictor of perioperative cardiac morbidity (PCM)
• Prior myocardial infarction (MI)	Significantly increased risk of perioperative MI in patients with prior MI, especially prior MI within 6 months
• Congestive heart failure (CHF)	A known predictor of PCM
• Peripheral or cerebral vascular disease	May themselves alter anesthetic management; associated with ASCAD
• History of rheumatic fever or valvular heart disease	May alter anesthetic management; will require antimicrobial SBE prophylaxis

Respiratory System

Much of anesthetic practice involves controlling and instrumenting the airway, assuring adequate oxygenation and ventilation, and delivering potent drugs via the lungs. Pulmonary status should be optimized prior to the patient's arrival in the operating room.

• Asthma	Potential for severe bronchospasm on intubation and extubation

- Emphysema

  Prone to bronchospasm; chronic hypoxemia and hypercarbia, if present, must be noted and compensated for

- Tobacco abuse

  Smokers have irritable airways, increased secretions, and elevated carboxyhemoglobin levels

Hepatic

As many of the drugs we administer are metabolized and detoxified in the liver, it is important to elicit a history of hepatic disease.

- Viral hepatitis

  If acute, a relative contraindication to elective surgery and anesthesia; may affect drug metabolism or distribution; if chronic active, may be treated with corticosteroids; represents a risk to the health care worker

- Hepatic cirrhosis

  May affect drug metabolism and distribution; if severe, may cause a coagulopathy

Renal

Not uncommonly we are called upon to anesthetize a patient with chronic renal failure. It is also important to be wary of the patient with nephrolithiasis, long-standing prostatic hypertrophy or hypertension, or recurrent pyelonephritis, as these patients may be on the brink of renal failure.

- Renal failure

  May be hypervolemic, or relatively hypovolemic after dialysis; note site of functioning A-V fistulae, type of dialysis, and date of last dialysis; beware of electrolyte abnormalities, especially elevated potassium levels; patients usually anemic

Gastrointestinal

The anesthesiologist's primary gastrointestinal concern is the risk of regurgitation and pulmonary aspiration of gastric contents. A history of peptic ulcer disease should be sought, as this may be associated with occult GI bleeding and anemia. The risk of regurgitation of gastric contents is increased in the following disorders:

- Hiatal hernia
- Diabetes with gastroparesis
- Obesity
- Pregnancy
- Upper GI bleeding
- Gastric outlet or small bowel obstruction
- Emergency cases

Central Nervous System

A number of CNS disorders may affect the choice of anesthetic:

• Seizures	Etiology, frequency, and drug therapy should be noted
• Stroke or TIA	May affect anesthetic, blood pressure management, and positioning
• Peripheral neurologic deficit	May affect positioning and choice of general or regional anesthesia
• Muscular dystrophies, Alzheimer's and Parkinson's diseases, myasthenia gravis, multiple sclerosis, para- or quadriplegia	All will affect anesthetic management in various ways
• Upper and lower motor neuron injuries	Contraindication to succinylcholine

Musculoskeletal

The primary musculoskeletal concerns are arthritides serious enough to compromise airway management or patient positioning.

- Osteoarthritis

  If cervical spine involved, intubation may be difficult; care in positioning

- Rheumatoid arthritis

  May affect intubation by involvement of TMJ, cricoidarytenoid joints, and cervical spine; may be corticosteroid treated; care in positioning

Endocrine

- Diabetes mellitus

  Insulin dependent or not? accelerated atherosclerosis and a high incidence of silent myocardial ischemia; sensory neuropathy and gastroparesis; may have renal insufficiency or failure; must decide on glucose and insulin management

- Thyroid disease

  Goiter may cause airway compromise; untreated hyperthyroid patients are at risk of thyroid storm; untreated hypothyroid patients are at risk of electrolyte disorders, hypothermia, and cardiomyopathy

- Adrenal disease

  Iatrogenic adrenal suppression; Cushing's disease may be associated with osteoporosis, glucose intolerance, and hypokalemic alkalosis; Addison's disease associated with hyperkalemia, hypothermia, weakness, and hypotension; symptoms suggestive of pheochromocytoma should be investigated

Hematology

The two main problems in this area that will confront the anesthesiologist are anemia and coagulopathy. A coagulapathy is a contraindication to some regional techniques, especially epidurals and subarachnoid blocks.

- Easy bruising or prolonged bleeding — May indicate previously undiagnosed bleeding diathesis
- Leukemia or myelodysplasia syndrome — May be associated with severe anemia and thrombocytopenia
- Sickle cell anemia — Requires careful pre-, intra-, and postoperative management to avoid a sickling crisis
- Liver disease — May be associated with a coagulation disorder and thrombocytopenia

Dental

Dental concerns relate primarily to intubation.

- Temporomandibular joint disorder — May make intubation difficult
- Loose or missing teeth and permanent or removable bridgework — Possibility of damage; should be removed before operation

Obstetric

It is not advisable to administer an anesthetic for an elective procedure during the first trimester of pregnancy because of the potential risk to the pregnancy.

- Contraceptive use and date of last menstrual period — To determine whether pregnancy is possible; if not certain, determination of β-hcG is advised
- Past obstetric history — Complications and anesthetic experience should be noted

Allergies

- Drug allergies

Avoid drugs to which a patient is allergic; distinguish between true allergy and simple side effect

Current Medications

With few exceptions, chronic medications should be continued throughout the perioperative period.

Tobacco, Alcohol, and Recreational Drugs

These common entities in today's society may affect the anesthetic in a variety of ways.

- Tobacco abuse

Note amount; common problems include chronic bronchitis, COPD, and coronary artery disease

- Alcohol abuse

Acute intoxication decreases, while chronic abuse increases, anesthetic requirements; also associated with hepatitis, cirrhosis, esophageal varices, coagulopathy, anemia, thrombocytopenia, gastritis, pancreatitis, and dementia

- Recreational drugs

Opioids: risk of withdrawal and increased perioperative narcotic requirement.
Cocaine: risk of arrhythmias, myocardial infarction, hypertension, tachycardia, hyperthermia, hypoglycemia, and psychosis
I.V. abuse: risk of local infection, sepsis, bacterial endocarditis, pulmonary emboli and infarction, hepatitis, HIV

Previous Medical History

- Previous operations

  What were they, what type of anesthetic, and any anesthetic complications

- Family history of anesthetic complications

  Main concerns are malignant hypothermia and pseudocholinesterase deficiency

Prior Medical Records

These records may be invaluable in clarifying details of a patient's medical condition. Prior anesthetic records should indicate ease (or lack of ease) of airway management, perioperative hemodynamic course, and whether or not there were any complications.

PHYSICAL EXAMINATION

General

- Vital signs, including rate and character of respirations
- Body habitus
- Inspect and/or palpate peripheral veins and arteries to assess them for ease of cannulation
- Inspect proposed sites of regional anesthetic for accessibility and infections
- Determine any movement limitations

Airway

Examination of the airway is vital. Examine the teeth and note on the record any loose teeth, caps, crowns, bridgework, or dentures. Explain to the patient the increased risk of dental damage these appliances (when permanent or not removed) present.

The mouth should ideally open at least three finger-breadths (50–60 mm). The posterior pharynx should be visible; if it is not, as is often the case in patients with large, thick tongues, it could be a harbinger of a difficult intubation.

The neck should flex easily chin to chest, and the head should readily extend at the atlanto-occipital joint. These two movements comprise the "sniffing position," which is the optimal position for endotracheal intubation.

Mandibular hypoplasia is often associated with difficult intubation. Two syndromes in which this is a feature are Treacher-Collins and Pierre-Robin. A useful clinical way to assess adequacy of mandibular length is to measure from the hyoid bone to the mandibular symphysis with the head extended. This distance should be about three fingerbreadths. If it is less than two fingerbreadths, visualization of the vocal cords may be difficult. Also, the distance from the lower border of the mandible to the notch of the thyroid cartilage, with the head extended, should be not less than 6 cm.

Assess the mobility of the larynx. A fixed, immobile larynx, as may be caused by radiation therapy, may also be associated with difficult intubation.

Cardiovascular and Respiratory

Auscultate the heart rate, rhythm, murmur, and gallops, and the lungs for rales (suggestive of CHF), rhonchi, or wheezes. Having the patient perform a forced expiration may help uncover otherwise inapparent wheezing and airflow obstruction.

Neurologic

Neurologic examination is especially important with the neurosurgical patient or those who are to have regional anesthesia.

• Neurological patients	Note preoperative mental status as well as the presence and severity of any focal deficits, so comparison with the postoperative state is possible
• Regional anesthesia patients	Note any preexisting motor or sensory deficits, to avoid having an existing deficit blamed on a regional anesthetic

DIAGNOSTIC TESTS

Diagnostic tests were originally ordered based on findings from the history and physical examination. Then, as multiphasic blood screens were developed, these were applied to large numbers of people in the hope that early detection of occult diseases might save lives. However, the problem of false-positive results (and the additional workup that they must generate in today's medicolegal climate) has swung the pendulum back in the other direction. Current recommendation is to restrict screening tests in healthy asymptomatic patients to

- Hemoglobin in all women and men over age 60
- Glucose and blood urea nitrogen in all patients over age 40
- Other laboratory tests as dictated by the results of the history and physical examination
- Chest roentgenogram in all patients over age 40 and in others as dictated by the history and physical examination
- Electrocardiogram in all patients over age 40 and in others as dictated by the history and physical examination

AMERICAN SOCIETY OF ANESTHESIOLOGISTS (ASA) CLASSIFICATION SCHEME

The ASA physical status rating, first described in the 1940s and revised since, represents an attempt to estimate anesthetic and surgical risk by stratifying patients according to the severity of their disease processes. It is as follows:

CLASS I	HEALTHY PATIENT
CLASS II	PATIENT WITH MILD, CONTROLLED, FUNCTIONALLY NONLIMITING SYSTEMIC DISEASE
CLASS III	PATIENT WITH SEVERE OR POORLY CONTROLLED SYSTEMIC DISEASE THAT IS FUNCTIONALLY LIMITING
CLASS IV	PATIENT WITH SEVERE SYSTEMIC DISEASE THAT IS A CONSTANT THREAT TO LIFE
CLASS V	MORIBUND PATIENT NOT EXPECTED TO SURVIVE 24 HOURS WITH OR WITHOUT SURGERY

Any of the categories above may have an "E" added when a patient requires an emergency operation. A V classification is by definition an emergency.

This physical status classification scheme is useful when anesthesiologists wish to communicate about such things as anesthetic techniques for certain types of patients or clinical studies in various patient populations. However, this classification scheme is at best only a gross predictor of outcome and cannot really be regarded as a gauge of anesthetic "risk."

CHOICE OF ANESTHETIC

The type of anesthetic to be used must be decided jointly by the anesthesiologist, patient, and surgeon. Few studies show increased safety of any one anesthetic technique over others (although it is important to note that anesthesiologists perform best when they use a technique with which they are familiar), so for any given patient, there usually are several options.

The anesthesiologist's primary job is to see the patient safely through the operation; a secondary (though still important) goal is to make the experience as pleasant and comfortable for the patient as possible. Facilitating the surgeon's task in any reasonable way possible is also important, which might mean avoiding an anesthetic technique with which the surgeon feels uncomfortable. For example, some surgeons feel very comfortable performing a carotid endarterectomy under local anesthesia with IV sedation, while others prefer a general anesthetic.

The patient should be told about the anesthetic options for the operation (such as general vs. regional vs. local) and, after a thorough explanation of what to expect from each, should be allowed to express a preference, which should be respected as long as it is not unreasonable or unsafe. The patient should be well informed about the events to occur, including NPO status, premedication (if planned), placement of IVs and any invasive monitors, and the postoperative events, including plans for pain management. Consent should be obtained for blood transfusion if deemed necessary. After a plan is arrived at and consent is obtained, a note to that effect should be written in the patient's chart.

EFFECTIVE USE OF CONSULTANTS

Frequently, patients have medical conditions that could affect their ability to tolerate anesthesia and surgery. Evaluation of these may be beyond the anesthesiologist's expertise. Some examples include the patient with functionally limiting COPD, the patient with disabling claudication and an abnormal ECG scheduled for femoral-popliteal bypass, and the elderly patient presenting for TURP who has an aortic systolic murmur, diminished upstroke of the carotid pulse, and left ventricular hypertrophy on ECG. These are times when an expert consultant can provide valuable information to help guide the anesthesiologist's planning. Additionally, routine evaluation by the patient's family physician or internist prior to elective surgery should be given serious consideration.

In the past, there have been two main problems with specialist consultations. All too often, consultants did not provide the information that was truly needed, and secondly, they sometimes overstepped the bounds of their expertise and began to make suggestions regarding the actual conduct of the anesthetic ("avoid hypotension and hypoxia"; "patient cleared for spinal"; "use intraoperative nitrates"; "close hemodynamic monitoring with PA catheter"). Much of the blame for this rests on the anesthesiologist or surgeon requesting the consultation. Some considerations for requesting a consultation are

1. Is the consultation necessary? Is it to manage a medical condition that can competently be managed by the surgeon or anesthesiologist (such as mild asthma, COPD, or NIDDM)? Is it anticipated that the information provided by the consultant will change the operative or anesthetic plan?

2. Ask an appropriate, specific question. Asking a cardiologist to "clear patient for surgery" is vague, at best, and is not as likely to result in a concise, helpful consult as a specific query such as: "Elderly man with systolic murmur, LVH by voltage criteria and history of near-syncopal episode. Please evaluate." Additionally, the consultant's function is not to appraise a patient's fitness for surgery, but rather to define the patient's medical condition and to suggest ways to optimize that condition.

PREANESTHETIC MEDICATION

The decision about how to premedicate a patient can be made easier by first asking two questions: (a) is premedication necessary or desirable in this patient? and (b) what are the goals of preoperative medication?

Studies have shown that most patients are anxious before

surgery, while others have demonstrated that a reassuring pre-operative visit by an anesthesiologist allays anxieties at least as effectively as preoperative sedatives do. A patient's emotional state can be assessed during the preoperative visit and a decision made about the necessity for preoperative anxiolytic medication. It may be unnecessary or unwise to premedicate certain types of patients: comatose patients don't need anxiolytics; patients with increased intracranial pressure may be harmed by preoperative depressant medications, as might patients at the extremes of age or those with decreased physiologic reserve.

Reasons to give preoperative medication are as follows:

1. Anxiolysis
2. Amnesia (also important in the anxious patient and in patients who will need many potentially unpleasant preoperative intravenous and monitoring line insertions)
3. Pain relief
4. Drying of secretions (important for anticipated difficult or fiberoptic intubations or for patients to be placed in the prone or lateral positions)
5. To increase gastric pH and decrease gastric volume (important for patients believed to be at increased risk of regurgitation and aspiration of gastric contents)
6. Attenuation of autonomic responses to stimuli
7. Reduction of anesthetic requirements

Commonly used preanesthetic drugs:

1. *Benzodiazepines* are useful in varying degrees for anxiolysis, sedation, and amnesia. They have a high therapeutic index and demonstrate minimal respiratory depression at usual clinical doses. They also help to minimize the incidence of emergence reactions following the use of ketamine, especially in adults.
   A. *Diazepam* is a very popular and effective premedicant, with good sedative, anxiolytic, and amnestic properties.
   B. *Lorazepam* produces heavy sedation and reliable amnesia. Its long duration of action makes it suitable primarily for long, inpatient cases.
   C. *Midazolam* is very useful because of its rapid onset of action and short half-life and duration of effect. Midazolam displays very good sedative and amnestic properties.

Drug	Route	Dose (mg/kg)	Elimination Half-life (hr)	Time to Peak Effect after Oral Dose (min)
Diazepam	IV, PO	0.1–0.2 (PO)	21–37	60–90
Lorazepam	IV, IM, PO	0.03–0.05 (PO)	10–20	120–240
Midazolam	IV, IM, PO	0.05–0.1 (IM)	1–4	30–60

2. *Barbiturates*

Secobarbital and pentobarbital are two barbiturates occasionally used as premedicants. They are given in doses of 50–200 mg/70 kg adult and provide reliable, safe sedation. They generally act longer and are not as specifically anxiolytic as the benzodiazepines. They have been largely supplanted by the benzodiazepines.

3. *Scopolamine*

This anticholinergic drug and antisialagogue crosses the blood-brain barrier and is a very effective sedative and amnestic agent when used IM in doses of 0.3–0.5 mg/70 kg adult. Its sedative and amnestic effects are greatly enhanced when it is used in combination with opioids. Some patients, particularly the elderly, may exhibit somnolence, confusion, or delirium, and this should be kept in mind if these symptoms occur postoperatively. This "central anticholinergic syndrome" can be treated with IV physostigmine, 0.25–2 mg/70 kg adult.

4. *Opioids*

Opioids are frequently used for premedication when analgesia is needed (e.g., a patient with a painful condition or one who will require potentially painful monitoring lines or regional anesthetic placement). They may also be used to achieve a basal state of analgesia when an N_2O/O_2/opioid anesthetic technique is planned. They are indicated in the opioid-dependent patient at risk for withdrawal. Many feel that preoperative opioids may produce dysphoria if used in the absence of pain or discomfort—a more specific anxio-lytic/sedative such as benzodiazepine being more appropriate in most patients. Dose reduction of opioids is appropriate in the elderly.

Side Effects of Opioids
Respiratory depression
Orthostatic hypotension
Nausea and vomiting
Pruritus
Potential for choledochoduodenal sphincter spasm
Bradycardia

A. *Morphine* is best given preoperatively IM 0.1–0.15 mg/kg. Peak effect is in 45–90 minutes, and duration of action is about 4 hours (half-life about 114 minutes). Morphine is often combined with scopolamine and a benzodiazepine for a "heavy" premedication. Caution is advised in the elderly, and O_2 supplementation via nasal cannula is advised, with vigilance for respiratory depression.

B. *Meperidine* is now used less frequently. Given IM 1–1.5 mg/kg, time to peak effect is approximately 1 hour. Duration of action is 2–4 hours; half-life is 3–4 hours. Meperidine is structurally similar to atropine and may cause mydriasis and a modest tachycardia. A principal metabolite is normeperidine, which may cause seizures after very large doses or with accumulation in patients with renal insufficiency.

5. Anticholinergics

These drugs are most commonly used preoperatively to dry oral secretions and possibly prevent periinduction vagally mediated bradycardia (most common in pediatrics). They are all well absorbed IM. Their principal side effects are similar to their therapeutic effects: tachycardia, unpleasant dry mouth, sedation and amnesia (which can progress to confusion and delirium in the elderly), inability to thermoregulate, and mydriasis, which infrequently causes an increase in intraocular pressure in patients with narrow-angle glaucoma.

A. *Atropine* is most effective at preventing reflex bradycardia in children if given at induction. Many anesthesiologists currently doubt whether atropine should be given routinely with modern anesthetics but prefer to give atropine postinduction or if needed. The IM dose is 0.01 mg/kg, with a maximum of 0.6 mg in adults.

B. *Scopolamine* may be used for sedation and amnesia, often in combination with a narcotic. It is also an effective antisialagogue. The dose is 0.3–0.5 mg/70 kg adult IM.

C. *Glycopyrrolate,* a quaternary ammonium ion, does not cross the blood-brain barrier and therefore does not produce sedation. Glycopyrrolate is a very effective antisialagogue and is indicated when a dry mouth is desired (e.g., when a difficult or fiberoptically assisted intubation is anticipated or when a position other than supine will be used). The dose is 0.2–0.3 mg/70 kg adult IM.

6. Prophylaxis against aspiration pneumonitis

Many patients presenting for operation may be at increased risk for regurgitation and aspiration of gastric contents. Studies have suggested (but not conclusively proven in humans) that the risk of adverse pulmonary sequelae is greater when gastric volume is greater than 0.4 ml/kg and pH is less than 2.5. The main drugs that have been proven useful in increasing gastric pH and reducing volume are the H_2 receptor antagonists and metoclopramide. Nonparticulate antacids are useful for reducing gastric acid (e.g., in obstetric patients).

A. *Cimetidine,* a H_2 receptor antagonist, is given in a dose of 3–4 mg/kg (as much as 7.5 mg/kg in infants or the obese patient) the night before and the morning of surgery to produce a reliable increase in gastric pH. It may be given PO, but if necessary can be given IV or IM. Side effects are rare and include confusion, especially in the elderly; bronchoconstriction in the asthmatic patient, due to unopposed H_1 receptor activity after the loss of H_2-mediated bronchodilation; and interference with the metabolism of drugs such as lidocaine, diazepam, propranolol, and theophylline, presumably due to inhibition of hepatic P-450 microsomal enzymes and possibly some reduction of hepatic blood flow.

B. *Ranitidine,* another effective H_2 antagonist, may be given in a dose of 150 mg/70 kg adult PO the night before and on the morning of surgery or IV or IM in a dose of 50 mg/70 kg adult. Due to structural differences, there is a much lower incidence of side effects than are seen with cimetidine.

C. *Famotidine,* a newer H_2 antagonist, is available in tablet, oral suspension, and IV formulations. The dose is 20–40 mg/70 kg adult PO or 10–20 mg/70 kg adult IV. Duration of action is 10–12 hours, so it is best given the night before and the morning of surgery.

D. *Metoclopramide* is a dopaminergic antagonist that stimulates gastric motility, thus speeding gastric emptying, and increases the tone of the lower esophageal sphincter, which should decrease the risk of passive regurgitation. Its effects at the lower esophageal sphincter are opposed by anticholinergics. It can be given by mouth 1–2 hours before induction and can also be given IV. The dose is 10–20 mg/70 kg adult. Metoclopramide may also be an effective antiemetic. Because of its antidopaminergic effects, extrapyramidal symptoms may occur.

Because metoclopramide does not alter gastric fluid pH and the H_2 antagonists do not alter gastric emptying, these two classes of drugs are most effective when used in combination. They do not, however, guarantee protection against regurgitation and aspiration.

E. *Nonparticulate antacids* like sodium citrate–citric acid combinations are effective in immediately increasing gastric pH, but the effect is short term. Ten to 30 ml can be given orally with other preoperative medications. Particulate antacids containing Mg or Al effectively raise gastric pH but may pose a risk of pulmonary injury if aspirated.

7. The patient's regular medication—what to give and what to omit:

It is common practice to continue all regular medications throughout the perioperative period. Exceptions include diuretics (unless they are required for adequate urine output), sucralfate, cholesterol-binding agents, and particulate antacids, which may present an increased risk of pulmonary damage if aspirated. The patient's usual medications may be given along with the other preoperative medications with a few sips of water. Three common classes of medication deserve special mention:

A. *β-Blockers*—Rebound hypertension and/or myocardial ischemia may occur when these drugs are abruptly stopped; therefore, they should be continued throughout the perioperative period. Intraoperative bradycardia may occasionally occur, but if hemodynamically significant, can be treated with atropine.

B. *Calcium channel blockers*—Myocardial ischemia may be associated with abrupt cessation of calcium channel blocking agents. They should be continued in their usual dose.

C. *Clonidine*—Abrupt cessation of clonidine is associated with severe rebound hypertension, with or without myocardial ischemia. Preoperative administration of this drug decreases the MAC of anesthetics and provides a more hemodynamically stable perioperative course. Bradycardia can be treated with atropine.

8. *Insulin*—There are many suggested perioperative insulin regimens for the insulin-dependent diabetic.

A. NPO after midnight, no IV fluids, half of usual morning subcutaneous insulin dose given. This common regimen is simple and non-labor-intensive, and it takes into account both the patient's NPO status and the fact that the insulin-dependent diabetic will probably need exogenous insulin even in the absence of food. Blood sugar is checked preoperatively, and intraoperative therapy is guided by intermittent blood sugar measurements. This plan assumes that the patient is scheduled for an early morning start to surgery.

B. NPO after midnight, no IV fluids, hold morning insulin. Blood glucose is monitored and treated as in the above regimen. This regimen is very simple and non-labor-intensive, and it is based on the presumption that short-term hypoglycemia is far more dangerous than short-term hyperglycemia. Obviously, this method does not allow "tight control," nor it is ideal for the brittle diabetic who is very prone to diabetic ketoacidosis.

C. NPO after midnight, IV dextrose-containing maintenance fluids at a fixed rate, and IV insulin infusion starting at about 1 unit/hour and adjusted according to fingerstick blood glucose determinations every 2 hours. This regimen is obviously more expensive and labor-intensive, but it is good for the brittle diabetic and allows tighter control of blood glucose perioperatively. Blood glucose measurements must be on schedule, since inadvertent hypo-glycemic episodes may occur.

Studies clearly demonstrating improved outcome of one regimen over another are lacking.

Suggested Readings

Clemency MV, Thompson NJ. "Do not resuscitate" (DNR) orders and the anesthesiologist: a survey. Anesth Analg 1993;76:394–401.

Fliesher LA, Barash PG. Preoperative cardiac evaluation for noncardiac surgery: a functional approach. Anesth Analg 1992;74:586–598.

Kaller SK, Everett LL. Potential risks and preventive measures for pulmonary aspiration: new concept in preoperative fasting guidelines. Anesth Analg 1993;77:171–182.

Mangano DT. Perioperative cardiac morbidity. Anesthesiology 1990; 72:153–184.

Rao TK, Jacobs KH, El-Etr AA. Reinfarction following anesthesia in patients with myocardial infarction. Anesthesiology 1983;59:499–505.

Chapter 2

Preoperative Preparation for Anesthesia

Proper preparation is required prior to beginning any type of anesthetic and should be done before the patient is brought into the operating room. The basic setup must be modified based on the type of anesthetic, monitors to be used, the patient's medical problems, and the location of the anesthetic (operating room, labor suite, radiology, etc.) A standard basic approach should be taken for all cases, since shortcuts may result in omissions and subsequent complications. The following is a basic approach to the preoperative preparation.

I. Machine checkout (see recommendation in Appendix)
     Record machine number on the anesthetic record and indicate that the anesthesia machine has been checked. This will allow investigation of the machine if there is an intraoperative problem.
II. Equipment to have available or know how to obtain
    A. Equipment to ventilate and oxygenate patient if the anesthesia machine or oxygen source should fail:
       Oxygen tank and regulator, self-inflating ventilation system (Ambu bag), tubing to connect tank and ventilation system
    B. Resuscitation equipment
       1. Emergency drugs—epinephrine, sodium bicarbonate, calcium chloride, glucose
       2. Defibrillator with external and internal paddles
    C. Emergency airway equipment if unable to ventilate or intubate the patient

1. Several sizes and shapes of masks
2. Selection of oro- and nasopharyngeal airways
3. Selection of laryngoscope blades and spare handle
4. Selection of endotracheal tubes of various sizes
5. Endotracheal tube stylet
6. Tube changer (Eschman or equivalent)
7. Fiberoptic laryngoscope or bronchoscope
8. High-pressure oxygen tubing and connectors to provide oxygen through a transtracheal catheter
9. Equipment for emergency tracheostomy or cricothyroidotomy

III. Equipment to have available for a general or regional anesthetic
   A. Airway equipment
      1. Working suction with wide-bore tubing—suction catheter and Yankauer suction
      2. Mask, endotracheal tube (cuff checked), laryngoscope (light checked), oropharyngeal airway, water-soluble lubricant, stylet, tongue blade, syringe for inflating cuff on ET tube
   B. Monitors should be turned on, calibrated, and verified for correct functioning
      1. Electrocardiogram—preferably two leads, II and V_5
      2. Blood pressure cuff
      3. Pulse oximeter with upper and lower alarm limits set
      4. Oxygen analyzer for anesthesia breathing circuit—calibrated and alarms set
      5. Capnograph or exhaled carbon dioxide detection device (mass spectography, infrared, etc.)
      6. Temperature monitor and probe
      7. Nerve stimulator if muscle relaxants will be used
      8. Precordial and esophageal stethoscope
   C. Drugs—all labeled with drug name, concentration
      1. Induction drug—thiopental, propofol, ketamine, etc.
      2. Muscle relaxant—succinylcholine or nondepolarizing drug
      3. Vasopressor as appropriate—ephedrine, phenylephrine, epinephrine, etc.

Table 2.1
Electrocardiography—Lead Placement

Standard ECG monitoring
GREEN—Right leg
WHITE—Right arm
RED—Left leg
BLACK—Left arm
BROWN—Precordial lead
    V_1—4th intercostal space, right of sternum
    V_2—4th intercostal space, left of sternum
    V_3—midway between V_2 and V_4
    V_4—5th intercostal space, left midclavicular line
    V_5—5th intercostal space, left anterior axillary line
    V_6—5th intercostal space, left midaxillary line

ECG lead	Positive	Negative
Bipolar leads		
I	LA	RA
II	LL	RA
III	LL	LA
Augmented unipolar leads		
aVR	RA	LA, LL
aVL	LA	RA, LL
aVF	LL	RA, LA

    4. Vasodilator if need is anticipated—intravenous nitroglycerin
    5. Anticholinergic agent
  D. Other equipment
    1. Gloves, both sterile and nonsterile for compliance with universal precautions
    2. Intravenous fluid and administration sets
    3. Intravenous catheters
    4. Skin antiseptics and dressings
    5. Tape to secure intravenous catheters and endotracheal tubes
    6. Blood and fluid warmers
    7. Heating blanket on operating table—turned on and appropriate temperature set
    8. Humidifier for inspired anesthetic gases
    9. Equipment for mask or nasal catheter oxygen supplementation prior to or after anesthesia

10. Central venous catheterization or regional block equipment trays

IV. Patient identification—Patients should be identified from their name bracelets and, if possible, by asking them to give their name, planned surgical procedure (operative side), and surgeon. The operative permit should be reviewed, new laboratory values and the most recent vital signs checked, and any recent progress notes checked for any changes from the preoperative evaluation. The NPO status of the patient should be verified. If blood for type and cross had been ordered, its availability should be checked.

V. Implementation of monitoring—As soon as contact with the patient has been made, monitoring should be initiated, especially if the patient has received or will receive sedating drugs. For intraoperative monitoring, the standards set forth by the American Society of Anesthesiologists should be followed as a minimum for all patients (Appendix) (see Table 2.1 for ECG lead placement). Baseline ECG tracings should be stored electronically or recorded on paper so that any intraoperative changes can be assessed.

VI. **Invasive monitoring** may be appropriate for the anesthetic care of some patients. The need for and choice of invasive monitors will depend on the patient's preexisting medical condition and the proposed surgical procedure. Before the induction of anesthesia, invasive monitors may be inserted with use of local anesthesia if baseline information is required or if it is felt that the patient's hemodynamic management would be improved by the information during the induction of anesthesia.

VII. The *anesthesia record* is a log of the occurrences of the case and must be carefully completed to document all treatments and responses. All blanks should be filled in, and there should not be time gaps without recordings. In addition to such basic information as vital signs, anesthetic gas flows, and drugs administered, appropriate patient care should be documented, including positioning, padding of pressure points, eye care, ongoing estimates of blood loss and fluid replacement, oxygen saturation, end-tidal CO_2

measurements, and documentation of adequate reversal of muscle relaxants at the end of the case, with evidence of full muscle strength. At the end of the case, the patient's condition and transfer to the PAU or to another qualified individual should be noted.

Chapter 3

Anesthetic Pharmacology

PRINCIPLES OF PHARMACOLOGY

Anesthesiology demands a thorough understanding of the principles of drug therapy.

Pharmacokinetics

Pharmacokinetics is branch of pharmacology concerned with evaluation of factors that influence the magnitude of drug effect as a function of time. The major principles of pharmacokinetics are drug *uptake, distribution,* and *elimination.*

1. **Uptake.** The routes of drug uptake have different advantages and disadvantages depending upon their ability to provide access to the bloodstream (Table 3.1).
2. **Distribution.** Once a drug has entered the blood compartment, the rate at which it penetrates tissues and other body fluids depends on *(a)* the rate of tissue perfusion, e.g. cardiac output; *(b)* tissue mass; *(c)* the extent of plasma protein and tissue binding; *(d)* regional differences in pH; and *(e)* the permeability characteristics of specific tissue membranes.

   Volume of distribution is a useful concept in loading doses to determine the quantity needed to achieve a desired blood or tissue concentration of a drug.

   A *multicompartment model* is often used in an attempt to reflect the different rates of blood flow to various tissues (Table 3.2).
3. **Elimination.** Ending the pharmacologic action of a drug is a function of both its rate of *biotransformation* or *metabolism* and its rate of *excretion.*

25

Table 3.1
Routes Most Commonly Used for Anesthetic Drugs

Inhalational
Intramuscular
Oral
Rectal
Intravenous
Transmucosal (e.g., nasal)
Transdermal

Table 3.2
Compartments

	Body Mass (%)	Cardiac Output (%)
Vessel-rich group (brain, liver, heart, kidneys, endocrine glands)	10	75
Muscle group	50	20
Vessel-poor group (bones, ligaments, cartilage, fat)	40	5

Clearance is the volume of plasma from which a drug is eliminated in unit time.

Zero-order elimination is the removal of a constant amount of a drug in unit time.

First-order elimination is the removal of a constant fraction of a drug in unit time.

Elimination half-life is the time for the concentration to fall by one half during elimination.

Pharmacodynamics

Pharmacodynamics is the study of uptake, binding, and interactions of drugs at their site(s) of action. Drugs used in anesthesia can achieve one or more of a number of desired and/or undesired (side) effects. The goals of anesthetic drug administration can vary, depending on the specifics of the situation and the patient to whom the agents are administered (Table 3.3).

"Physiologic homeostasis" is a broad expression referring to the manipulation of the body's response to perioperative stimuli (e.g., endotracheal intubation, surgical incision, and visceral

Table 3.3
Desired Effects of Anesthetic Pharmacology

Anxiolysis
Hypnosis
Amnesia
Muscle relaxation
Analgesia
Maintenance of physiologic homeostasis
Reversal of anesthetic effects

traction). Pharmacologic interventions may be triggered by monitoring the patient's responses to such stimuli or by anticipation of commonly observed phenomena.

Classically, the inhalational anesthetics have been used to achieve most of the desired goals of anesthetic pharmacology. Increasingly, there is a trend to achieve specific goals with receptor-specific agents in the hope of rendering improved results, i.e., returning the patient to a preoperative level of physiologic function as quickly and as safely as possible.

SPECIFIC DRUGS USED IN ANESTHESIOLOGY

Antiarrhythmics

Abnormal cardiac rhythms are a common occurrence in patients under general anesthesia. Reversible causes should be quickly searched for and corrected after weighing the side effects of the dysrhythmia against those of the specific agent. Treatment of life-threatening ventricular tachycardia or fibrillation should be based on the latest ACLS protocol (Appendix). Table 3.4 concentrates on IV agents most commonly used for acute therapy.

Antihypertensive Agents

Blood pressure is the product of cardiac output (CO) and systemic vascular resistance (SVR). Cardiac output is a function of the heart rate (HR) and the stroke volume (SV). Stroke volume is affected by preload, afterload, and contractility. The mechanism listed for each drug defines its most prominent action (Table 3.5).

Table 3.4
Antiarrhythmics

Agent	Indication	Dosage (IV)	Mechanism
Atropine	Sinus bradycardia	0.01–0.02 mg/kg	Anticholinergic/ increase SA node rate
Isoproterenol (Isuprel)	Brachycardia, sinus or sinus arrest	Bolus:0.02–0.06 mg infusion:5 μg/min	β-Receptor stimulation/may produce hypo- or hypertension
Esmolol (Brevibloc)	Paroxysmal supraventricular tachycardia (PSVT)	Bolus: 0.25–1 mg/kg Infusion: 50–250 μg/kg/ min	Short-acting β-blockade/ metoprolol 1–5 mg would be longer acting alternative to infusion
Verapamil (Calan, Verelan)	PSVT (not WPW); atrial fibrillation/flutter with rapid ventricular response (AFRVR)	5–10 mg IV, may be repeated in 30 min	Calcium channel blockade/ decreases A-V nodal conduction/ significant hypotension due to negative inotropic effect (may respond to IV calcium)
Diltiazem (Cardizem)	PSVT; AFRVR	Bolus: 0.15–0.25 mg/kg Infusion: 5–15 mg/hr	Calcium channel blockade/decrease A-V nodal conduction; less negative inotropic effect than verapamil
Adenosine	PSVT	6-mg rapid	Slows A-V nodal

Induction Agents

Intravenous agents for induction of anesthesia possess the desirable characteristics of rapidly producing sleep (generally in a single arm to brain circulation time), having a limited duration, and having a minimal affect on the cardiovascular system. The choice of an induction agent may be affected by the patient's age and physical status as well as the volume status. The dose of induction agent may also be affected by the potency of the premedication and/or by the coadministration of other agents such as short-acting narcotics (Table 3.6).

Table 3.4 (*continued*)
Antiarrhythmics

Agent	Indication	Dosage (IV)	Mechanism
(Adenocard)		IV bolus; 12-mg bolus in 1–2 min if not converted	conduction/transient heart block can occur; half-life < 10 sec
Digitalis (Digoxin, Lanoxin)	Atrial fibrillation/flutter; PSVT	0.25–0.5 mg over 5 min; 0.125–0.25 mg in 4 & 8 hr	Slows A-V nodal conduction/onset 5–30 min; positive inotropism helpful; low therapeutic index
Lidocaine (Xylocaine)	Premature ventricular contractions (PVCs); ventricular tachycardia(VT)	1 mg/kg slow IV; then 0.5 mg /kg in 5 min; then infusion 10–50 μg/kg/min	Raises threshold for action potential generation; toxicity causes tinnitus, circumoral paresthesias, seizure; decrease dose in CHF (25–50%)
Procainamide (Pronestyl)	PVCs, VT unresponsive to lidocaine	7–10 mg/kg, given as 100-mg boluses q 5 min	Fast sodium channel blockade; hypotension, prolonged Q-T
Bretylium (Bretylol)	VT, ventricular fibrillation	Bolus: 5 mg/kg initial, double if no response Infusion: 1–2 mg/min	Inhibits norepinephrine release ("chemical sympathectomy")/postural hypotension, nausea and vomiting

Inhalational Agents

Volatile liquids taken up via the alveolar-bloodstream interface were the first forms of anesthetics used. They have been the primary method of providing anesthesia for over a century and still best meet the goals of anesthesia as noted above. Several pharmacokinetic principles must be clearly understood to safely and effectively use the inhalational agents. While similar in their effects

Table 3.5
Antihypertensive Agents

Agent	Bolus (IV)	Infusion	Onset	Duration	Action(s)	Mechanism
Esmolol (Brevibloc)	0.5–1 mg/kg	50–500 μg/kg/min	1–2 min	10 min	↓HR, SV	Selective β_1-blockade
Propranolol (Inderal)	0.5–1 mg	—	2–6 min	30–60 min	↓HR, SV	Nonselective β-blockade
Metoprolol (Lopressor)	1–2 mg	—	2–6 min	1–3 hr	↓HR, SV	Selective β_1-blockade
Labetalol (Trandate, Normodyne)	2.5–5 mg	0.2–2 mg/kg/hr	2–5 min	40–90 min	↓HR, SVR	α-Blockade + non-selective β-blockade
Nicardipine (Cardene)	N/R	1–2 μg/kg/min	2–5 min	30 min	SVR	Calcium channel blockade
Enalaprilat (Vasotec)	1.25 mg	—	5–10 min	1.5–4 hr	↓SVR	ACE[a] inhibitor
Hydralazine (Apresoline)	2.5–5 mg	—	5–15 min	2–4 hr	↓SVR	Direct vasodilator (?EDRF[b])
Nitroglycerin (Tridil,Nitro-Bid)	50–100 μg	0.25–2 μg/kg/min	30–60 sec	20–40 min	↓Preload	Venodilation
Nitroprusside (Nipride)	10–50 μg	0.1–0.5 μg/kg/min	15–30 sec	2–5 min	↓↓SVR	Potent vasodilator (?EDRF[b])
Trimethaphan (Arfonad)	Infusion only	0.3–6 mg/min	2–5 min	10–30 min	↓HR, SVR	Ganglionic blockade

[a] ACE, angiotensin converting enzyme.
[b] EDRF, endothelial relaxing factor.

Table 3.6
Induction Agents

	Thiopental	Etomidate	Ketamine	Midazolam	Propofol
Dose: Healthy (III, co-ad.)	3–5 mg/kg IV (2–3 mg/kg)	0.3–0.4 mg/kg IV (0.2–0.3 mg/kg)	1–3 mg/kg IV	0.2–0.3 mg/kg IV (0.1–0.2 mg/kg)	1.5–3 mg/kg IV (1–2 mg/kg)
Alt. route	10 mg/kg rectal	—	5–10 mg/kg IM	—	—
Onset	One circ. time IV; 5–8 min rectal	One circ. time	IV, 30–60 sec IM, 5–8 min	1–3 min	One circ. time
Duration	5–15 min	7–14 min	10–15 min	12–60 min	2–5 min
Cardiovascular depression	++	+	+	+	++(+)
Contraindications	Allergy, Porphyria	Adrenal insufficiency?	Increased ICP/IOP[a] High BP?	Benzodiazepine allergy	Hypovolemia
Other	Caution in hypovolemia	Myoclonic movements can occur	Consider amnestic to counter CNS side effects	Can be reversed with flumazenil	Pain on injection (30%)

[a] ICP, intracranial pressure; IOP, intraocular pressure

on consciousness, their differences in potency, speed of uptake, and distribution, and their varying side-effect profiles are some of the reasons a variety of choices continues to exist.

Pharmacokinetics

The pharmacokinetics of the inhalational agents determine whether the goal of attaining a partial pressure of the anesthetic agent in the brain is achieved. Four phases of the uptake and distribution of volatile agents are

$$INSPIRED \rightarrow ALVEOLAR \rightarrow BLOOD \rightarrow TISSUE$$

The inspired concentration is affected by the *concentration effect* and the *second gas effect* (usually the simultaneous use of nitrous oxide and another agent).

The alveolar concentration is most affected by the alveolar ventilation; i.e., increasing the rate and depth of ventilations causes a more rapid induction.

The blood concentration, a reflection of the uptake of the anesthetic agent from the lung, is affected by the *solubility* (most often expressed as the blood/gas partition coefficient), the *cardiac output,* and the *alveolar-to-arterial partial pressure difference.*

Table 3.7
MAC

Factors that increase MAC	
Hyperthermia	
Chronic alcohol abuse	
MAO inhibitors	
Hypernatremia	
Factors that decrease MAC	
Hypothermia	
Acute alcohol abuse	
Severe hypoxia	
Metabolic acidosis	
Pregnancy	
Medications that decrease MAC	
Opioids	Benzodiazepines
Pancuronium	Barbiturates
Propofol (infusion)	Clonidine
Ketamine	Lidocaine

The tissue concentration of anesthetics is affected by *tissue blood flow, tissue solubility* (often expressed as the tissue/blood partition coefficient), and the *blood-tissue partial pressure gradient.*

Recovery from anesthesia is affected by the same factors that govern induction. Metabolism of the anesthetic agent is only clinically important at very low concentrations of halothane, which is metabolized by the liver.

Pharmacodynamics

The pharmacodynamics of the inhalational agents arise from their unique route of administration (via the alveolar-blood interface) and interface with the pharmacokinetics of the agents via comparisons of their potency. The usual means of comparing the agents today is commonly referred to as *MAC,* or *minimum alveolar concentration.* By definition, MAC is the alveolar concentration (now clinically measurable with end-tidal agent monitoring) that prevents movement in response to a surgical incision in 50% of subjects at one atmosphere. Achieving a 95% "success rate" requires approximately 1.3 MAC (also known as the AD95). Increments of MAC can be mathematically approximated (e.g., 70% N_2O would be 70/104, or 0.67 MAC), as well as accumulated (e.g., 70% N_2O + 1% isoflurane = 1.5 MAC). Many physiologic and pharmacologic factors increase or decrease MAC (Table 3.7).

Two useful derivatives of MAC are known as MAC-BAR, the alveolar concentration required to block the sympathetic response to incision (approximately 1.5 MAC), and MAC-awake, the dose at which the response to the verbal command "open your eyes" occurs (approximately 0.3–0.5 MAC); MAC-awake is thought to be a reliable index of amnesia.

Inhaled anesthetics (Table 3.8) are used today as sole anesthetics for induction and maintenance, as maintenance agents after intravenous induction, and/or in combination with opioids, muscle relaxants, and other adjuvants to achieve what is commonly called *balanced anesthesia.* Balanced anesthesia seeks to take advantage of "small" doses of numerous agents to achieve specific goals, while avoiding the disadvantages of large doses of a single agent; for example, using the vagotonic activity of the short-acting opioids (e.g., fentanyl) to "counter" the

Table 3.8
Inhalation Anesthetics

	N₂O	Halothane	Enflurane	Isoflurane	Desflurane	Sevoflurane
Vapor pressure	39,000	243	175	239	664	160
Mol. wt.	44	197	184	184	168	200
Solubility (oil/gas)	1.4	224	98	98	18.7	53.4
Blood/gas	0.47	2.3	1.8	1.4	0.42	0.6
Brain/blood	1.1	2.6	2.6	3.7	1.3	1.7
Metabolized	Inert	20%	2%	0.2%	0.02%	2–3%
MAC						
in 100% O_2	104%	0.77%	1.68%	1.15%	6.0%	1.7%
in 70% N_2O	—	0.29%	0.57%	0.50%	2–3%	0.65%
Dose-dependent effect on						
Cardiovascular system	Inconsistent; can stimulate sympathetic nervous system	↓BP by myocardial depression; little/no HR Δ; slight ↓SVR	↓BP by myo. depr./↓SVR (40% @ 1 MAC)	↓BP(< H < E); myo. depr. < H,E; ↑HR, ↓SVR; CO nl @ 1 MAC	Similar to isoflurane, but more dose-dependent effect on ↑HR	HR effects like halothane, but may have SVR effect of isoflurane
Pulmonary	May ↑PVR	Least pungent	Most CO_2 ↑	? < effect on HPV	? Similar to isoflurane	Nonirritating

PaCO$_2$ @ 1 MAC	42	46	60	48	?	?
CNS	Modest increase in CSF pressure due to cerebral vasodilation	Effect on CMRo$_2$: H < E < I; cerebral vasodilation H > E > I	Can produce high voltage, repetitive-spiking activity on EEG; no Δ in seizure risk	?Enhanced preservation of cerebral O$_2$ supply-demand relationship	? Similar to isoflurane	? Similar to isoflurane
Skeletal muscle relaxation	All potentiate the effects of nondepolarizing muscle relaxants, with order of potentiation I = E > H > N$_2$O; desflurane and sevoflurane probably similar to isoflurane					
Other/advantages	Low solubility speeds induction—good for second gas effect	Pleasant odor for inhalation induction (pediatric); good uterine relaxation	Potent coronary vasodilator without evidence of coronary steal	Most stable on cardiovascular, pulmonary, cerebral systems	Low solubility means most rapid recovery of halogenated agents available	Nonirritating, favorable solubility, may replace halothane for mask induction
Warnings	Bone marrow toxicity? Closed air spaces (may ↑ in size)	"Halothane hepatitis" esp. with repeat administration; arrhythmogenesis (epi.)	Fluoride ion production concern for renal toxicity	?"Coronary steal"—ischemia	Requires special pressurized vaporizer; O$_2$ monitoring essential	Metabolism/degradation concerns delaying release in U.S.

tachycardia often produced by pancuronium or isoflurane. The elegance of the techniques of balanced anesthesia is intimately connected, however, to a thorough understanding of the pharmacology of all of the agents being used.

Neuromuscular Blockers

(See Table 3.9.) Since curare was introduced into anesthetic practice some 50 years ago, development of new neuromuscular blocking agents has focused on improvements in speed of onset, duration of action, and side effects. Monitoring neuromuscular blockade with twitch response is essential to their safe use and termination of action before emergence. The agents in Table 3.9 are listed in order of increasing duration of action. The first, succinylcholine, is the only commonly used depolarizing agent; the remainder are nondepolarizers. Because of the risk of hyperkalemia in pediatric patients with unrecognized neuromuscular disorders, succinylcholine should only be used in emergency airway situations in children less than 13 years of age.

Opioids

(See Table 3.10.) Opioid receptor stimulation results in dose-dependent analgesia, respiratory depression, suppression of cough reflex, and drowsiness. These drugs also produce nausea and vomiting, urinary retention, constipation, and, in high doses, muscular rigidity. One of their most useful aspects is their minimal effect on cardiovascular function, even at high doses. It is controversial whether the short-acting fentanyl analogues can provide "anesthesia"; while MAC can be reduced by 25–75%, intraoperative recall has been reported when they are used without hypnotics or amnestics (e.g., inhalational agents, benzodiazepines). Recent years have seen the expansion of opioids to direct use in the neuraxis (i.e., epidural and intrathecal) as well as in intranasal and transdermal preparations.

Because specific receptors for opioids exist, they can be classified in three groups based on pharmacokinetics, potency, and agonist/antagonist activity: the **classical agonists,** the **fentanyl analogues,** and the **partial or mixed agonists/antagonists.**

The dosing schedules of opioids are considerably broad, depending on their specific settings, routes of administration, and specific patient parameters. **Premedication** and **postoperative** intermittent doses are very similar for the "classical" agonists, such as morphine. Intravenous administration as part of a **"balanced"** or **"nitrous-narcotic-relaxant"** technique must be accompanied by a thorough understanding of the pharmacokinetics of the agent used to avoid respiratory depression at the conclusion of the case. **Epidural** administration for labor analgesia or postoperative pain may be either intermittent or continuous, with emphasis on appropriate monitoring for side effects. Use of opioids often allows reduction in the concentration of local anesthetics, thereby reducing the associated motor blockade. Intrathecal dosages are often single-use, administered just before or after completion of the surgical procedure.

Fentanyl Analogues

(See Table 3.11.) Synthetic agonists have been (and continue to be) developed that combine high potency with low half-lives to limit postoperative respiratory depression. Most produce bradycardia and suppress the hormonal and metabolic stress responses at "cardiac" doses (those most commonly used for cardiac surgery). They are also being increasingly used during monitored anesthesia care (MAC) cases, combined with local anesthesia or conduction blocks. A similar dosing schedule is used for acute postoperative pain in the Post Anesthesia Care Unit (PACU). Another common usage of these agents is in suppressing the hemodynamic response to intubation (hypertension/tachycardia) in patients with ischemic heart disease or intracranial pathology.

Partial Agonists and Agonist-Antagonists

(See Table 3.12.) A thorough description of the opioid receptors (currently μ, δ, κ, and σ) is beyond the scope of this book; suffice it to say that the exploitation of agents with differential effects at these receptors is responsible for the release of a class of opioids designed to maximize analgesia while minimizing undesirable side effects such as respiratory depression. They are most commonly used as preoperative or postoperative analgesic medications, although some are used for labor analgesia or as components of MAC.

Other Agents

Table 3.13 covers some miscellaneous drugs used in perioperative period.

Table 3.9
Neuromuscular Blockers

Agent	Intubating Dose	Onset (min)	Duration (min) 95% Recovery Time	Maintenance Infusion Bolus	Comments
Succinylcholine (Anectine, Quelicin)	1 mg/kg (1.5–2.0 mg/kg after pret.)[a]	0.5–1	3–5	10–100 μg/kg/min (repeat bolus NR)	Best for rapid sequence induction; avoid in pseudocholinesterase deficiency, burns, hyperkalemia, open eye injury, malignant hyperthermia-susceptible patient; side effects: bradycardia, muscle pains; avoid phase II block (twitch monitoring)
Mivacurium (Mivacron)	0.15 mg/kg	2–4	8–15	8 μg/kg/min; 1–2 mg	Histamine release may produce hypotension; avoid in pseudocholinesterase deficiency
Vecuronium (Norcuron)	0.1 mg/kg	2.5–3	45	1–2 μg/kg/min; 0.01–0.015 mg/kg	Duration increased 40–60% in hepatic/renal disease; minimal cardiovascular effects; minimal histamine release
Atracurium (Tracrium)	0.4 mg/kg	3–5	64	6–8 μg/kg/min; 0.08–0.10 mg/kg	Hoffman elimination/ester hydrolysis; mild histamine release @ large doses; minimal cardiovascular effects; no change in hepatic/renal disease

Drug	Intubating dose	Onset (min)	Duration (min)	Maintenance	Comments
Tubocurarine (Curare)	0.6 mg/kg	4–6	120–180	2 μg/kg/min; 1.5–3 mg	Significant histamine release, autonomic ganglia blockade (hypotension); dosages reduced 50% by inhalational agents; duration 2–3$\times$ in renal failure
Metocurine (Metubine)	0.4 mg/kg	4–6	40–80	N/R .04–.08 mg/kg	Mild histamine, autonomic ganglia blockade; low-dose hemodynamically stable
Pancuronium (Pavulon)	0.1 mg/kg	3–6	45–90	N/R 1 mg	Significant vagolytic effect producing tachycardia; histamine release minimal
Doxacurium (Nuromax)	0.05 mg/kg	5–7	100 (40–240)	N/R 1 mg	Minimal cardiovascular side effects; significant prolongation in hepatic/renal failure
Pipecuronium (Arduan)	0.10–0.15 mg/kg	5–7	120–180	N/R 1–2 mg	Same as doxacurium

[a]Pretreatment: administration of small dose of nondepolarizer (e.g., tubocurarine 3 mg) 2–3 min before intubating dose; with succinylcholine, this attenuates fasciculation and postoperative myalgias. May also refer to use of small dose of intubating agent (e.g., vecuronium 1–2 mg) to facilitate rapid intubating conditions ("priming" or "timing" principle).

Table 3.10
Classical Opioid Agonists

Agent	Equipotent Dose	Pre/post Medication Dose	Duration of Action	"Balanced" Anesthesia Dose (IV)	Postoperative Epidural Dose	Postoperative Intrathecal Dose	PCA Dosing Schedule	Comments
Morphine (M.S.)	10 mg	0.1 mg/kg IM or SC 0.05–0.1 mg/kg IV	3–5 hr	0.2–0.3 mg/kg	4–10 mg q 12–24 hr infusion: 0.5–1 mg/hr[a,b]	0.25–1 mg q 12–24 hr[a]	1–2 mg q 10–15 min	Histamine release common (pruritus)
Meperidine (Demerol)	80–100 mg	1 mg/kg IM 0.2–0.7 mg/kg IV	3–5 hr	2–5 mg/kg	50–100 mg q 8–24 hr infusion: 5–10 mg/hr[a,b]	25–50 mg q 12–24 hr[a,c]	10–25 mg q 10–15 min	Tachycardia more common than M.S.
Hydromorphone (Dilaudid)	1.5 mg	0.01–0.02 mg/kg IM or SC 0.007–0.01 mg/kg IV	2–4 hr	0.02–0.04 mg/kg	0.5–1 mg q 8–24 hrs infusion: 0.05–0.1 mg/hr[a,b]	N/R	0.5–1 mg q 10–15 min	Oral dose 2–4 mg p 4–6 hr

[a]Preservative-free recommended.
[b]May be combined with local anesthetic (e.g., bupivicaine 0.0625–0.25%).
[c]Not FDA-approved for this usage.

Table 3.11
Fentanyl Analogues

Agent	Equipotent Dose	"MAC"/PACU Dose (IV)	Maintenance Infusion Rates	"Hemodynamic Suppression" Dose	"Cardiac Surgery" Doses	Epidural Doses	Other
Fentanyl	100 μg	1–2 μg/kg q 10–30 min	0.5–5 μg/kg/hr	5–8 μg/kg	50–100 μg/kg	Bolus: 50–100 μg Infusion: 10–80 μg/hour	Transdermal available 25–100 μg/hr
Sufentanil	15 μg	0.1–0.3 μg/kg q 10–30 min	0.1–1 μg/kg/hr	1–2 μg/kg	8–30 μg/kg	Bolus: 5–20 μg Infusion: 2–10 μg/hr	Controversial effects on CNS
Alfentanil	750 μg	8–16 μg/kg + 0.25–1 μg/kg/min	1–1.5 μg/kg/hr	50–150 μg/kg	150–250 μg/kg + 0.5–1.5 μg/kg/min	N/R	Few data in children

Table 3.12
Partial/Mixed Agonists/Antagonists

Agent	Equipotent Dose (compare to MS 10 mg)	Duration of Action	Comments
Buprenorphine (Buprenex)	0.3–0.4 mg IM or IV	6 hr	Partial μ-agonist with action very similar to morphine; binds tightly to receptors, increasing its duration of action; poorly reversed with naloxone
Butorphanol (Stadol)	1 mg IV 2–3 mg IM 1–2 mg intranasal (IN)	3–4 hr IV 4–5 hr IM 3–4 hr IN	κ-Receptor agonist, mixed effects at μ-receptors; significant psychomimetic effects (sedation, dysphoria); "ceiling" effect on MAC reduction (10–15%)
Dezocine (Dalgan)	10 mg IV or IM	2–4 hr	More effective than other mixed agonists/antagonists in reducing MAC (up to 65%)
Nalbuphine (Nubain)	10 mg IV, IM, or SC	3–5 hr	κ-Receptor agonist, moderately potent μ-receptor antagonist; less sedation than others; initial dose same resp. depression as morphine, but no increase with additional doses
Pentazocine (Talwin)	20–40 mg IV, IM, or SC	3–4 hr	κ-Receptor agonist; can increase BP; significant dysphoria at high doses (>30 mg)

Table 3.13
Other Agents Used during Anesthesia

Agent	Indication/Usage	Dosage/Route	Notes
Droperidol (Inapsine)	Antiemetic; neuroleptic	0.625–2.5 mg IV (antiemetic) 2.5–10 mg IV (neuroleptic)	Can cause hypotension; sedation can delay discharge with large doses; oculogyric crisis rare
Ondansetron (Zofran)	Antiemetic	4 mg PO; 4–8 mg IV	Very effective without sedation
Promethazine (Phenergan)	Antiemetic; sedative	12.5–50 mg IM 12.5–25 mg slow IV 12.5, 25, 50 mg PR	Slight antihistamine, anticholinergic effects; significant sedation
Ketorolac (Toradol)	Nonsteroidal antiinflammatory drug	10 mg PO 15–60 mg IM	Very good analgesic adjuvant without respiratory depression
Furosemide (Lasix)	Loop diuretic	10–40 mg IV	Can cause hypovolemia, hypokalemia
Bumetanide (Bumex)	Loop diuretic	0.5–1 mg IV	Slightly faster/shorter duration of action than furosemide
Hydrocortisone (Solu-Cortef)	Corticosteroid: prevention/treatment of adrenal insufficiency	100 mg IM or IV	Watch for fluid retention, steroid myopathy, etc.
Sodium bicarbonate	Treatment of metabolic acidosis	Calculated on base deficit (BD): or 1–2 mEq/kg IV	Also adjunct in life-threatening hyperkalemia

Premedicants

(See Table 3.14.) Used in conjunction with the preoperative visit, premedications are used with one or more of the following goals:

Sedation	Antisialogogue (drying of secretions)
Anxiolysis	Reduction of vagal activity
Analgesia	Decreased gastric volume
Amnesia	Increased gastric pH
Prevention of allergic phenomena	Attenuate stress response

Caution should be exercised when administering premedicants to certain patients, including:

Children under 1 year of age
Elderly
Patients with intracranial pathology
Critically ill or hypovolemic patients

Reversal Agents

The use of receptor-specific agonists in anesthesiology has led to the increasing use of agents specifically designed to reverse their effects. Table 3.15 lists the agents most commonly used as specific reversal agents.

Sympathomimetic Agents

Drugs used to increase blood pressure, heart rate and/or cardiac output play a vital role in perioperative care. Modulation of the autonomic nervous system during anesthesia coexists with the assessment of anesthetic depth as the hallmarks of patient management. A thorough understanding of autonomic receptors is important for appropriate use of this powerful class of agents. (Table 3.16)

Table 3.17 lists the sympathomimetics used to increase cardiac output (CO) or preload (PL) through enhanced venous return or to modulate heart rate (HR) or peripheral vascular resistance (PVR) to influence blood pressure.

Table 3.14
Agents Used in the Preoperative Period [a]

Agent	Dosage	Purpose	Advantages	Disadvantages
Atropine	0.01–0.02 mg/kg IM or IV	Antisialogogue ↓vagal activity (bradycardia)	Superior cardiac vagal blockage	Can have CNS effect; tachycardia; urinary retention
Glycopyrrolate (Robinul)	0.1–0.3 mg IM or IV	Same as above	Less CNS effect; less tachycardia	Less effective than atropine at ↑HR
Scopolamine	0.2–0.6 mg IM or IV or patch—behind ear night before surgery	Antisialogogue; antiemetic; amnestic	Less tachycardia; amnestic effect useful with morphine	Delirium; miosis
Diphenhydramine (Benadryl)	25–50 mg PO or IM	Sedation; antisialogogue; H₁-blocker	Antiemetic; antitussive	Mild anticholinergic-like side effects; No gastric effects
Cimetidine (Tagamet)	300 mg PO or IV	↑Gastric pH; ↓gastric volume	H₂-blocker	Confusion (rare) Hypotension (rare) Hepatic enzyme inhibition
Ranitidine (Zantac)	150 mg PO 50 mg IV	Same as above	Longer acting H₂-blocker	Thrombocytopenia (rare)
Famotidine (Pepcid)	20–40 mg PO 20 mg IV	Same as above	Longest acting H₂-blocker	
Diazepam (Valium)	0.05–0.15 mg/kg PO	Sedation; anxiolysis	Good amnesia; long acting (20–40 hr) anticonvulsant	Active metabolites can extend sedation; Painful IV injection
Lorazepam (Ativan)	0.05/kg PO	Same as above	Better amnesia; long acting (10–20 hr)	Slower onset (1–2 hr)

Midazolam (Versed)	0.04–0.08 mg/kg IM 0.02–0.05 mg/kg IV 0.2–0.5 mg/kg PO 0.2–0.8 mg/kg IN ÷	Same as above	Superior amnesia; short acting (2–4 hr)	Respiratory depression, especially when combined with narcotics
Metoclopramide (Reglan)	5–20 mg PO or IM 10 mg IV	Antiemetic; aspiration; prophylaxis	Increases gastric emptying	Dystonic reactions rare; gastric effects negated by narcotics
Clonidine	0.2–0.4 mg PO	Sedation (mild); antisialogogue; attenuate S.R.	Decreases MAC, blood pressure (4–8 hr)	Use with caution in elderly, hypovolemic, children

[a]Narcotics are often used as premedicants, alone or in combination with the above agents, for dosage schedule, see the opioids chart
[b]Intranasal

Table 3.15
Reversal Agents

Agent	Type of Drug Reversed	Dosage	Evaluation of Effect	Cautions/Side Effects
Flumazenil (Romazicon)	Benzodiazepine	0.2 mg/min up to 1 mg q 20 min—max 3 mg/hr	Increased arousal, return to consciousness	Resedation if used to reverse longer-acting agents such as lorazepam or diazepam; withdrawal seizures in benzodiazepine-dependent patient
Physostigmine (Antilirium)	Anticholinergic (e.g., atropine)	0.5–1 mg IV or IM; repeat × 1 10–30 min	Decreased delirium; anxiety, hallucinations	Too rapid administration can cause bradycardia, vomiting, salivation
Naloxone (Narcan)	Opioid—respiratory depression, sedation; pruritus, nausea	0.6–1 μg/kg/min up to 10 μg/kg/min; 20–100 μg/hr infusion for pruritus, nausea	Increase in respiratory rate, increased response to stimulation (e.g., endotracheal tube)	Nausea, vomiting, tachycardia, hypertension; seizures can occur with too rapid administration; observe carefully for return of narcosis
Edrophonium (Enion)	Neuromuscular blocking agents	0.5–1 mg/kg + atropine 7 μg/kg	Return of train-of-four; increase in respiratory depth; sustained head lift, hand grip; negative inspiratory force >20 cm H_2O	Fastest onset of action (0.8–2 min); fewer muscarinic side effects[b] than others
Neostigmine		40–70 μg/kg + atropine 15 μg/kg[a]		Intermediate onset (3–11 min)
Pyridostigmine		0.15–.25 mg/kg + atropine 15 μg/kg[a]		Slowest onset (4–16 min) but longest duration

[a]Can use glycopyrrolate 4–10 μg/kg (not recommended with edrophonium).
[b]Bradycardia, salivation, lacrimation.

Table 3.16
Sympathetic Nervous System Receptors

Receptor	Locations	Effect of Stimulation
α_1	Heart, vascular smooth muscle	Increased contractility; vasoconstriction
α_2	Adrenergic nerve endings, central nervous system (presynaptic); kidney; platelets	Inhibits norepinephrine release; inhibits renin release; platelet aggregation
β_1	Heart; adipose tissue	Increased heart rate, conduction, contractility, coronary vasodilation; lipolysis
β_2	Bronchial and vascular smooth muscle; liver; skeletal muscle; pancreas	Relaxation; gluconeogenesis, glycogenolysis; insulin release

Table 3.17
Sympathomimetic Agents

Agent	Bolus Dose	Infusion Dose	Site of Activity — α₁ art	α₁ ven	β₁	β₂	CO	HR	PVR
Isoproterenol	100 µg	0.02–0.15 µg/kg/min	0	0	++++	++++	↑↑	↑↑	↓↓
Dobutamine	N/R	2–30 µg/kg/min	0	0	+++	++	↑↑	0,↑	0
Dopamine (LD = low dose) (HD = high dose)	N/R	2–5 (LD); 5–30 (HD) µg/kg/min	LD +++ / +++ HD +++	LD +++ / HD +++	+++ / +++	++++	↑↑↑–→	0,↑ / ↑↑	0,↑ / ↑↑
Ephedrine	5–10 mg	N/R	+		+++	++	↑↑	↑	↑
Epinephrine	10–100 µg	0.01–0.05 (LD) 0.05–0.15 (ID) 0.15–0.30 (HD) µg/kg/min	+ (LD) / + ID +++ / +++ HD +++	+++ / +++	+++ / +++ / +++	+++ / +++ / +++	↑↑ / ↑– / ↑–→	↑ / ↑↑ / ↑↑↑	↑ / ↑↑ / ↑↑↑
(ID = intermediate dose)									
Norepinephrine	N/R	0.1–0.4 µg/kg/min	++++	++++	++++	+	↑–	↑–	↑↑↑
Phenylephrine	50–100 µg	0.10–0.75 µg/kg/min	++++	+	0	0	–→	–↓	↑↑
Amrinone	0.75 mg/kg	5–10 µg/kg/min	A noncatecholamine, phosphodieserase inhibitor that increases intracellular cAMP; Combines increased inotropy with arterial vasodilation to increase cardiac output, often with reflex increase in heart rate; bolus over 2–5 minutes						
Calcium salts: chloride, gluconate	2–10 mg/kg	1.5 mg/kg/min (max 1 gm)	Used to improve myocardial contractility after hypothermic cardioplegia, massive infusion of citrated blood, or hypotension from calcium channel blockers; may ↑ risk of vent. fibrillation						

Chapter 4

Perioperative Fluid Management

Management of the surgical patient's fluid status is a dynamic process that begins with preoperative assessment, includes intra-operative evaluations and intervention, and continues into the PACU or intensive care unit. Correction of preoperative de-rangements in volume status should result in a smoother hemo-dynamic course intraoperatively.

DISTRIBUTION OF BODY WATER AND ELECTROLYTES

Total Body Water (TBW)

Estimated Volume

Adult: 50–60% body weight (wt) in kg (e.g., 35–42 liters in a 70-kg adult)

Infant (< 1 year): 80–85% wt

Infant (> 1 year): 70–75% wt

Decreased 5–10% in obese, female, elderly

Distribution of TBW

Intracellular fluid (ICF) = 30–40% wt or 60% TBW

Extracellular fluid (ECF) = 20% wt or 40% TBW

  Plasma volume = 5% wt or 25% ECF

  Interstitial fluid = 15% wt or 75% ECF

Estimated Blood Volume (EBV)

Adult male: 7.5% body weight (i.e., 75 ml/kg)*

Adult female: 7.0% body weight*

Neonates and infants: 8.5% body weight

Premature infant: up to 100 ml/kg body weight

  *with obesity reduce percentage in calculation by 0.5–1%

Table 4.1
Distribution of Electrolytes in Body Compartments

	Sodium	Potassium	Calcium	Magnesium
ECF Concentration (mEq/liter)	140	4.5	5	2
ICF Concentration (mEq/liter)	10	150	1	40

Maintenance Fluid Requirements in Healthy Individuals Not Having Conditions Resulting in Large Losses of Fluid

1. Adult
   2–3 liters per day (100–125 ml/hr)
   Insensible loss $\approx$ 1 liter
   Urine output $\approx$ 1–2 liters
2. Infants and children (three acceptable formulas) (also see Chapter 19)
   a. 1500 ml/M^2 body surface area *per day*
   b. 100 ml/kg for first 10 kg body weight *per day*
      + 50 ml/kg for second 10 kg body weight *per day*
      + 25 ml/kg for each kg > 20 kg *per day*
      For example, 22-kg child:
      (100 ml/kg $\times$ 10 kg) + (50 ml/kg $\times$ 10 kg) + (25 ml/kg $\times$ 2 kg) = 1550 ml/24 hours or 65 ml/hr
   c. "4–2–1" rule for *per hour* basis:
      4 ml/kg for first 10 kg
      + 2 ml/kg for 11–20 kg
      + 1 ml/kg for each kg$\geq$21 kg
      For example, 22 kg child:
      (4 ml/kg $\times$ 10 kg) + (2 ml/kg $\times$ 10 kg) + (1 ml/kg $\times$ 2 kg) = 62 ml/hr
3. Patients with normal renal function will usually tolerate large variations in daily fluid intake and losses.

Electrolytes (Table 4.1)

Sodium

Total body Na^+ content is 40–45 mEq/kg

1. Major ECF cation

2. $Na^+ + Cl^- + HCO_3^-$ responsible for 90% of ECF solutes and osmotic pressure
3. Daily requirement 1–2 mEq/kg/day; normal renal function can compensate for variance between 0.25 and 6 mEq/kg/day intake
4. Serum concentration $[Na^+]$ regulated by several mechanisms
   a. Left atrial stretch receptors
   b. Central baroreceptors
   c. Renal afferent baroreceptors
   d. Aldosterone via renal reabsorption
   e. Atrial natriuretic factor
   f. Renin-angiotensin system
   g. Antidiuretic hormone affecting free water clearance by kidney
   h. $[Na^+]$ changes usually are due to change in TBW; 3 mEq/liter decrease represents $\approx$ 1 liter extra TBW
5. Hyponatremia may be produced by a total body Na^+ deficit or by an excess of TBW (Table 4.2).
   a. Calculation of NA^+ deficit if TBW is normal:

   $$Na^+ \text{ deficit (mEq)} = (\text{desired } Na^+ - \text{present } Na^+) \times TBW$$

   b. Chronic hyponatremia can usually be corrected slowly by restriction of free water intake.
      i. Mild hyponatremia can be corrected with 0.9% NS infusion if the patient's intravascular volume status is not increased.
      ii. ¼ of Na^+ deficit given slowly as 3% saline (only necessary if patient is symptomatic)
      iii. Not > 10–12 mEq/liter change in 24 hours because more rapid correction may cause permanent CNS abnormalities (central pontine myelinolysis)

Potassium (Table 4.2)

1. 98% of total K^+ is intracellular
2. Daily requirement of 1–3 mEq/kg/day (minimum 0.6 mEq/kg/day)
3. Serum $[K^+]$
   a. A decrease in serum $[K^+]$ of 1 mEq/liter represents a total body deficit of 100–200 mEq.

Table 4.2
Common Electrolyte Disturbances

	Laboratory Data	Causes	Signs/Symptoms	Treatment
Hyponatremia	Na$^+$ > 135 mEq/liter	Excess Na loss Renal GI Skin ↓ H$_2$O excretion Renal Hepatic Cardiac SIADH ↑ H$_2$O intake Absorption (TURP) Psychogenic	Altered mental status Seizures Weakness Muscle cramps Nausea, vomiting	Acute: Diuresis 0.9–3% NS Long-term: H$_2$O restriction for SIADH ↑ water loss
Hypernatremia	Na$^+$ > 145 mEq/liter	↑ Water loss Renal GI Skin ↓ Water intake	Mental status changes Myoclonus Edema	↑ Water intake ↓ Na$^+$ intake ↑ Na$^+$ excretion
Hypokalemia	K$^+$ < 3.5 mEq/liter	Excess excretion ↑ pH Diuretics Renal tubular acidosis ↓ Intake Intracellular movement Drugs pH status	ECG signs U waves ST depression Potentiates digitalis toxicity arrhythmias Muscle cramps Weakness Mental status changes	KCl po IV (0.25 mEq/kg over 30–60 min) *max.* 1 mEq/kg/hr IV with ECG monitor
Hyperkalemia	K$^+$ > 5.5 mEq/liter	Renal failure Iatrogenic	ECG signs Peaked T wave Prolonged PR Absent P wave Wide QRS Sine wave Heart block Weakness Confusion	↑ Excretion Diuresis Dialysis Redistribution Insulin/glucose (10–20 units, 25–50 gm) ↑ pH with NaHCO$_3$ ↓ PaCO$_2$ (0.5 mEq/liter/10 torr ↓) Physiologic reversal of effects Ca^{2+} slowly IV

b. Acid-base effects on $[K^+]$
  i. Acidosis increases $[K^+]$; H^+ moves intracellularly in exchange for K^+; 0.1 unit decrease in pH results in 0.6 mEq/liter increase in $[K^+]$.
  ii. Alkalosis decreases $[K^+]$ in a similar ratio.
c. Drugs
  i. α-Adrenergic agents increase $[K^+]$.
  ii. β-Adrenergic agents and some diuretics (furosemide, thiazides) decrease $[K^+]$; insulin/glucose drive K^+ into cell
d. Iatrogenic
  i. NG suction
  ii. Inadequate supplementation to IV fluids
  iii. Renal tubular damage from nephrotoxins

4. Chronic hypokalemia often does not produce clinical neurophysiologic effects if the ratio of intra- to extracellular $[K^+]$ is maintained. Treatment of hypokalemia should not be too rapid because acute increases in extracellular K^+ may be catastrophic. KCl is very irritating to peripheral veins and should not be given at concentrations above 40 mEq/liter in a peripheral IV.

Calcium

1. 99% contained in bone
2. Major functions related to anesthesia care
  a. Neuromuscular junction
  b. Cardiac muscle contractility
  c. Coagulation
3. Ionized form active (value related to pH and plasma protein concentration, primarily albumin)
4. Daily requirement 0.1 mEq/kg/day
5. Abnormal levels
  a. Hypercalcemia (total serum calcium > 10.5 mg/dl or ionized > 1.3 mM)
    i. Causes
      • Excess intake and GI absorption
      • Parathyroid hormone (PTH) excess
      • Redistribution
        Immobilization

       Malignancies

       Adrenal insufficiency

  ii. Signs and symptoms
- Coma or obtundation
- Weakness
- Muscle cramps
- Renal failure

 iii. Treatment—increased $[Ca^{2+}]$ is worsened by volume contraction
- IV/hydration with 0.9% NS
- Diuresis with furosemide
- Correction of underlying condition (e.g., malignancy)

b. Hypocalcemia (ionized calcium < 1 mM)

   i. Causes
- Inadequate absorption due to vitamin D or PTH deficiency
- Redistribution
  Alkalosis $2°$ hyperventilation
  Citrate infusion $2°$ massive blood transfusion
  Hypermagnesemia
- Hyperphosphatemia

  ii. Signs and symptoms
- Mental status changes (e.g., dementia, depression
- Muscle cramps
- Paresthesias
- Arrhythmias
- Chvostek and Trousseau signs
- Weakness, fatigue
- Prolonged QT interval
- Depressed myocardial contractility—CHF

 iii. Treatment
- $CaCl_2$ 15 mg/kg IV slowly (1 gm $CaCl_2$ = 13.6 mEq Ca^{2+})

  or
- Calcium gluconate 15–30 mg/kg IV slowly (1 gm = 4.5 mEq Ca^{2+})
- Administration of large doses of calcium should be monitored by ECG to assess for heart block or ventricular fibrillation. Calcium increases dig-

italis toxicity. Calcium cannot be given in fluids containing HCO_3^- because precipitates will form.

Magnesium

1. 50% is stored in bone
2. Imbalance often parallels calcium or potassium level
3. Necessary for neuromuscular junction function and cardiac muscle excitability
4. Daily requirement 0.04 mEq/kg/day
5. Abnormal levels
   a. Hypermagnesemia ($[Mg^{2+}] > 2.5$ mg/dl)
      i. Causes
         - Excess intake
         - Iatrogenic
         - Antacids
         - Renal failure
         - Addison's disease
         - Lithium use
      ii. Signs and symptoms
         - Weakness (potentiates nondepolarizing muscle relaxants)
         - ECG changes (prolonged PR and QT intervals, conduction delays, heart block)
         - Decreased deep tendon reflexes, respiratory insufficiency
         - Mental status changes, somnolence
      iii. Treatment
         - IV hydration and diuresis
         - Calcium (5–10 mEq) antagonizes effects
         - Dialysis
   b. Hypomagnesemia ($[Mg^{2+}] < 1.7$ mg/dl)
      i. Causes
         - Alcoholism
         - Malnutrition
         - Burns
         - Acute pancreatitis
         - Diuretics
      ii. Signs and symptoms

- Mental status changes, lethargy, depression seizures
- Weakness, muscle spasms
- ECG changes (wide QRS, peaked T, prolonged PR and QT, ST depression)
- Dysrhythmias

iii. Treatment

- $MgSO_4$ 2–3 gm IV slowly, plus infusion up to 10 gm over 5–6 hours (for $MgSO_4$, 1 gm = 8 mEq Mg^{2+})

PREOPERATIVE ASSESSMENT OF VOLUME STATUS

Intravascular volume status may not correlate with total body fluid status. For example, a patient with liver failure may have excess total body Na^+ and water (as manifested by peripheral edema and ascites) but have a low intravascular volume. Na^+ and water homeostasis may be independently controlled; therefore, serum Na^+ concentration may not be an accurate measure of intravascular volume.

Hypovolemia

1. Causes of decreased intravascular volume in the preoperative period:

Anorexia, vomiting
Diarrhea or preoperative bowel preparation
Fever (1°C rise increases fluid needs by 10%)
Bleeding (may not be apparent with trauma such as retroperitoneal, pelvic, or long bone fracture)
Chronic hypertension (treated and untreated)
Bowel obstruction
Sepsis
Diuresis due to hyperglycemia, radiologic contrast media, diuretics

2. Signs and symptoms (see Chapter 16 for signs of acute blood loss)

Tachycardia
Hypotension or orthostatic BP changes
Dry mucous membranes

Weight loss
Cutaneous vasoconstriction and diminished distal pulses
Poor capillary refill
Cool skin
Poor to no pulse on pulse oximeter
Poor skin turgor
Flat neck veins (low CVP)
Low urine output (< 1 ml/kg/hr)
Mental status changes

   3. Laboratory tests—support diagnosis, but insensitive for making the diagnosis

↑ Serum osmolality (concentration of solute in osmoles/liter water) molecules that dissociate contribute more than 1 osm (e.g., 1 mole NaCl yields 2 osm)
↑ Serum sodium
↑ BUN (normally BUN/creatinine in serum is 10/1 but may be higher with dehydration)
↑ Hemoglobin
Acidosis 2° poor perfusion

Hypervolemia

1. Causes

Renal failure
Cardiac failure
Iatrogenic

2. Signs and symptoms

Increase in weight
Edema
Dyspnea (especially when supine)
Hypertension
Jugular venous distension
Rales on chest auscultation
S_3 gallop

3. Diagnostic tests

Measurement of CVP or PCWP
Chest x-ray for increased pulmonary vasculature or signs of pulmonary edema

FLUID THERAPY IN THE PERIOPERATIVE PERIOD

The goal of fluid administration is adequate tissue perfusion with oxygen delivery and waste elimination. Signs of adequate fluid replacement include

- Appropriate HR and BP
  < 10% loss of EBV without effect
  15% loss of EBV results in resting tachycardia or orthostatic hypotension
  > 20% loss of EBV results in hypotension
- Urine output 0.5–1 ml/kg/hr
- Normal or improving acid base status (initially pH may decrease as perfusion improves, because of lactic acid that accumulated during less than adequate perfusion)
- Mixed venous Po_2 > 35 mm Hg (65% saturation)
- Appropriate CVP and/or pulmonary capillary wedge pressure

- Appropriate cardiac index (2.0 liter/min/M^2)

Solutions Available for Replacement Therapy—Crystalloids, Colloids, and Blood

Crystalloids (Table 4.3)

Perioperative fluid losses vary in source and therefore in electrolyte composition. For example, fluid lost from the stomach has a lower sodium content (60–100 mEq/liter) and higher potassium content (10–20 mEq/liter) than bile (Na^+, 135–145 mEq/liter; K^+, 5–10 mEq/liter) or small intestine (Na^+, 120–140 mEq/liter; K^+, 5–10 mEq/liter). Therefore different replacement solutions may be needed to maintain electrolyte balance. Tissue trauma that occurs with surgery leads to an isotonic shift of intravascular fluid into a "third space," an extravascular, nonfunctional sequestration site from which the fluid is no longer accessible to the circulation and must be replaced to maintain normovolemia. Crystalloids are usually used to replace deficits from overnight fasts, intraoperative maintenance, and initial fluid resuscitation.

Colloids (Table 4.4)

Colloid solutions contain natural or synthetic macromolecules that are less permeable to the intact vascular endothelium.

Table 4.3
Commonly Used Crystalloids

Solution	Na$^+$ (mEq/liter)	K$^+$ (mEq/liter)	Cl$^-$ (mEq/liter)	Lactate (mEq/liter)	Osmolarity (mosm/liter)	pH	Glucose (mg/dl)	Ca^{2+} (mEq/liter)
LR	130	4	109	28	273	6.6		2
D$_5$LR	130	4	109	28	525	4.9	50	2
0.45% NS	77		77		146	4.3		
0.9% NS	154		154		308	5.0		
D$_5$W					252	4.5	50	

Table 4.4
Commonly Used Colloids

Product	Na$^+$ (mEq/liter)	Cl$^-$ (mEq/liter)	K$^+$ (mEq/liter)	Ratio of Volume Administered: Volume Added/ Vascular Volume
5% Albumin	145	145		1:1
25% Albumin	150	150	1	1:4.5
6% Hydroxyethyl starch* in NS	154	154		1:1.2

*Because of potential effects on clotting and RE cells, infusions should be limited to 1 liter/24 hours.

These molecules remain in the intravascular space for a longer time and maintain or increase the plasma colloid oncotic pressure, decreasing fluid movement out of the vascular volume into the interstitial space.

Comparison of Crystalloids and Colloids (Table 4.5)

Controversy remains regarding which type of solution is best for replacement therapy.

Perioperative Fluid Requirements

Maintenance Requirements

Patients for elective surgery have been NPO for 8–12 hours, may have had bowel preparations, and have had other fluid losses before arrival in the operating room. Preoperative fluid administration should begin to replace these losses. Half of the remaining deficit can be replaced in the first hour of surgery, and the rest over the next two hours. In addition, hourly maintenance requirements (based on formulas given above) should be continued throughout the procedure. There may be increased maintenance requirements in patients who are febrile or who have other ongoing losses of body fluids.

Blood Loss

Blood loss must be replaced continuously but not necessarily with blood. The **allowable blood loss** should be calculated for each pa-

Table 4.5
Crystalloid versus Colloid

	Crystalloid	Colloid
Advantages	Inexpensive Promotes urinary flow ($\uparrow$ intravascular volume) Fluid of choice for initial resuscitation of trauma/hemorrhage Expands intravascular volume ($1/4$ volume given retained intravascularly) Restores third space losses	More sustained intravascular volume increase (1/3 still intravascular at 24 hr) Maintains or $\uparrow$ plasma colloid oncotic pressure Requires smaller volume for equal effect Less peripheral edema (more fluid remains intravascular) May lower intracranial pressure
Disadvantages	Dilutes colloid osmotic pressure Promotes peripheral edema ? Higher incidence of pulmonary edema Requires large volume Effects are transient	Expensive May produce coagulopathy (dextrans and hetastarch) With capillary leak may potentiate fluid loss to the interstitium Impairs subsequent cross-matching of blood (dextrans) Dilutes clotting factors and platelets $\downarrow$ Platelet adhesiveness (absorption onto platelet membrane receptor) Potential blocking of renal tubules and reticuloendothelial cells in the liver Possible anaphylactoid reaction with dextrans

tient before surgery. This is the blood loss that can be replaced with fluids not containing RBCs to keep the patient euvolemic and with a hematocrit above a predetermined value (H_1).

$$\textbf{Allowable blood loss} = (EBV)(H_0 - H_1)/H_{ave}$$

EBV = estimated blood volume in ml

H_0 = original hematocrit (expressed as %)

H_1 = lowest acceptable hematocrit

$H_{ave} = (H_0 + H_1)/2$

Table 4.6
Rates of Fluid Administration to Replace Third Space Losses

Fluid Shift	Example of Operation	Rate* (Crystalloid)
Minor	Tendon repair	0–3 ml/kg/hr
	Tympanoplasty	
Moderate	Hysterectomy	6 ml/kg/hr
	Inguinal hernia	
Major	Total hip replacement	9 ml/kg/hr
	Abdominal case with	
	peritonitis	

*Includes 2 ml/kg/hr maintenance but not usual 3 ml crystalloid/ml blood loss if blood not replaced with blood.

In some patients with low starting Hct, allowable blood loss is 0, and blood is replaced as soon as blood loss begins. Otherwise, blood loss can initially be replaced with three times the volume of crystalloid such as LR or NS. This is continued until the allowable blood loss is reached, when blood or packed RBCs are given. When blood loss equals 10% of EBV but is below the allowable blood loss, some practitioner choose to give colloid in a volume equal to blood loss. In the latter case, colloid is used until the allowable blood loss is reached.

Third Space Loss

The volume of fluid replacement for third space loss is estimated from the type of surgery (Table 4.6) and is usually given as LR or NS. The estimates may not be accurate when procedures are very long (> 4 hr).

INTRAOPERATIVE ASSESSMENT—INDICATIONS FOR MONITORING

In some situations, the estimates for fluid replacement are inadequate, and clinical signs must be supplemented with information from invasive monitoring. Some limitations to these monitoring techniques may make them invalid for assessing volume status in certain patients. Table 4.7 lists monitors in order of increasing invasiveness.

Table 4.7
Volume Status Monitors

Monitor	Limitations	Indications
Blood pressure (noninvasive)	Peripheral vasoconstriction due to • peripheral vascular disease • ↓ Temperature • Vasoactive drugs Inaccessible site	All patients
Heart rate	Chronotropic drugs • β-Blockers • Epinephrine Conduction delays and blocks	All patients
Hematocrit	Time for equilibration Unknown baseline value	Serial for hemodilution Undetermined blood loss
Urine output	Renal insufficiency/failure Diuretics Glycosuria due to osmotic effect	Prolonged cases (≥ 4 hr) Anticipated blood loss Large 3rd space losses
Intraarterial catheter	Access	Need for beat-to-beat monitoring as with vasoactive-drug drips (e.g., SNP, epi) or anticipated or current instability
Central venous pressure (CVP)	Measures pressure not volume Moderate-to-severe pulmonary disease • COPD • Pulmonary hypertension Cardiac compromise	Rapid volume infusion anticipated 3rd space loss Large blood loss
Pulmonary artery catheter (PCWP)	Inability to place properly	CVP not adequate reflection of volume status (see CVP limitations)

Table 4.8
Indications for Transfusion

Condition	Laboratory Value	Component
Anemia	Hgb < 8 in healthy patient Hgb < 10 for those needing ↑ oxygen-carrying capacity such as angina, CHF, elderly; 1 ml/kg increases Hct 1.5%	PRBCs
Coagulopathy	PT > 1.5 × normal	Vitamin K for patients on Coumadin preoperatively FFP in emergency
	PTT > 1.5 × normal	FFP
	↓ Fibrinogen	Cryoprecipitate
Thombocytopenia	Platelet count < 100,000	1 unit platelets/10 kg body weight

BLOOD AND BLOOD COMPONENT THERAPY

Indications for Transfusion (Table 4.8)
Avoiding Homologous Transfusion

Techniques are available to decrease transfusion of banked blood, which reduces the risks of infection transmitted via blood or blood product and of transfusion reaction.

1. Preoperative autologous donation; limitations—emergency surgery, anemia, religious beliefs
2. Preoperative hemodilution; limitations—need to maximize O_2-carrying capacity (e.g., cardiac and pulmonary compromise, sickle cell disease) or religious beliefs
3. Controlled hypotension; limitations—cardiac disease, carotid disease, previous stroke
4. Regional anesthesia cannot be used if patient or procedure is not amenable
5. Intraoperative blood salvage (cell saver); contraindications—infection, cancer cells, religious beliefs

Suggested Readings

James MF. Clinical use of magnesium infusions in anesthesia. Anesth Analg 1992;74:129–136.

Wong KC, Schafer PG, Schultz JR. Hypokalemia and anesthetic implications. Anesth Analg 1993;77:1238–1260.

Zaloga GP, Prough DS. Fluids and electrolytes. In: Barash PG, Cullen BF, Stoelting RK, eds. Clinical Anesthesia. 2nd ed. Philadelphia: JB Lippincott, 1992:203.

Chapter 5

Airway Management

Oxygen is the single most important element involved in energy production, and without it, cells will begin to die within minutes. This fundamental reality demands that the primary responsibility of those engaged in airway management is to deliver oxygen to the patient by whatever means is necessary. Adequate oxygenation can be maintained via several techniques, although hypercarbia may persist.

GOALS OF AIRWAY MANAGEMENT

Desirable goals of airway management include oxygenation, ventilation, airway patency, airway protection, and pulmonary toilet or suctioning.

Oxygenation

Adequacy of arterial oxygen content depends on the concentration of inspired oxygen (FIO_2), transport to the alveoli, diffusion across membranes into the blood, and hemoglobin concentration.

FIO_2

When there is possible airway compromise, the initial FIO_2 should be high, approaching 1.0 (100%). After the airway has been established and hemodynamic parameters stabilized, the FIO_2 may be weaned, based on laboratory values and clinical evidence that the basic oxygenation goals are being met.

Oxygen Delivery to Tissues

Tissue oxygenation requires oxygen transport from the lungs, and delivery is a function of the oxygen content of the blood and the cardiac output.

Oxygen Content

The oxygen content of 100 ml of blood can be calculated by the formula:

$$\text{Content (ml)} = (1.34 \times \text{Hemoglobin} \times \% \text{ Saturation}) + (0.003 \times \text{PaO}_2)$$

Because the hemoglobin concentration and the oxyhemoglobin saturation are two important parameters in this formula, practical goals for adequate oxygen delivery are to keep the hemoglobin concentration above 7–8 gm/dl and the oxyhemoglobin saturation above 90%.

Cardiac Output

An adequate volume of oxygenated blood must be delivered by the heart to the tissues. This usually requires a cardiac index (cardiac output/body surface area) above 2.0 liters/min/m^2. Cardiac index may be augmented with intravascular volume adjustment, inotropes, or vasoactive drugs.

Oxygen Utilization and Availability

Many factors affect oxygen utilization and availability such as hemoglobin type, temperature, pH, and metabolic rate. Adequacy of global oxygen saturation is ensured when the mixed venous oxygen saturation (sampled from the pulmonary artery) is greater than 65%.

Ventilation

The goals of ventilation are to deliver oxygen to the alveoli and to remove carbon dioxide. Often, patients can ventilate themselves, but if this is inadequate, artificial ventilation by natural or artificial airway should be initiated. After the primary goal of delivering oxygen to the lungs has been achieved, the secondary goal of ventilation is to rid the body of CO_2, to maintain normal pH. The success of ventilatory intervention can be assessed by measuring an arterial blood gas, with goals of $PaO_2 > 60$ mm Hg and pH between 7.35 and 7.45.

Airway Patency

A basic goal of airway management is to establish an avenue through which oxygen can be delivered to and CO_2 can be evacuated from the lungs. In a sedated or obtunded patient breathing spontaneously, ventilation may be adequate or may require only simple changes in head position, but in apneic patients or those with airway obstruction, instrumentation may be necessary to establish an airway (Table 5.1).

Airway Protection

After the airway is established, it must be protected to ensure that vomit, blood, and secretions do not reach the lungs. Airway protection is best achieved by placing a properly sized tube into the trachea. In the adult patient, a cuff on the distal end of the tracheal tube can be inflated to form a seal to protect the lungs. In a child less than 7–8 years old, an uncuffed endotracheal tube is commonly used, and the size of the tube should be such that it forms a fair seal at the level of the cricothyroid cartilage, the narrowest portion of the pediatric airway. Tracheostomy is usually performed in patients who have had endotracheal tubes for several days and who will need intubation for more than 7–14 days.

Pulmonary Suctioning

The goals of tracheal-bronchial suctioning are to evacuate secretions, plugs, clots, etc., from the lower airway as well as to

Table 5.1
Clinical Situations Requiring Airway Management

Ventilatory arrest
Inadequate ventilatory effort
Inadequate oxygenation
Cardiac arrest
Airway trauma (disruption, hematoma, burns)
Airway tumors
Airway infections
Hyperventilation to treat increased intracranial pressure
Pulmonary toilet
Airway protection (obtunded patients)

induce coughing when appropriate. These maneuvers promote pulmonary toilet and help keep larger, lower airways open. Suctioning can be performed easily in patients with endotracheal tubes or tracheostomies. In these instances, suctioning is necessary because coughing may be ineffective.

NORMAL LARYNGEAL ANATOMY

Adult

1. Located at C4–6
2. Anterior boundary of larynx is epiglottis
3. Vocal cords extend from the thyroid cartilage to the arytenoid cartilages
4. Narrowest part of larynx is the space between the vocal cords (rima glottidis)

Infant

1. At birth, glottis at level of C3, and by age 3, is at C4–5
2. Narrowest part of larynx is at the cricoid cartilage
3. Vocal cords angled in relation to axis of trachea

Innervation

1. Branches of vagus for both sensory and motor function
2. Internal branch of the superior laryngeal nerve—sensation to level of vocal cords
3. External branch of the superior laryngeal nerve—cricothyroid muscle
4. Recurrent laryngeal nerves—sensation below cords and other laryngeal muscles
   a. With bilateral partial injury of recurrent laryngeal nerves, the vocal cords will be positioned near the midline and the airway will likely be obstructed
   b. With bilateral transection of recurrent laryngeal nerves, the vocal cords will be in a midposition and the airway will likely be adequate because there will be both adductor and abductor muscle palsy

TOPICAL ANESTHESIA FOR THE AIRWAY

An antisialogogue should be given IM 30–45 min before topical anesthesia of the airway because secretions can limit local anesthetic contact with the mucosa.

Nasal Passages

Because of the vascularity of the nasal mucosa, topical anesthesia for nasal intubations should contain vasoconstrictors such as phenylephrine, which can be mixed with 4% lidocaine and sprayed or applied with pledgets or cotton-tipped applicators. Cocaine 4% is an alternative because it provides both anesthetic and vasoconstrictor effects.

Pharynx, Vocal Cords, and Trachea

1. Aerosolization of 4 ml of 4% lidocaine over 5 minutes usually provides adequate anesthesia to the entire airway.
2. Tongue
   a. Spray with 4% or 10% lidocaine or apply with pledgets.
   b. Bilateral glossopharyngeal nerve blocks will produce anesthesia for the posterior third of the tongue and the posterior pharynx and will eliminate the gag reflex.

3. Larynx
   a. Topical spray with 4% lidocaine
   b. Superior laryngeal nerve blocks
      i. Percutaneously at the thyrohyoid membrane above the cornu of the hyoid cartilage with 2% lidocaine
      ii. Permucosally at the lateral border of the piriform fossae with pledgets soaked with 4% lidocaine (Krause forceps)

4. Trachea and carina
   a. Translaryngeal injection (at cricothyroid membrane) of 3–5 ml of 2–4% lidocaine
   b. Injection of 3–5 ml of 2–4% lidocaine directly through the glottis via tubing or fiberoptic bronchoscope

PREDICTING THE DIFFICULT AIRWAY

In assessing the patient with a need for airway management, it is important to evaluate airway anatomy because abnormalities may necessitate use of special techniques. When facing a difficult airway, it's best to call for help early, because an assistant may be necessary.

Table 5.2
Obvious Airway Abnormalities

Trauma to the face, head, or neck
Upper airway infection
Obstruction, foreign body
Stridor
Craniofacial abnormalities
Tumor in the mouth, face, or neck
Burns

Table 5.3
Occult Causes of Difficult Airways

Inability to extend the neck (1)
Short neck
Short jaw
Receding mandible (overbite) (2)
Temporomandibular joint dysfunction
Inability to visualize the uvula, oral pharynx, or soft palate in an awake
    patient asked to open the mouth and stick out the tongue (large tongue)
    (3)

Airway Abnormalities (Predicting the "Difficult Airway")

Even for the new house officer, it is often easy to predict
whether an airway is normal or abnormal. Table 5.2 lists conditions that should immediately signal the possibility of an difficult airway. Specific attention to anatomic features may help
predict difficulties in airway management, as listed in Table 5.3.

Inability to Extend the Neck

Normal neck extension from the horizontal plane is approximately 35 degrees. If neck extension is limited, the line of sight
from the mouth to the glottis is more acute, and the vocal cords
may be difficult to visualize with a laryngoscope. Neck extension, as well as rotation and flexion, should be examined before
undertaking airway instrumentation. In cases of head and neck
trauma, stability of the cervical spinal column *must be documented*
before the head and neck are moved.

Short Neck

If the distance from the thyroid cartilage to the mental prominence is less than 6 cm with the neck extended, the glottis may be difficult to visualize. The vocal cords will appear to be in an "anterior" position, and placement of the endotracheal tube through the cords could be difficult.

Short Jaw

The distance from the tip of the chin to the mandibular angle is less then 9 cm in patients who may be difficult to intubate.

Temporomandibular (TM) Joint Dysfunction

Mouth opening may be limited by temporomandibular joint dysfunction. Mouth opening should be at least 3 cm between the front teeth or gums. If opening is limited, a laryngoscope cannot be placed properly, and visualization will be grossly impaired. Some awake patients have limited TM mobility as a result of pain, which may normalize after induction of anesthesia or with use of muscle relaxants. Although TM mobility may improve, it is often best to err on the conservative side and base clinical management on the distance of "awake" mouth opening.

Assessment of Tongue Size

Mallampati et al. have described a classification of the upper airway based on ability to visualize pharyngeal structures (3). Sitting upright with the head in a neutral position, the patient is asked to fully open the mouth and to maximally stick out the tongue. In class I patients, the soft palate, uvula, and anterior and posterior tonsillar pillars can be visualized. With class II, all of the preceding can be seen except the tonsillar pillars, and with class III, only the base of the uvula can be visualized. In class IV, only the anterior portion of the soft palate can be seen. Difficult direct vision of the vocal cords is likely in class IV patients, but difficult intubation may occur in class II or III as well.

AIRWAY EQUIPMENT (Table 5.5)

Oxygen Source

Oxygen is supplied either from an individual tank (Fig. 5.1) or from a wall outlet that uses the hospital's central oxygen tanks. In the United States, oxygen tanks, flowmeters, and tubing for oxygen are colored green. A full "E" cylinder has 640 liters of oxygen pressurized to 2200 p.s.i. at standard temperature. Since oxygen is a compressed gas in an "E" cylinder, the volume of gas remaining is proportional to the pressure in the tank. A regulator is necessary to reduce the pressure of oxygen coming from the cylinder before it enters the flowmeter and leaves via a connector or nipple.

Suction Apparatus

Equipment for suctioning the mouth and pharynx should be immediately available. Vomit, blood, or saliva may be present in the mouth and obscure the glottis. The suction apparatus should be equipped with either a flexible plastic catheter or rigid Yankauer tip, depending on the situation. Both pieces of equipment should be immediately available.

Oral and Nasal Airways

In a sedated or unresponsive patient, an oral airway (Fig. 5.2) can be inserted to lift the tongue anteriorly away from the pharyngeal wall if mask ventilation is obstructed. Alternatively, a nasal airway (Fig. 5.3) can be inserted so that its tip passes between the tongue and pharyngeal wall, thus creating a passage for oxygen. Neither airway guarantees an open channel, though both may help in certain circumstances. Although a nasal airway is better tolerated in an awake or lightly sedated patient, traumatic insertion may cause bleeding from the nose into the pharynx, which will produce coughing or gagging.

Anesthesia or Resuscitation Mask

An anesthesia or resuscitation mask is designed to be connected to an anesthesia circuit or resuscitation bag (Fig. 5.1) and then held over a patient's nose and mouth to create an airtight seal. (Fig. 5.4) This system can be used for positive pressure or spontaneous ventilation. There are many sizes and shapes of masks

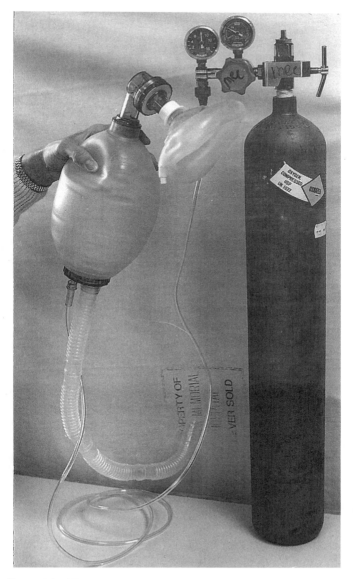

Figure 5.1. "E" cylinder oxygen tank connected to self-inflating resuscitation bag.

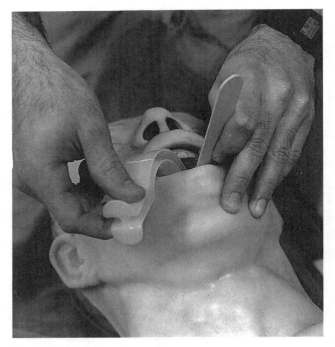

Figure 5.2.   Insertion of an oral airway.

to accommodate all patients. Ventilation and oxygenation can be performed in most cases via mask, but in this situation, the airway is not protected from aspiration.

Self-Inflating Resuscitation Bag

A self-inflating resuscitation bag fills for positive pressure ventilation even when no supplemental gas flow (oxygen) is being delivered. Under these circumstances, ventilation is with room air ($FIO_2 = 0.21$). When oxygen is delivered to the bag and a reservoir "tail" is used (Fig. 5.1), a high FIO_2 can be delivered to the patient. Many self-inflating resuscitation bags have valves that permit both spontaneous and positive pressure ventilation (Fig. 5.4).

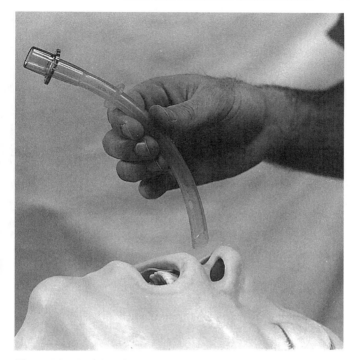

Figure 5.3.   Insertion of a nasal airway.

Laryngoscope

A laryngoscope (Fig. 5.5) is an instrument that is designed to illuminate the upper airway as well as to displace the soft tissue of the mouth so that the vocal cords can be visualized directly. The scope has two basic parts: *(a)* a handle containing batteries and *(b)* the blade containing the light source, which is inserted into the mouth. Blades may be of various sizes and shapes to permit visualization of the glottis. In general, curved blades are used to indirectly lift the epiglottis; straight blades displace the epiglottis directly.

Endotracheal Tube

Endotracheal tubes (Fig. 5.6) may be made of any of several nontoxic materials and can be placed either through the

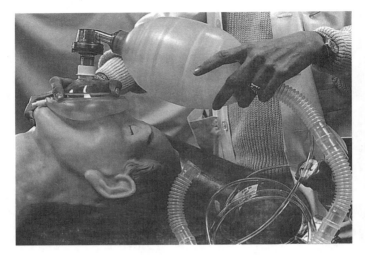

Figure 5.4. Self-inflation resuscitation bag attached to an anesthesia mask. This system can be used for efficient bag-mask ventilation and oxygen.

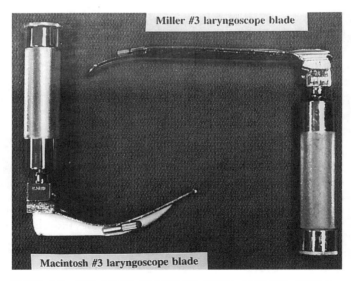

Figure 5.5. Two popular laryngoscope blades, commonly called a straight blade (Miller) and a curved blade (Macintosh).

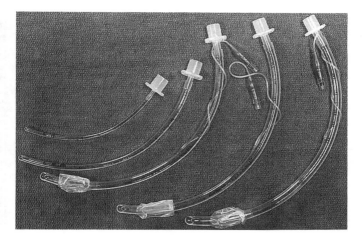

Figure 5.6. Variously sized endotracheal tubes. Smaller, pediatric tubes are uncuffed.

mouth or nose into the trachea. When positioned properly, the distal tip of the tube should be below the vocal cords and the carina. A cuffed endotracheal tube should be inserted far enough so that the cuff is below the larynx, because cuff pressure may injure the vocal cords or submucosal nerves.

BASIC TECHNIQUES OF AIRWAY MANAGEMENT

Mouth-to-Mouth (Mouth-to-Mouth-Nose) Ventilation (4)

This simplest form of ventilation has the advantage of being readily available but is used only in emergency situations when airway equipment is not accessible. Its disadvantages are that a relatively low FIO_2 (exhaled O_2) can be delivered and the risk of patient/operator cross-contamination.

After establishing that the patient is not breathing and that obstruction in the upper airway has been cleared, the patient's airway is opened by lifting the chin anteriorly. Slight neck extension, if not contraindicated, may help improve airway patency. The patient is ventilated by the operator, who breathes into the mouth (with the nose pinched closed) of the adult patient or into the mouth and nose of a pediatric patient. Breaths are coordinated with chest compressions if circulatory

Table 5.4
CPR in Adults and Children (4, 5)

	Compression Rate (compressions/ min)	Ventilation Rate (breaths/ min)	Compression to Ventilation Ratio	Depth of Compression (inches)	Hand Position
Infant	At least 100	20	5:1	0.5–1.0	1 fingerbreadth below nipples
Child (1–8 years)	80–100	15	5:1	1.0–1.5	2 fingerbreadths above xiphoid
Adult	80–100	12	5:1	1.5–2.0	2 fingerbreadths above xiphoid

Reproduced with permission from Finucane BT, Santora AH. Principles of Airway Management. Philadelphia: FA Davis, 1988:227.

resuscitation is being performed. The ratio of breaths to chest compressions is listed in Table 5.4. Care should be taken to provide little neck manipulation if cervical spine injury is suspected.

Mouth-To-Mask Resuscitation

Devices are available that allow the operator to breathe through a protective valve and ventilate the patient via a mask (Fig. 5.7). The advantages of this system are that supplemental oxygen can be provided and the chance for infection is significantly diminished. Equipment for emergency mouth-to-mask ventilation should be available on every resuscitation cart as well as throughout the hospital.

Mask-Resuscitation Bag Ventilation

Mask-resuscitation bag ventilation is very efficient and effective and protects against oral contamination of the operator. The components include an anesthesia-type mask that is applied to the patient's face (over the nose and mouth), a self-inflating resuscitation bag, an oxygen reservoir, and oxygen tubing that connects to a 10–15 liter/minute oxygen source.

The mask is applied tightly to the patient's face and held

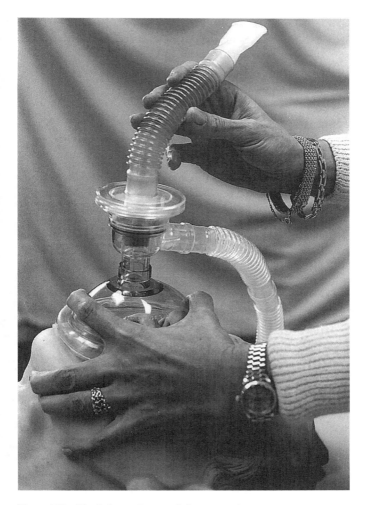

Figure 5.7.   Mouth-to-mask resuscitation apparatus.

in place with the left hand. The mask is secured by applying downward pressure with thumb and index finger. The other fingers engage the mandible and provide the chin lift. The patient is ventilated by squeezing the resuscitation bag with the right hand. The patient should be observed to ensure that there is an adequate chest rise and fall with each ventilation. The bag should be allowed to self-inflate slowly to maximize the FIO_2.

Endotracheal Intubation

Oral Intubation

Most commonly, the trachea is intubated by direct vision, with the tube inserted through the mouth. Patients to be intubated are usually anesthetized or unresponsive. With general anesthesia, muscle relaxants are often used to facilitate intubation. Patients should be adequately oxygenated before laryngoscopy and intubation. Required equipment is a laryngoscope with appropriately sized blade, suction apparatus, an endotracheal tube, and a 10-ml syringe to inflate the cuff, if the tube is so equipped (Table 5.5).

First, the patient's head is placed in the "sniff" position, elevated 1–2 inches with cushion or folded sheets, with slight

Table 5.5
Endotracheal Tube, Laryngoscope Blade, Oral Airway, Nasal Airway and Suction Catheter Sizes

Age (years)	Endotracheal Tube Size (I.D. in mm)	Laryngoscope Blade Size and Type	Oral Air-way (mm)	Nasal Air-way (FR)	Suction Catheter (FR)
Premature	2.5–3.0	Miller 0[*]	40	12–14	5
Neonate	3.0–3.5	Miller 0	40	14	6
Neonate–1.5	3.5–4.5	Miller 1	40	14–18	8
1–2	4.0–4.5	Miller 1–1$1/2$	60	14–18	8
2–6	4.5–6.0	Mac 2[**]	60	16–18	10
6–12	6.0–6.5	Mac 2	80	18–24	12
12–16	6.5–7.5	Mac 2–3	90	24–28	14
16–adult	7.0–8.0	Mac or Miller 3	100	28–30	14
Large adult	7.5–8.0	Mac 4	100	30	14

[*]Miller: straight blade. [**]Mac: Macintosh—curved blade.

neck extension. Next, the operator holds the laryngoscope in the left hand. The mouth is opened with the right hand, either by pushing downward on the chin or by compelling the mouth to open by placing the thumb and finger on the teeth or gums and "prying" gently. The laryngoscope blade is then directed down the right side of the tongue, allowing the flange of the blade to displace the tongue toward the left side of the mouth. The blade is advanced until the epiglottis is visualized. If a curved blade is used, the tip of the blade is placed above (anterior) the epiglottis into the vallecula. If a straight blade is used, the tip of the instrument is advanced under the epiglottis. Once the blade is positioned, the epiglottis is displaced by lifting on the laryngoscope handle at a 30–45 degree angle. The glottic structures should come into view. The operator next passes the endotracheal tube through the vocal cords approximately 3–4 cm or until the cuff passes the cords. The cuff is inflated with 4–5 ml of air. The 15-mm adaptor on the distal end of the tube is then connected to a self-inflating resuscitation bag or anesthesia circuit, and the patient is ventilated. The tube's position should be confirmed by auscultating the patient's chest and by observing for bilaterally equal chest rise with ventilation. If capnography is available, the presence of CO_2 is the best sign of endotracheal intubation.

If the glottis cannot be adequately visualized, it is sometimes possible to blindly insert a blunt-tipped "tube changer" into the trachea. The tube changer can then be used as a guide, with the endotracheal tube placed over it and pushed gently into the trachea. The tube changer can then be removed.

"Rapid Sequence Intubation"

"Rapid sequence intubation" is a technique to decrease the likelihood of aspiration of stomach contents upon airway manipulation. Conditions that may place patients "at risk" for aspiration include pregnancy, obesity, bowel obstruction, decreased airway reflexes, and probable or known "full stomachs." The purposes of the "rapid sequence intubation" are to insert the endotracheal tube after muscle relaxation, to prevent gastric distension, and to prevent gastric contents from reaching the pharynx. The steps in rapid sequence intubation are described in Chapter 16 on trauma and burns. Rapid sequence intubation and muscle relaxants should not be used when difficulty with intubation is anticipated.

Nasal Intubation

1. Direct Vision.

In some situations, it is desirable to pass a tube through the nose into the trachea. To perform this technique under direct vision, the endotracheal tube is inserted through the nose until the tip of the tube can be seen in the oral pharynx. Laryngoscopy is performed, and the endotracheal tube is advanced until the tube passes into the trachea. Sometimes it is necessary to have an assistant apply downward pressure on the thyroid cartilage to align the glottis with the endotracheal tube as it is advanced. The tip of the tube can be directed toward the glottis with a Magill forceps. To prevent nasal bleeding, vasoconstrictors can be used on the nasal mucosa, a relatively smaller tube can be selected, and the tube softened by immersion in warm water.

2. "Blind" Intubation.

The trachea can be intubated by passing the endotracheal tube "blindly" through the nose into the glottis. The endotracheal tube should be well lubricated and advanced through the nose into the oropharynx. With the patient breathing spontaneously, the tube is advanced while breath sounds can be heard through the tube. If it should enter the esophagus, the tube is withdrawn slightly and redirected. If the patient is not breathing, the tube is advanced to the 26-cm mark, and the patient is ventilated. Tube placement is confirmed by auscultation or identification of CO_2.

CRICOTHYROTOMY

Occasionally, standard management techniques may not be successful establishing an airway, i.e, the patient cannot be ventilated by mask and cannot be intubated (See Appendix, ASA Difficult Airway Algorithm). Other methods (e.g., cricothyrotomy) must be used. Since these are invasive techniques usually performed under emergent conditions, they can result in significant morbidity or the death of the patient if done improperly. (See Appendix for ASA Algorithm for Management of the Difficult Airway.)

Emergency "Surgical" Cricothyrotomy.

Emergency cricothyrotomy requires a knife blade and a small (3.0–5.0 mm I.D.) endotracheal tube. A Kelly clamp or large hemostat is also useful to have on hand. The cricothyroid membrane is identified by placing the index and third fingers over the thyroid and cricoid cartilages. After disinfecting the skin, a skin incision is made over the cricothyroid membrane, and the knife blade is advanced into the trachea through the membrane. An opening into the trachea is created by twisting the knife blade to the side or by sliding the hemostat to create a gap through which the endotracheal tube is passed. The endotracheal tube may be inserted along the knife blade if a hemostat has not been used. The endotracheal tube can then be used to ventilate the patient with 100% oxygen. High inflating pressures may be required because a small tube creates rather high resistance to gas flow.

It is critical to ensure that the endotracheal tube is inserted into the trachea rather than anteriorly into the mediastinum. Breath sounds should be present with proper placement. Positive pressure ventilation through a tube in the mediastinum can result in mediastinal air and pneumothorax. With proper use of cricothyrotomy, the patient can often be successfully oxygenated until a more formal airway is established.

Needle Cricothyrotomy

The trachea can be cannulated with a small catheter inserted through the cricothyroid membrane. Oxygen can be delivered through the cannula to provide adequate oxygenation. If a high-pressure jet ventilator is available, the system is very efficient for both oxygenation and ventilation.

To perform the technique, the cricothyroid membrane is located as described above. A 14- or 16-gauge needle/catheter (such as a standard intravenous needle/catheter) is attached to a 20-ml syringe and advanced through the membrane at a slight caudad angle (Fig. 5.8). When the needle/catheter passes into the trachea, air can be aspirated. The needle/catheter is passed a few more millimeters into the trachea, then the catheter is slid off the needle and should be positioned in the trachea. The catheter can then be attached to a jet ventilator. Short (0.5–1.0

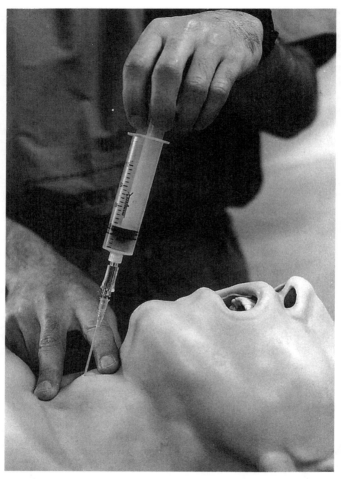

Figure 5.8. Needle cricothyroidotomy. Insertion of a 16-gauge needle/catheter through the cricothyroid membrane.

sec) bursts of 50 p.s.i. oxygen are delivered to the patient at a rate of 10/min. Chest rise should be used to ensure an adequate tidal volume, and the chest should fall after each inspiration, indicating exhalation through a patent airway. Barotrauma may result if exhalation does not occur or if gas from the catheter tip should dissect through the tracheal mucosa.

If a jet ventilator is not available, the catheter can be interfaced with a self-inflating resuscitation bag in two ways. First, a 3-ml syringe with the plunger removed is connected to the catheter. Then, the connector from a 7.5-mm I.D. endotracheal tube is inserted into the open end of the syringe. The resuscitation bag can then be attached to the connector. Alternatively, the adaptor from a 3.0-mm I.D. endotracheal tube is directly inserted into the catheter hub (Figs. 5.9, 5.10).

The thin-walled IV catheter may kink easily, obstructing gas flow. Some authors recommend that a thick-walled catheter, such as a vessel dilator, be inserted into the trachea (6). This technique is more involved and requires the temporary placement of a guide wire, over which the dilator is passed, into the trachea.

The primary complication of the transtracheal techniques is barotrauma. The techniques should be performed under the direction of an experienced individual.

FIBEROPTICALLY DIRECTED INTUBATION

Fiberoptically directed intubation can be used to intubate even very difficult or compromised airways. It is often useful in the circumstances listed in Table 5.6. Excessive secretions or the presence of blood make the technique very difficult or impossible. In elective situations, an anticholinergic drying agent should be administered to dry secretions. If fiberoptic intubation is being used to secure the airway after failure of other techniques, it should be used before the airway becomes bloody from traumatic laryngoscopy. In emergent situations, fiberoptic laryngoscopy can be performed while an assistant provides ventilation via a catheter in the cricothyroid membrane. (7, 8)

Tube Depth

The "depth" to which the tube is advanced into the trachea can be measured from the teeth or gums. The average depth at

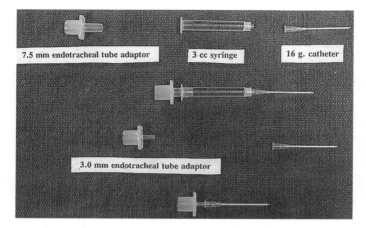

Figure 5.9. Two methods of connecting an IV catheter to an endotracheal tube adaptor.

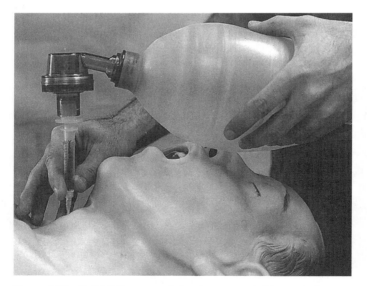

Figure 5.10. Self-inflating resuscitation bag connected to a cricothyroidotomy catheter.

Table 5.6
Situations in Which Fiberoptically Directed Intubation Should Be Considered

---

Airway trauma
Airway burns
Airway infections or tumors
Abnormal airway anatomy
Cervical spine injury

Table 5.7
Laryngeal Mask Airway

Mask Size	Patient Weight (kg)	Cuff Volume for Inflation (ml)
1	<6.5	2–5
2	6.5–20	7–10
3	30–70	15–20
4	> 70	25–30

which to tape or secure the tube can be estimated by the following formula:

$$\text{Depth (cm)} = 12 + (\text{age}/2) \text{ (up to 22 cm in adults)}$$

In the newborn or premature infant, this formula might estimate a depth that is actually too deep, resulting in a main stem intubation. Therefore, in these patients, the tube should be positioned as follows:

Depth
  Premature: 6–10 cm
  Term neonate: 8–10 cm

If the patient is nasally intubated, add 2–4 cm to the depth estimated by the formula above.

LARYNGEAL MASK AIRWAY (LMA) (9)

For anesthetized patients, the LMA can be used to assist ventilation when mask ventilation is not possible. The LMA can also be used to maintain the airway in anesthetized patients breathing spontaneously. Pulmonary aspiration is not prevented by the LMA if gastric reflux should occur. Also, a properly positioned LMA can be used as a guide for fiberoptic intubation. There are four sizes for use in infants through large adults (Table 5.7).

References

1. White A, Kander Pl. Anatomical factors in difficult direct laryngoscopy. Br J Anaesth 1975;47:468–473.
2. Bellhouse CP, Dore C. Criteria for estimating likeihood of difficulty of endotracheal intubation with the Macintosh laryngoscope. Anaesth Intensive Care 1988;16:329–337.
3. Mallampati SR, Gatt SP, Gugine LD, et al. A clinical sign to predict difficult tracheal intubation: a prospective study. Can Anaesth Soc J 1985;32:429–434.
4. Emergency Cardiac Care Committee and Subcommittees, American Heart Association. Guidelines for cardiopulmonary resuscitation and emergency cardiac care. JAMA 1992;268:2172–2298.
5. Finucane Bt, Santora Ah. Principles of Airway Management. Philadelphia: Fa Davis, 1988:227.
6. Boyce JR, Peters G. Vessel dilator circothyrotomy for transtracheal jet ventilation. Can J Anaesth 1989;36;350–353.
7. Benumof JL. Management of the difficult adult airway with special emphasis on awake tracheal intubation. Anesthesiology 1991;75:1087–1110.
8. American Society of Anesthesiologists Task Force on Management of the Difficult Airway. Practice guidelines for management of the difficult airway. Anesthesiology 1993;78:597–602.
9. Pennant JH, White PF. The laryngeal mask airway. Its uses in anesthesiology. Anesthesiology 1993;79:144–163.

Chapter 6

Regional Anesthesia

Advantages of regional anesthesia include the ability to perform surgery on an awake patient with decreased postoperative somnolence and less risk of pulmonary aspiration. It may be associated with better postoperative analgesia and a decrease in the physiologic stress response to surgery. Sympathectomy following regional anesthesia is useful in patients with peripheral vascular disease, with better graft patency following surgery. Total hip arthroplasty under regional anesthesia is associated with a reduction in intraoperative blood loss. Some patients do not wish to be awake during surgery, even if sedated, and for them regional anesthesia is undesirable.

LOCAL ANESTHETICS

Concentrations Used for Anesthesia

Drug	Epidural (%)	Spinal (%)	Peripheral (%)	Topical (%)
Lidocaine	1.5–2	5	0.5–2	4–10
Mepivacaine	2	—	1–2	
Bupivicaine	0.5–0.75	0.5–0.75	0.25–0.5	
Chloroprocaine	3	—	1–3	
Tetracaine	—	1	—	
Etidocaine	1–1.5	—	—	
Ropivicaine	0.5–1.0	—	0.25–0.5	

Mechanism of Action

Local anesthetics alter sodium ion permeability in neural membranes, preventing membrane depolarization and producing a reversible blockade of nerve conduction.

	Chemical Configuration			Physicochemical Properties				Biologic Properties		
Agent	Aromatic Lipophilic	Intermediate Chain	Amine Hydrophilic	Molecular Weight (Base)	pK_a (25°C)	Partition Coefficient[b]	Percent Protein Binding	Equieffective Anesthetic Concentration	Approximate Anesthetic Duration (min)	Site of Metabolism
Esters										
Procaine	$H-N(H)-$(ring)$-$	$COOCH_2CH_2-N$	$(C_2H_5)(C_2H_5)$	236	8.9	0.02	5.8	2	50	Plasma
Chloroprocaine	N_2N-(ring, Cl)$-$	$COOCH_2CH_2-N$	$(C_2H_5)(C_2H_5)$	271	8.7	0.14	—	2	45	Plasma
Tetracaine	$H_9C_4N(H)-$(ring)$-$	$COOCH_2CH_2-N$	$(CH_3)(CH_3)$	264	8.5	4.1	75.6[c]	0.25	175	Plasma
Amides										
Prilocaine	(ring, CH_3)	$NHCOCH(CH_3)-N$	$(H)(C_3H_7)$	220	7.9	0.9	55 approx	1	100	Liver, lung
Lidocaine	(ring, CH_3, CH_3)	$NHCOCH_2-N$	$(C_2H_5)(C_2H_5)$	234	7.9	2.9	64.3[d]	1	100	Liver
Mepivacaine		$NHCO$	(piperidine) $N-CH_3$	246	7.6	0.8	77.5[d]	1	100	Liver
Bupivacaine		$NHCO$	(piperidine) $N-C_4H_9$	288	8.1	27.5	95.6[d]	0.25	175	Liver
Ropivacaine		$NHCO$	(piperidine) $N-C_3H_7$	274	8.0	6.1	94	0.3	150[f]	Liver
Etidocaine		$NHCOCH(C_2H_5)-N$	$(C_2H_5)(C_3H_7)$	276	7.7	141	94[d]	0.25	200	Liver

Bupivacaine	288	8.1	27.5	95.6[e]	0.25	175	Liver
Ropivacaine	274	8.0	6.1	94	0.3	150[f]	Liver
Etidocaine	276	7.7	141	94[e]	0.25	200	Liver

[a]Reproduced with permission from Denson DD, Mazoit JX. Physiology, pharmacology, and toxicity of local anesthetics: adult and pediatric considerations. In: Raj PP, ed. *Clinical Practice of Regional Anesthesia*. New York: Churchill Livingstone, 1991: 75.

[b]pH corresponds to 50% ionization.

[c]*n*-Heptane/pH 7.4 buffer.

[d]Data derived from rat sciatic nerve blocking procedure.

[e]Plasma protein binding, 2 μg/ml.

[f]Nerve homogenate binding.

[g]Guinea pig sciatic nerve.

Physical Properties (Table 6.1)

1. Lipid solubility (determines potency)
2. Protein binding (determines duration of action)
3. pKa (determines amount ionized compound and thus the speed of onset)

   pKa = pH at which 50% of the drug is ionized

   pKa = pH + log[cation/base]
4. Three-part structure (determines method of metabolism and elimination)
   a. Aromatic chain
   b. Intermediate chain (with either an ester or amide linkage)
   c. Amino group

Amides all undergo biotransformation in the liver (oxidation, dealkylation, hydrolysis, conjugation) to an inactive compound excreted by the body. Ropivicaine is the newest amide and is an effective alternative to bupivicaine. It is less cardiotoxic with slightly shorter duration.

   Esters undergo hydrolysis by plasma cholinesterases.

Factors Affecting Neural Blockade

Fiber Size and the Presence of Myelin. Generally, smaller nerve fibers are more easily blocked than larger ones, but myelination enhances the ability of local anesthetics to block nerve conduction.

Diffusion. Motor blockade often precedes sensory blockade, since the peripheral location of the motor fibers in the outer mantle of the nerve bundle permits blockade initially as local anesthetic diffuses into nerves. The peripheral location of motor fibers also allows more rapid systemic absorption of local anesthetics. Thus motor fibers are the first to be blocked and the first to recover.

Dose. Increases the duration of blockade.

Epinephrine. Epinephrine 1:200,000 (5 μg/ml) increases the duration of local anesthetic blockade by local vasoconstriction, delaying absorption from the injection site and lower systemic levels. It should not be used near terminal arteries (e.g., digits) because of risk of necrosis. Intrathecal epinephrine 0.2–0.3 mg

(200–300 μg) or neosynephrine 2 mg may be added to prolong the duration of intrathecal local anesthetics (spinal anesthesia).

Acid/Base Status (pKa). Most local anesthetics are weak bases (pKa > 7.4) prepared in acid solutions as ionized, water-soluble, hydrochloride salts. Alkalinization increases the free base (un-ionized form), allowing passage across the lipophilic axonal membrane and quicker onset. Once inside, the drug dissociates and the charged, ionized form blocks neuronal conduction via sodium channel alteration. For this reason, local anesthetics are less effective when injected into infected acidic tissue.

Protein Binding. The percentage of protein binding correlates with the duration of action of local anesthetics. Protein binding varies with the pH, so acidosis results in an increase in available active drug. Only the unbound portion is active.

Local Anesthetic Toxicity

Toxicity results from elevated systemic concentrations of local anesthetics. Intercostal blocks have the highest systemic levels, followed by caudal > epidural > brachial plexus > femoral/sciatic blocks.

CNS Irritability. Caused by blockade of cortical inhibitory pathways, CNS irritability usually precedes cardiac symptoms and is worsened by acidosis, increased PCO_2, and hypoxia. The amygdala portion of the brain is most reactive to local anesthetics.

Symptoms:

Lidocaine levels > 5 μg/ml: tinnitus, drowsiness, numbness of lips and tongue, and blurred vision

Lidocaine levels > 10 μg/ml: seizures, unconsciousness, and apnea

Cardiac Irritability. Conduction block of cardiac sodium channels results in abnormal conduction and contractility, peripheral vasodilation and ultimately cardiovascular collapse. Symptoms are usually seen with higher levels than those required for CNS toxicity (e.g., lidocaine levels > 20 μg/ml). Bupivicaine is more potent and more cardiotoxic than lidocaine, but although it is equipotent with ropivicaine, it has greater toxicity. Cardiac toxicity is increased by acidosis, hypoxia, hyperkalemia, and pregnancy.

Methemoglobinuria. Following large (>10 mg/kg) doses of prilocaine, *o*-toluidine may accumulate, resulting in the oxidation of Hgb to MetHgb. Treatment is with reducing agents (methylene blue, ascorbic acid).

Allergic Reactions. Ester local anesthetics are metabolized to PABA (*p*-aminobenzoic acid) derivatives, which may result in an allergic reaction. There is no cross reactivity between esters and amides. Allergy to amides is extremely rare, and most cases have been attributed to the methylparaben preservative.

Treatment of Local Anesthetic Toxicity

1. Adequate ventilation with 100% oxygen by face mask.
2. Small doses of IV barbiturate (thiopental 50–100 mg) or benzodiazepine (midazolam 1–2 mg or diazepam 5–10 mg) for treatment of seizures if cardiovascular status permits.
3. Intubate and ventilate if refractory. Succinylcholine may be necessary to abolish muscle activity.
4. Cardiovascular toxicity may require epinephrine for support of BP and heart rate. Bretylium is probably preferred for treatment of ventricular arrhythmias.

NEURAL BLOCKADE: CENTRAL

Epidural Anesthesia

Indications

Central neural blockade is indicated for surgical anesthesia for lower abdominal and lower extremity operations; postoperative analgesia for thoracic, upper and lower abdominal and lower extremity procedures; and chronic pain syndromes.

Surface landmarks for placement include

Vertebra prominens	C7
Inferior angle scapula	T7
Posterior superior iliac crest	L4

Contraindications

Contraindications to epidural/spinal anesthesia include

Absolute
a. Patient refusal
b. Infection at the puncture site

c. Local anesthetic allergy
d. Hypovolemic shock
e. Uncorrected coagulopathy/full anticoagulation

Relative
a. Generalized infection
b. Progressive neurologic deficit
c. Increased intracranial pressure
d. Fixed stroke volume (aortic stenosis, IHSS)

Technique

Hydration
    Administer fluid bolus intravenously to ensure adequate intravascular volume
Monitoring
    Frequent blood pressure and heart rate checks for 20 minutes following local anesthetic bolus
    Attention to fetal heart rate in pregnant patient
    Have airway equipment and resuscitation drugs available
Patient position
    Sitting
    Lateral decubitus
Needle placement
    Midline
    Paramedian
Loss of resistance
    Air
    Saline
Hanging drop technique
Test dose (rule out intravascular or intrathecal injection)
    Local anesthetic— (e.g. lidocaine 45 mg) look for signs of systemic local anesthetic injection and intrathecal blockade
    Epinephrine— (15 μg) check for tachycardia
    Air— 1 ml can be detected by precordial Doppler
Administration of local anesthetic: (Table 6.2)
Incremented bolus doses or infusion
Follow anesthetic level by dermatome and record progress (Fig. 6.1)

Table 6.2
Agents for Epidural Blockade [a]

Agent	Usual Concentration (%)	Usual Onset (min)	Usual Duration of Surgical Anesthesia	Main Clinical Use
Chloroprocaine	2–3	5–15	30–90	Obstetrics
Lidocaine	1–2	5–15	60–120	Obstetrics Surgery
Mepivacaine	1–2	5–15	60–150	Surgery
Prilocaine	1–3	5–15	60–150	Surgery
Bupivacaine	0.25–0.75	10–20	120–140	Obstetrics Surgery
Etidocaine	1–1.5	5–15	120–240	Surgery

[a] Reproduced with permission from Covino BG, Lambert DH. Epidural and spinal anesthesia. In: Barash PG, Cullen BF, Stoelting RK, eds. *Clinical Anesthesia*. Philadelphia: JB Lippincott, 1989: 775.

Complications

Headache
Hypotension
Nausea
Back pain
Dural puncture
Local anesthetic toxicity

Neurologic (rare)
Direct needle trauma (neuropathy)
    Anterior spinal artery syndrome
    Arachnoiditis
    Infection/abscess
    Hematoma
    Not related to anesthetic technique
        Positioning
        Tourniquet/cast ischemia
        Preexisting disease
        Surgical retraction

Characteristics of Complications seen with Epidural Blockade

a.   *Hypotension*
        Sympathetic blockade produces decreased venous return, decreased cardiac output, and hypotension
        Blockade of T1–T4 (cardiac accelerator fibers) produces bradycardia
        May be associated with nausea
    Treatment
        Ensure adequate ventilation and oxygenation
        Bradycardia: atropine 0.4 mg

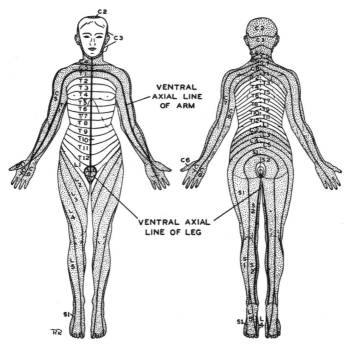

Figure 6.1. Dermatome chart with new patterns in the extremities based on single nerve root syndromes for use in determining spinal anesthetic levels. (From original of Figure 2 by Drs. J. Jay Keegan and F.D. Garrett. From Keegan JJ. The segmental distribution of the cutaneous nerves in the limbs of man. Anat Rec 1948;102:409.)

Hypotension: Increase venous return (fluid bolus, leg elevation)
Ephedrine 5–10 mg
Neosynephrine 50–100 μg

b. *Dural puncture*
   i. *Postdural puncture headache*
      Onset: 24–48 hours following dural puncture
      Etiology: CSF leak causing retraction on the pain-sensitive intracranial structures
      Characteristics
      Frontal and/or occipital

Positional (worse with sitting or standing)
Photophobia
Diplopia
Tinnitus
Associated factors
Increased incidence with
Larger needles (larger dural defect)
Younger patients
Female patients
Lower incidence with tapered needles (Whitacre)
Therapy
First 24–48 hours
Bedrest
Abdominal binders
Intravenous or oral hydration
Oral analgesics
Caffeine (500–100 mg IV)
Epidural saline (if catheter already in place)
If that fails
Epidural blood patch at level of dural puncture with
10–20 ml fresh autologous blood

    ii. *Severe hypotension with respiratory arrest* is usually due to intrathecal injection of a large dose of local anesthetic intended for the epidural space. Respiratory arrest is usually due to medullary ischemia and requires intubation, ventilation, and hemodynamic support with early use of epinephrine. Sensory blockade above T7 affects the intercostal and abdominal muscles and is not tolerated in patients with severe pulmonary disease who depend on their accessory muscles for respiration.

c. *Local anesthetic toxicity:* see above (Table 6.2)
d. *Neurologic*
    i. *Nerve trauma*
Acute onset
Pain or paresthesias during catheter insertion or injection
Numbness in a dermatomal distribution
Recovery likely within 3 months.
    ii. *Anterior spinal artery syndrome*
Acute onset

Characterized by painless paraplegia

Associated with severe peripheral vascular disease and intraoperative hypotension

Due to compromise to the anterior spinal artery of Adamkiewicz

iii. *Epidural hematoma*

Acute onset

Severe backache with rapidly progressive neurologic deficit

Requires surgical evacuation within 12 hours

iv. *Arachnoiditis*

Insidious onset (up to 1 week)

Variable painful neurological deficit

Cauda equina syndrome

v. *Epidural abscess*

Insidious onset

Progressive neurologic deficit over 3 days

Most are associated with endogenous infection

Severe backache and tenderness associated with fever and elevated white cell count

Requires immediate surgical evacuation

Spinal Anesthesia

Indications

Spinal anesthesia is indicated for surgical anesthesia for lower abdominal, perineal, and lower extremity procedures.

Factors Affecting the Spread of Local Anesthetics in Spinal Anesthesia

CSF volume

Site of injection

Local anesthetic characteristics (Table 6.3)

  Baricity

  Dose (mg)

Patient position

CSF Volume. Smaller CSF volumes result in greater spread. Large differences in height and increased intrabdominal pressure resulting in venous engorgement affect the CSF

Table 6.3
Guidelines for Employing Hyperbaric and Isobaric Solutions in Spinal Anesthesia[a]

Surgical Site	Solution	C[b](%)	Usual Dose (mg)	Usual Volume (mL)	Usual Duration No EPI[b] (hr)	Usual Duration 0.2 mg EPI (hr)
Above L-1	Hyperbaric					
	Bupivacaine	0.75	10–15	1.5–2	2	2
	Tetracaine	0.5	10–15	2–3	2	3
	Lidocaine	5.0	50–75	1–1.5	1	1
Below L-1	Isobaric					
	Bupivacaine[c]	0.5	15	3	3–4	4–6
	Tetracaine	0.5	15	3	3–4	4–6
	Lidocaine[c]	2.0	60	3	1–2	2–3

[a]Reprinted with permission from Resident & Staff Physician (September 1987) by Romaine Pierson Publishers, Inc.
[b]EPI, epinephrine; C, concentration.
[c]Isobaric solutions of bupivacaine and Lidocaine are not yet approved by the FDA for spinal anesthesia. However, this use has been reported in numerous publications. Solutions intended for spinal anesthesia should not contain any preservatives or antioxidants, such as methylparaben, sodium bisulfite, or sodium metabisulfite.

volume. The CSF volume is reduced above L2 where the spinal cord occupies a greater portion of the subarachnoid space.

Local Anesthetic Characteristics. *Density* is the weight (gm) of 1 ml of a solution at a specified temperature. The density of CSF is 1.0003 at 37°C. Specific gravity and baricity are ratios. *Specific gravity* of water is 1.0000 and the baricity of CSF is 1.0000. *Baricity* is the ratio of the density of a local anesthetic to the density of CSF at a specified temperature. The baricity of hyperbaric local anesthetic solutions is >1.0000, isobaric is 1.0000, and hypobaric <1.0000.

To make a drug	*add*
Hyperbaric:	glucose
Isobaric:	saline (preservative free) or CSF
Hypobaric:	water (preservative free)

Dose. The total dose (mg) of local anesthetic appears to have more effect on the spread than the volume or concentration of the drug. However, dose, volume, and concentration of a local anesthetic are all integrally related.

Patient Position. Patient position affects the spread of anesthetics more with hypo- and hyperbaric solutions than with isobaric solutions. Hyperbaric local anesthetic solutions injected intrathecally will give a denser block on the dependent side, while hypobaric solutions produce a denser block on the nondependent side.

Complications

Headache (from dural puncture)
Hypotension (level of sympathetic blockade is higher than for epidural anesthetic at the same dermatone level)
Nausea
Back pain
Persistent paresthesias
Cauda equina syndrome (continuous spinal microcatheters)

Caudal Blockade

Indications: perineal, perianal analgesia
Complications: similar to those with epidural/spinal anesthesia as

well as rectal perforation, trauma to fetal head in pregnant patients

NEURAL BLOCKADE: PERIPHERAL

Contraindications. Infection at the site and patient refusal are contraindications.

Equipment. Short beveled block needle (preferably insulated), variable output nerve stimulator with alligator clips, ECG electrode, control syringe, and extension tubing (immobile needle) are needed. With the nerve stimulator, the "black-to-block" rule (needle as cathode) is used in which the black clip is attached to the block needle and the red clip to the ECG electrode attached to the patient. This enables nerve stimulation at a lower current than if the needle were the anode.

Monitoring. Basic monitoring includes pulse oximetry, BP, and ECG; *always* give a test dose prior to bolus. Airway equipment and resuscitation drugs should be available.

Drugs. Bupivicaine 0.25–0.5%, Mepivicaine 1–2%, Lidocaine 2% are used; epinephrine 1:200,000 is often added to increase duration.

Cervical Plexus

Anatomy: Anterior primary rami of C2–4; C1 is motor only.
Indications: Thyroid surgery, carotid endarterectomy, superficial neck surgeries
Complications: Intrathecal/epidural blockade, intravascular injection, stellate ganglion block; caution with bilateral blocks because of phrenic nerve blockade with resulting respiratory insufficiency

Brachial Plexus blockade (Fig. 6.2)

Anatomy. The brachial plexus is comprised of the ventral rami of C5–T1, with some contribution from C4 and T2. It supplies all the motor and most sensory function for the upper extremity. The upper shoulder and neck is supplied by the cervical plexus.

Indications. Brachial plexus blockade is used for shoulder, arm or hand surgery, sympathetic blockade of the arm for chronic

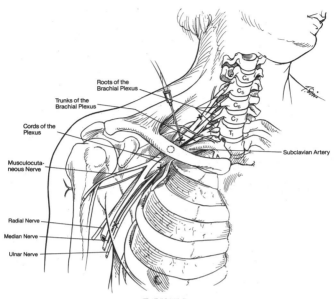

Figure 6.2. Anatomy of the brachial plexus. The needle is placed on the brachial plexus *(X)* with the supraclavicular approach. The other *X marks* denote the interscalene, infraclavicular, and axillary approaches. (Reproduced with permission from Raj PP, Pai U, Rawal N. Techniques of regional anesthesia in adults. In: Raj PP, ed. *Clinical Practice of Regional Anesthesia.* New York: Churchill Livingstone, 1991: 282.)

pain, and shoulder manipulations under anesthesia. The intercostobrachial nerve must be blocked separately because it is a branch of the intercostal nerve and not in the sheath with the brachial plexus.

1. Interscalene approach

Advantages
Shoulder anesthesia
Arm position is unimportant
Cervical plexus anesthetized
Less risk pneumothorax
Complications
Phrenic nerve block
Intravascular injection

Disadvantages
Lower trunks missed (C8T1)
Caution in patients with
    chronic lung diseases

Epidural or intrathecal injection

Stellate ganglion block

Recurrent layngeal nerve block

Pneumothorax

2. Supraclavicular

Advantages

Quick onset

Low volume required (15–25 ml)

Difficult technique

Arm position unimportant

Plexus most compact

Complications

Pneumothorax (0.5–6% incidence)

Intravascular injection

Hematoma (subclavian a.)

Horner's syndrome

Phrenic nerve block

Disadvantages

More reliable with paresthesias

3. Subclavian perivascular

Advantages

Anesthesia for entire arm

Complications

Pneumothorax

Intravascular injection (subclavian a.)

Nerve trauma

Phrenic n. block

Stellate ganglion block

Recurrent laryngeal n. block

Disadvantages

May miss inferior trunk (C8T1)

4. Axillary block

Advantages

Good for forearm and hand surgery

Few complications

Easy technique

No risk of pneumothorax

Continuous blockade easily performed

Disadvantages

Arm positioning required

May miss muscultaneous and axillary nerves

Complications
Toxicity (due to large doses
 ($\geq$ 40 ml) of local anes-
 thetic)
Intravascular injection
Hematoma
Nerve trauma
Techniques
  Fascial click
  Transarterial (radial nerve
    is posterior to artery)
  Paresthesias
  Nerve stimulator
5. Infraclavicular Block

Advantages
No positioning required
Less risk pneumothorax

Disadvantages
Difficult localization
May miss musculocutaneous
  and axillary nerves
Long needle, uncomfortable

Complications
Intravascular injection
Nerve trauma
6. Testing brachial plexus block
Motor
  Radial n: extension of elbow, wrist and fingers, arm supina-
    tion
  Ulnar n: opposition of thumb and 5th finger
  Median n: opposition of thumb and middle or index fin-
    gers, arm pronation
  Musculocutaneous n: flexion of elbow
Sensory
  Radial n: dorsal lateral hand and thumb
  Ulnar n: medial 4th finger and 5th finger
  Median n: ventral 2nd, 3rd and lateral 4th fingers
  Musculocutaneous n: lateral forearm

**Blocks for Specific Nerves of the Upper Extremity
(Rescue Blocks) (Fig. 6.3)**

Indications: Supplementing brachial plexus blocks, diagnostic
blocks for neuropathic pain

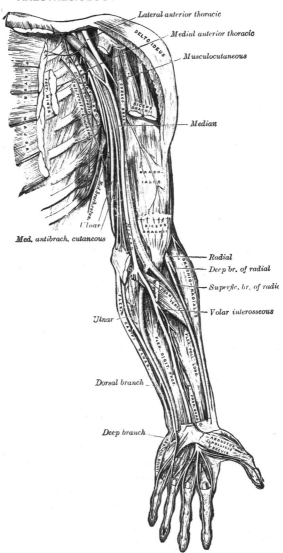

Figure 6.3. Nerves of the upper extremity. (Reproduced with permission from Raj PP, Pai U, Rawal N. Techniques of regional anesthesia in adults. In: Raj PP, ed. *Clinical Practice of Regional Anesthesia.* New York: Churchill Livingstone, 1991: 296.

Doses: 3–5 ml local anesthetic (1–2% lidocaine, 0.25–0.5% bupivicaine with or without epinephrine 1:200,000); paresthesias or nerve stimulators may be used; if unable to get either, a field block in the area of the nerve may be used

1. **Radial nerve** (Fig. 6.4)
   At spiral groove: block as it wraps around the midhumerus before coursing over the lateral epicondyle
   At elbow: 1 cm lateral to the biceps tendon, medial to the brachioradialis muscle
   At wrist: (superficial radial), block with subcutaneous ring of lateral half of the wrist.
2. **Ulnar nerve** (Fig. 6.5)
   At elbow: 2 cm proximal to the groove at the medial epicondyle of the humerus with elbow flexed about 30°
   At wrist: block just lateral to the flexor carpi ulnaris tendon at the level of the styloid process.
3. **Median nerve** (Fig. 6.6)
   At elbow: medial to the brachial artery 1 cm above the line joining the two epicondyles
   At wrist: between the tendons of the palmaris longus and the flexor carpi radialis.
4. **Musculocutaneous nerve**
   Choracobrachialis muscle: needle remains at same site as for axillary block; withdraw to the skin, then inject 5–10 ml of drug into the belly of the choracobrachialis muscle, superior to the axillary artery
   At elbow: lateral to the biceps tendon and medial to the radial nerve at the intercondylar line
5. **Intercostobrachial nerve**
   Innervates the skin of the inner aspect of the upper arm and must be blocked after an axillary block if a tourniquet is to be used; at the level of the axillary artery, inject 5–10 ml of local anesthetic subcutaneously as a ring extending inferiorly toward the axilla. This may be done following an axillary block by partially withdrawing the needle and redirecting inferiorly toward the axilla.
6. **Digital nerve blocks of finger**
   Insert needle on lateral sides of the base of the digits bilaterally. No epinephrine. Inject the drug at both the dorsal and lateral sides of the finger.

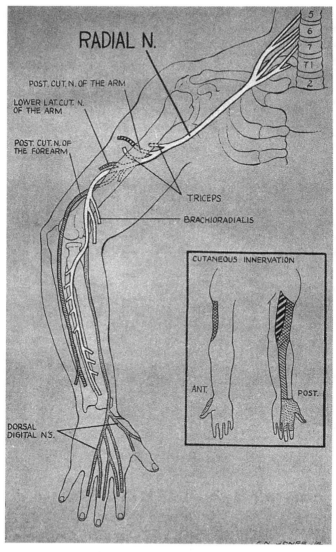

Figure 6.4. General anatomic course of the radial nerve. (Courtesy EA Rovenstien.)

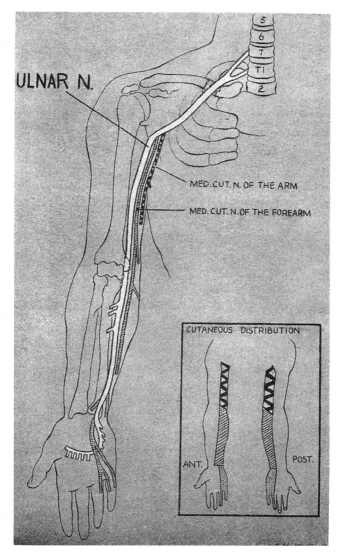

Figure 6.5. General anatomy and course of the ulnar nerve in the arm. (Courtesy E.A. Rovenstine.)

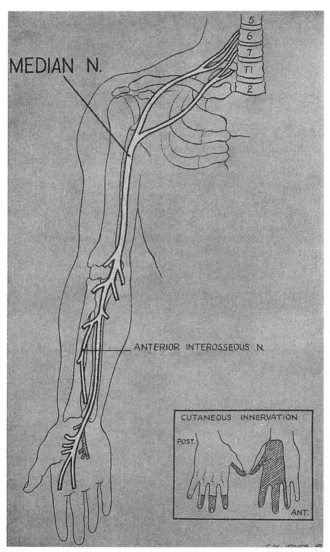

Figure 6.6. General anatomy and course of the median nerve in the arm. (Courtesy E.A. Rovenstine.)

Intercostal Nerve Block

Indications: Postoperative analgesia for abdominal surgery, chronic abdominal pain, postherpetic neuralgia

Anatomy: ventral rami of T1–T11, T12 is subcostal. There are 4 branches: gray rami communicans, posterior cutaneous branch, lateral cutaneous branch, and anterior cutaneous branch. The lateral cutaneous branch arises anterior to the midaxillary line, sending cutaneous fibers anteriorly and posteriorly to the chest and abdominal wall. It must therefore be blocked medial to the midaxillary line, prior to the division.

Complications
   Pneumothorax
   Epidural blockade
   Intravascular injection
   Nerve trauma

Lower Extremity Blocks (Figs. 6.7, 6.9)

Leg innervation
   Femoral n.
   Sciatic n.
   Obturator n.
   Lateral femoral cutaneous n.
Knee innervation
   Femoral n.
   Sciatic n.
   Obturator n.
Ankle innervation
   Femoral n. (saphenous)
   Sciatic n. (tibial, sural, peroneal)

1. Lateral femoral cutaneous block

Anatomy: L2–3; innervates lateral thigh

Indications: anesthesia of graft donor site; meralgia paresthetica (pain due to injury of the lateral femoral cutaneous nerve).

Complications: nerve trauma

2. Femoral nerve block

Anatomy: L2–4; divides into anterior and posterior branches at inguinal ligament.

Anterior branch: skin over anterior thigh

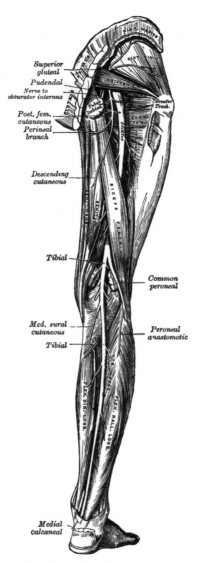

Figure 6.7. Anterior nerves of the lower extremity. (Reproduced with permission from Raj PP, Pai U, Rawal N. Techniques of regional anesthesia in adults. In Raj PP, ed. *Clinical Practice of Regional Anesthesia*. New York: Churchill Livingstone, 1991: 306.

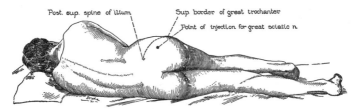

Figure 6.8. Position used in blocking the sciatic nerve by the classic technique. (From Labat G. Regional Anesthesia: Its Technic and Clinical Application. 2nd ed. Philadelphia: WB Saunders, 1928.)

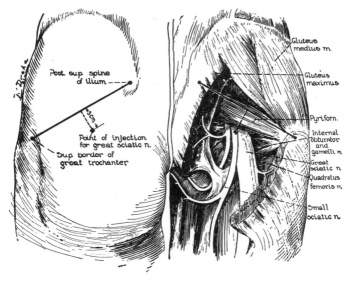

Figure 6.9. Sciatic block. Shown are superficial landmarks to the *right* and the anatomic structures to the *left*. (From Labat G. Regional Anesthesia: Its Technic and Clinical Application. 2nd ed. Philadelphia: WB Saunders, 1928.)

Posterior branch: quadriceps muscle, knee

Saphenous nerve: medial calf and medial malleolus

Indications: supplemental surgical anesthesia of thigh and knee, postoperative analgesia for knee surgery

Contraindications: prior vascular graft surgery involving the femoral artery

Complications
    Hematoma
    Nerve trauma
    Systemic toxicity/intravascular injection
3. Obturator nerve block
Anatomy: L2–4; innervates lower medial thigh, proximal to knee
Indications: supplement femoral, lateral femoral cutaneous, and sciatic block for anesthesia of the knee
4. Sciatic nerve block (Figs. 6.8 and 6.9)
Anatomy: L4–S3, sensory innervation to posterior thigh and below the knee, except for medial calf (femoral)
Indications
    Combine with femoral, lateral femoral cutaneous, or obtura-
        tor block for surgical anesthesia of leg
    Surgery on foot not requiring a tourniquet
    Postoperative analgesia
    Chronic pain
Technique
    Posterior approach (classic approach of Labat)
    Posterior approach (Raj)
    Anterior approach
    Lateral approach
    Distal sciatic block at the knee (tibial and peroneal)
Complications
    Nerve trauma
    Systemic toxicity
5. Ankle Block (Fig. 6.10)
Indications: surgeries on the foot not requiring a tourniquet; requires 5 ml local anesthetic per injection
Anatomy
    Tibial n.: divides into posterior tibial and sural
    Sural n.: between the lateral malleolus and the Achilles ten-
        don; innervates lateral foot and lateral malleolus
    Posterior tibial n.: between the medial malleolus and the achil-
        les tendon; innervates sole of foot and heel
    Common peroneal n. (superficial and deep): superficial extends
    and innervates over dorsum of the foot; *deep* lies lateral to the
    extensor hallucis longus and deep to the extensor retinacu-
    lum and supplies the web between the 1st and 2nd toes
    Saphenous n.: superior to the medial malleolus; inervates me-
    dial foot above the medial malleolus

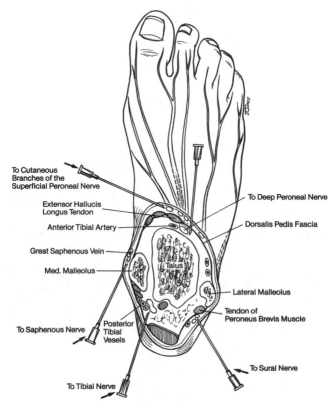

To Cutaneous
Branches of the
Superficial Peroneal Nerve

To Deep Peroneal Nerve

Extensor Hallucis
Longus Tendon

Anterior Tibial Artery

Dorsalis Pedis Fascia

Great Saphenous Vein

Med. Malleolus

Talus

Lateral Malleolus

Tendon of
Peroneus Brevis Muscle

To Saphenous Nerve

Posterior
Tibial
Vesels

To Sural Nerve

To Tibial Nerve

Figure 6.10. Position of needle placement at the ankle for blocking the five nerves of the foot. (Reproduced with permission from Raj PP, Pai U, Rawal N. Techniques of regional anesthesia in adults. In Raj PP, ed. *Clinical Practice of Regional Anesthesia.* New York: Churchill Livingstone, 1991: 317.)

Blocks of the Lower Abdomen and Pelvis

1. Ilioinguinal/iliohypogastric block

Anatomy: T12, L1; ilioinguinal n. supplies base of penis, scrotum (males) and labia majora (females); hypogastric n. supplies lower abdomen above inguinal ligament

Indications: Analgesia for inguinal herniorraphy, chronic pain following herniorraphy

Complications: neuralgia, infection

2. **Genitofemoral block**

   Anatomy: L1, L2; supplies medial thigh and scrotum (males) and labia majora (females)

   Indications: chronic pain in labia, groin

   Complications: neuralgia, infection

Intravenous Regional Anesthetic (Bier Block)

Advantages	Disadvantages
Easy	Only good for short cases (< 1 hr)
Reliable	
Rapid onset and recovery	Toxicity risk with tourniquet failure or release
Excellent relaxation	Tourniquet required (painful)
	Rapid recovery, no postoperative analgesia

Drugs

Prilocaine: rapidly metabolized, nonirritating, fewer CNS side effects, but methemaglobinemia in doses > 600 mg caused by metabolite, *o*-toluidine

Lidocaine: most commonly used (50 ml of 0.5% solution; max 3 mg/kg); rapidly metabolized, slight burning with injection, moderate CNS side effects

Bupivicaine: more profound blockade, but higher associated toxicity

Chlorprocaine: rapidly metabolized, low toxicity profile, but high incidence of thrombophlebitis (possibly due to the methylparaben preservative)

NEURAL BLOCKADE: SYMPATHETIC

Stellate (Cervicothoracic) Ganglion Block

Anatomy: fusion of the lower cervical and first thoracic ganglion; lies opposite C7 anterior to the longus colli muscle; however C6 (Chassaignac's tubercle) is more prominent and is used as the landmark for blocks

Indications: sympathetically maintained pain, vascular impairment (atherosclerotic, vasospasm, embolic) involving the upper extremities

Complications
   Recurrent laryngeal nerve block
   Horner's syndrome, hematoma
   Phrenic n. block
   Intravascular injection—CNS/cardiac toxicity
   Brachial plexus block
   Epidural injection

Lumbar Sympathetic Block

Anatomy: L1–3, anterolateral to the vertebral bodies and anterior to the psoas muscle
Indications: sympathetically maintained pain, peripheral vascular disease
Complications
   Intravascular/intrathecal/epidural injection
   Somatic nerve blockade (L2) with/without neuralgia
   Hypotension

Celiac Plexus block

Anatomy: receives innervation from T5–12 (greater, lesser, and least splanchnic nerves) to innervate the abdominal viscera
Indications: abdominal pain from pancreatic or other abdominal cancers; chronic benign abdominal pain
Complications
   Intravascular/epidural/subarachnoid injection
   Intraosseous/intrapsoas injection
   Hypotension
   Retroperitoneal hematoma
   Abscess
   Punctured viscus
   Following neurolytic block
      Sexual dysfunction
      Paralysis
      Neuritis
      Diarrhea

Suggested Readings

Cousins MF, Bridenbaugh PO. *Neural Blockade in Clinical Anesthesia and Management of Pain.* 2nd ed. Philadelphia: JB Lippincott, 1988.

Greene, N. Distribution of local anesthetic solutions within the subarachnoid space. Anesth Analg 1985;64:715–730.

Holmes CM. Intravenous regional anesthesia. Lancet 1963;1:245.

Lambert DH, Covino BG. Hyperbaric, hypobaric and isobaric spinal anesthesia. Res Staff Physician 1987;33:79.

Scott DB. *Techniques of Regional Anesthesia.* Appleton & Lange. Norwalk, CT: 1989.

Symposium on Local Anesthetics. Regional Anesthesia, April–June 1977.

Chapter 7

Intraoperative Complications

TACHYCARDIA (Table 7.1)

Several factors may contribute to intraoperative tachycardia.

Tachycardic episodes from **light anesthesia** may be minimized by ensuring an appropriate anesthetic depth before potent stimulation such as laryngoscopy or incision occurs. A sudden increase in the intensity of surgical stimulation (e.g., periosteal manipulation or visceral traction) may increase the heart rate even if the level of anesthesia was previously adequate. Opiates, because of their vagotonic effects, are particularly useful to slow the heart rate. Alternatively, esmolol 0.5–1 mg/kg temporarily lowers the heart rate during the stress of intubation or emergence from anesthesia.

Hypovolemia, anemia, hypoxia, and hypercarbia may also cause tachycardia. Patients who are debilitated or who have had extensive bowel preparations may have circulating volume deficits of 1 liter or more. Rehydration with crystalloid may reveal an underlying anemia that requires blood transfusion.

Tachycardia may reflect an **increased metabolic rate** in a patient who is febrile, hyperthyroid, or experiencing malignant hyperthermia (see section on malignant hypothermia below). An increased heart rate may be the first sign that a patient on chronic β-blocker or clonidine therapy has not received their morning medication.

BRADYCARDIA (Table 7.2)

In general, a patient's heart rate is less important than the hemodynamic consequences of the heart rate. A patient with idiopathic hypertrophic subaortic stenosis may benefit from an an-

Table 7.1
Differential Diagnosis of Intraoperative Tachycardia

I. Increased oxygen consumption
    A. Fever/sepsis
    B. Malignant hyperthermia
    C. Hyperthyroidism
II. Decreased oxygen supply
    A. Hypoxemia
    B. Anemia
    C. Hypovolemia
III. Increased sympathetic stimulation
    A. Inadequate anesthesia
    B. Hypercarbia
    C. Hypovolemia
        1. $\downarrow$ Blood volume from losses
        2. Relative $\downarrow$ blood volume
            a. Pulmonary embolus
            b. Pericardial tamponade
            c. Tension pneumothorax
            d. Surgical mechanical maneuvers that $\downarrow$ venous return or obstruct the vena cava
            e. Vasodilation
                i. Drugs
                ii. Sepsis
                iii. Allergic
    D. Bladder distention
    E. Antihypertensive "rebound"
    F. Pheochromocytoma, carcinoid
    G. Anaphylaxis
    H. Congestive heart failure
IV. Drug-related
    A. Volatile anesthetics—isoflurane, enflurane
    B. Muscle relaxants—succinylcholine, pancuronium, gallamine
    C. Anticholinergics—atropine, glycopyrrolate, scopolamine
    D. Miscellaneous—thiopental, meperidine, tricyclic antidepressants, aminophylline, ketamine, catecholamines, vasodilators
V. Tachyarrythmias—A fib, PAT, etc.

---

esthetic technique that lowers the pulse to 50, while a patient with aortic regurgitation may experience a decreased cardiac output if the pulse drops from 90 to 70. Pulse rates in the 40s are often seen in healthy, young persons.

Bradycardia is a late sign of hypoxia; pulse oximetry documents that even profound hypoxia may occur without a change in heart rate.

Table 7.2
Causes of Bradycardia

Healthy "trained" heart
Hypoxia (late after tachycardia)
Anesthetic drugs, narcotics
β-Adrenergic blockade
Vagal reflexes (e.g. oculocardiac)
Myocardial ischemia, inferior wall
Increased intracranial pressure
Digitalis toxicity
Bradyarrhythmias (A-V nodal, heart block, etc.)

A slow heart rate may reflect the adequacy of therapy in patients receiving β-blockers to treat coronary artery disease or hypertension. The pulse rate may decrease even further, particularly if halothane or narcotics are administered for anesthesia or a drug other than pancuronium is used for paralysis. Observation alone is appropriate if the slow heart rate does not compromise cardiac output or blood pressure. If hypotension occurs, ephedrine 5–10 mg or atropine 0.2–0.4 mg IV usually restores pulse and pressure. Patients receiving large doses of long-acting β-blockers may require isoproterenol, epinephrine, or temporary pacing to maintain hemodynamic stability.

Laryngoscopy and traction on extraocular muscles, viscera, or the brainstem all can cause reflex bradycardia. These reflexes are not blocked by anticholinergic premedication, but stopping the stimulation allows the heart rate to normalize. Atropine or glycopyrrolate should be given only if hemodynamically significant bradycardia persists, because its use may precipitate more serious dysrhythmia.

HYPOTENSION (Table 7.3)

Blood pressure is related to cardiac output and systemic vascular resistance, and thus, hypotension may result from decreases in either cardiac output or vascular resistance.

Many surgical patients are hypovolemic. Since most general anesthetic agents are both myocardial depressants and vasodilators, hypotension is common following induction. Either benzodiazepines or opioids alone do not decrease myocardial con-

Table 7.3
Causes of Hypotension

1. Decreased cardiac output
   Anesthetic drugs
   Hypovolemia
   Dysrhythmia
   Acidosis
   Hypocalcemia
   Myocardial ischemia
   Pneumothorax
   Pulmonary embolus
   Cardiac tamponade
2. Decreased vascular resistance
   Anesthetics
   Anaphylactoid response
   Sympathetic blockade (with spinal/epidural)
   Sepsis
   Other drugs—nitroprusside, nitroglycerin, histamine releasing agents

tractility, but their use in combination frequently results in hypotension.

A patient's normal, preoperative blood pressure must be considered before treating hypotension. A fall greater than 20–30% from the patient's baseline mean blood pressure should be corrected. Serious hypotensive episodes may be minimized by fluid infusion before induction and by careful titration of anesthetic agents. If hypotension does occur, it can be managed with further fluid administration, vasopressors, or noxious stimulation (laryngoscopy or incision). Phenylephrine 50–100 μg intravenously is a direct-acting α-agonist that increases vascular resistance without increasing the heart rate. Ephedrine, 5–10 mg IV has both α- and β-adrenergic properties, resulting in higher blood pressure, pulse rate, and vascular resistance.

If the fall in pressure is severe or if repeated doses of vasopressors or large amounts of fluid are required to maintain blood pressure, alternate diagnoses must be considered. Auscultation of the heart and lungs, evaluation of pulmonary compliance and cardiac filling pressures, inspection of the ECG as well as arterial blood gas, electrolytes, and hemoglobin analyses may reveal a previously unsuspected cause of hypotension.

HYPERTENSION (Table 7.4)

Wide fluctuations in blood pressure increase the risk of myocardial ischemia. Chronically hypertensive patients have hypertrophied arteriolar smooth muscle and diminished circulating volume. This combination results in high blood pressure peaks during stimulation, followed by hypotension when stimulation ceases or if the hypertension is treated too aggressively. Patients with elevated blood pressure preoperatively, untreated "borderline" hypertension, or elevated blood pressure on admission (labile hypertensives) may be predicted to have greater hemodynamic lability intraoperatively.

Hypertensive episodes may be minimized by anticipating noxious stimuli and deepening anesthesia with thiopental, opioids, or volatile agents before stimulation. If the blood pressure elevation persists, additional causes should be considered and the anesthetic depth reassessed. Opioids may not blunt autonomic reflexes adequately; volatile agents block sympathetic reflexes at doses above those necessary to produce unconsciousness. Therefore, patients who are hypertensive despite "adequate" levels of anesthesia should be treated with antihypertensive medication. This approach should minimize hypertension and tachycardia that occurs after anesthesia as the patient returns to consciousness while shivering, in pain, and coughing on an endotracheal tube. Several antihypertensive

Table 7.4
Causes of Intraoperative Hypertension

Light anesthesia
Essential hypertension
Hypercarbia
Bladder distention
Tourniquet pain
Absorption of epinephrine, phenylephrine applied to surgical field
Antihypertensive rebound
Ketamine, pancuronium
Drug interaction:
    MAO inhibitor and opioid (meperidine)
    Droperidol and epinephrine
Pheochromocytoma
Increased intracranial pressure

Table 7.5
Antihypertensive Therapy[a]

Labetalol	2.5–10 mg IV bolus
β-Adrenergic Blockers:	
Propranolol	0.5–1 mg
Metoprolol	1–2 mg
Esmolol	0.5–1 mg/kg bolus
	50–250 μg/kg/min infusion
Hydralazine	2.5–5 mg IV
Nitroglycerin	0.5 μg/kg/min infusion
Nifedipine	10 mg sublingual
Nitroprusside	0.5–1 μg/kg bolus
	0.5–3 μg/kg/min infusion
Verapamil	1.25–2.5 mg
Enalaprilat	250–500 μg
Phentolamine	0.5–1 mg bolus
	2.5–5 μg/kg/min infusion
Trimethaphan	1–5 mg bolus
	10–100 μg/kg/min infusion

[a] Suggested initial doses, must titrate to effect.

medications may be administered in the operating room (Table 7.5). Selection of a specific drug must take into account the desired duration of action and the patient's preexisting medical condition. A nitroglycerin drip, for example, is easily titrated to the patient's blood pressure and may protect against myocardial ischemia in patients with coronary artery disease.

β-Blocking drugs are noteworthy for several reasons. Abrupt discontinuation of a β-blocker prior to surgery may result in a hyperadrenergic crisis, manifested by hypertension, tachycardia, and angina. It is treated (or prevented) with intravenous propranolol or metoprolol. Esmolol is a β-blocker with a brief, 14-minute half-life. It may be administered as a bolus or by continuous infusion. Labetalol is a very useful drug with both α- and β-blocking effects. An initial dose of 2.5–10 mg IV lowers blood pressure and heart rate while maintaining cardiac output.

Clonidine, 0.1–0.4 mg given orally 60 minutes preoperatively, controls the wide blood pressure fluctuations in poorly controlled hypertensive patients. In addition to providing greater hemodynamic stability, clonidine produces a dry mouth and sedation. Anesthetic requirements are reduced by as much as half. Patients on chronic clonidine therapy also may experience a rebound hyperadrenergic state if they do not receive clonidine on the day of surgery. The hypertension is best treated with a vasodilator followed by β-blockade to lower heart rate. In this instance, β-antagonism prior to α-blockade leads to vasoconstriction, greater increases in blood pressure, and possible left ventricular failure. Clonidine is also available in a continuous-release patch. This preparation maintains a constant blood level for 7 days. Once the patch is applied, there is a 2–3 day lag before therapeutic blood levels are reached. After the patch is removed, however, clonidine levels decline within 12 hours.

Tourniquet pain is a poorly understood phenomenon that manifests as gradually increasing blood pressure after an extremity tourniquet has been inflated 45–60 minutes. Patients with otherwise satisfactory regional blocks begin to complain of a dull, aching discomfort at the tourniquet site. For patients having general anesthesia, tourniquet pain does not require therapy if the blood pressure remains physiologic or can be treated with short-acting antihypertensive drugs or increased concentrations of volatile agents. Since the blood pressure falls immediately after tourniquet release, the concentration of volatile agent should be lowered 5–10 minutes before tourniquet deflation. Patients undergoing spinal anesthesia with bupivacaine, experience less lower extremity tourniquet pain than patients receiving tetracaine.

RHYTHM DISTURBANCES (Table 7.6)

Ventricular Arrhythmias

Premature Ventricular Contractions (PVCs)

Most PVCs occurring under anesthesia are benign and require no treatment. They are frequently due to light anesthesia, especially in the presence of hypercarbia, and often occur after intubation. Deepening anesthesia with thiopental, lidocaine, or opioid or volatile agents and ventilation with oxygen usually restores normal sinus rhythm. Hyperventilation should be avoided; the resultant alkalosis shifts potassium and magnesium intracellularly, increasing ventricular irritability. PVCs may also appear as an escape rhythm if the sinus rate drops below the

Table 7.6
Causes of Dysrhythmias

Inadequate anesthesia
Electrolyte abnormalities
  K^+
  Mg^{2+}
Hypercarbia
Hypocarbia
Preexisting cardiopulmonary disease
Myocardial ischemia
Ventricular escape rhythm
Sympathetic stimulation
Catecholamines (e.g., epinephrine and halothane)

intrinsic ventricular rate. Atropine 0.2–0.4 mg IV increases the sinus rate and corrects the dysrhythmia.

Causes of PVCs

1. Low serum potassium and magnesium levels result in ventricular ectopy. Factors predisposing to potassium and magnesium depletion include critical illness, malnourishment, alcoholism, diarrhea, nasogastric suction, and diuretic use. If electrolyte abnormalities exist, an infusion of KCl 10 mEq and $MgSO_4$ 1–2 gm may be given over 30–60 minutes. Potassium is irritating to peripheral veins when given in concentrations above 40 mEq/liter. Higher concentrations may be given via a central venous catheter, but fatal dysrhythmia may occur if the potassium is infused too rapidly. Magnesium is a vasodilator that may cause transient hypotension. Nondepolarizing muscle relaxants are potentiated by high magnesium levels.

2. Patients with ischemic heart disease and chronic PVCs often revert to normal sinus rhythm following anesthetic induction because of decreases in sympathetic activity and improved oxygen delivery. Conversely, the onset of PVCs in a patient with coronary artery disease may herald the development of myocardial ischemia.

Treatment of PVCs

1. When PVCs occur intraoperatively, oxygenation, ventilation, electrolytes, and the ECG should be assessed. More than five

PVCs per minute, R-on-T PVCs, multifocal PVCs, or couplets should be treated. Lidocaine 1.0–1.5 mg/kg IV followed by a 20–50 μg/kg/min infusion is usually effective.

2. **Ventricular tachycardia** (see Appendix for treatment protocol) **Torsades de pointes** is a variety of ventricular tachycardia in which the ECG complexes twist around a central axis; it occurs in patients with prolonged Q-T interval (congenital, antiarrhythmic drugs, electrolyte abnormalities such as K^+, Mg^{2+}, Ca^{2+}, or subarachnoid hemorrhage). Instead of administering the usual antiarrhythmic drugs, treatment should be directed at correction of the underlying electrolyte problem, pacing for bradycardia, or cardioversion.

3. **Ventricular fibrillation** (see Appendix for treatment protocol)

Atrial Dysrhythmias

Atrial dysrhythmias are common in patients with underlying cardiac or pulmonary disease, especially if they are hypocarbic. Atrial ectopy is frequent in patients taking large doses of bronchodilators. These dysrhythmias are rarely of hemodynamic significance and no special therapy may be indicated if oxygenation, ventilation, and electrolytes are normal.

Conduction Abnormalities

Left or Right Bundle Branch Block

Complete left or right bundle branch block or hemiblock of the left bundle usually does not produce hemodynamic dysfunction. Insertion of a pulmonary artery catheter may produce a right bundle branch block, usually reversible after removal of the catheter, and can result in complete heart block in a patient with preexisting left bundle branch block. Therefore, some practitioners insert only pulmonary artery catheters with pacing capability in patients with left bundle branch block.

Heart Block

1. **First degree** (P-R interval >200 msec) block results from prolongation of the impulse across the AV node and does not require treatment.

2. **Second degree**
   a. **Type I** block occurs when there are progressively longer P-R intervals until a P wave is not followed by a QRS. It can be seen with myocardial ischemia or with an acute inferior myocardial infarction but may be found in some patients without cardiac disease.
   b. **Type II** block represents disease in the conducting bundles and is diagnosed by constant P-R intervals with some impulses regularly nonconducted to the ventricles.
3. **Third degree (complete AV) block** means that no impulses cross the AV node and results in either asystole or ventricular escape beats. Atropine or β-adrenergic drugs should be used to maintain the ventricular rate until a pacer can be placed.

MYOCARDIAL ISCHEMIA

Perioperative myocardial infarction (MI) has a high mortality rate. Therefore, intraoperative ischemic episodes must be prevented, if possible, and treated promptly should they occur. Evidence continues to accumulate that ischemic ECG changes occur intraoperatively without apparent changes in myocardial oxygen supply or demand. These episodes are believed to be manifestations of silent ischemia, which is common in patients with coronary artery disease. Intraoperative ischemia may reflect the inadequacy of preoperative antianginal therapy, emphasizing the important role the primary physician plays in treating myocardial ischemia aggressively before hospital admission.

Treatment is directed toward optimizing myocardial oxygen delivery while minimizing oxygen demand. Tachycardia has deleterious effects on both supply and demand. Neither general nor regional anesthetic techniques have been clearly shown to be superior in decreasing cardiac morbidity. Likewise, no drug or combination of drugs used for general anesthesia is superior in the patient with coronary artery disease, as long as wide swings in heart rate and blood pressure do not occur. Opioids, which slow the heart rate and tend to maintain blood pressure, are frequently supplemented with volatile agents to decrease myocardial oxygen consumption.

The use of **isoflurane** in patients with ischemic heart disease is controversial, because of the potential for intracoronary steal.

Isoflurane is a potent coronary vasodilator. Since coronary artery segments distal to stenoses may already be maximally dilated, the use of isoflurane may decrease resistance in normal vessels and shunt blood away from the ischemic zone. Intracoronary steal may occur in a minority of patients, but if isoflurane is selected, the lowest effective concentration should be used. The clinician must be alert to ischemic ECG changes.

If myocardial ischemia does occur, the oxygen supply:demand ratio must be optimized. Arterial oxygenation must be assessed and 100% oxygen given. Nitroglycerin should be infused at a rate of 0.5–2 μg/kg/min. Intravenous propranolol 0.5–1 mg, metoprolol 1–2 mg, or esmolol 0.5–1 mg/kg should be titrated to lower the heart rate. The liquid contents of a nifedipine capsule may be placed under the patient's tongue. These measures may decrease the blood pressure, which should be supported by intravenous fluids, transfusion to a hematocrit of 30% or phenylephrine infusion. A pulmonary artery catheter may help optimize filling pressures.

Hypertension and tachycardia during emergence should be minimized by the use of nitroglycerin and β-blockade.

HYPOXEMIA (Table 7.7)

Routine **pulse oximetry** has greatly facilitated the early detection of hypoxemia. However, pulse oximetry may not accurately measure hemoglobin saturation after the injection of various dyes, if the patient is wearing nail polish, or if there is poor peripheral perfusion caused by vasoconstriction, decreased cardiac output, or peripheral vascular disease. Carboxyhemoglobin absorbs light at the same wavelengths used by pulse oximeters, so oxygen saturation measurements may not be accurate in cases of carbon monoxide poisoning. Patients with significant lung disease require a room air blood gas or saturation measured by pulse oximeter before administration of any sedatives, so that the adequacy of postoperative oxygenation may be assessed more easily.

Unrecognized **esophageal intubation** remains a common cause of hypoxemia. Indirect signs of tube placement (auscultation, visualization of chest rise, or "fogging" of the tube during exhalation) are unreliable. Even a tube that has been seen to lie between the vocal cords or one that has been placed using fi-

Table 7.7
Causes of Hypoxemia

Low FiO_2
Shunt
  Endobronchial intubation
  Blunted HPV from anesthesia vasodilation, etc.
  Esophageal intubation
V/Q mismatching
Hypoventilation
  Inadequate VT
  Disconnect
Venous desaturation
Diffusion barrier

---

beroptic visualization of the carina may become dislodged. The only reliable indicator of tracheal location is the continued presence of CO_2 in exhaled gases. There may be no exhaled CO_2, even with a correctly positioned tube, if there is not pulmonary blood flow (e.g., cardiac arrest or a massive pulmonary embolus).

Hypoxic gas mixtures (low FIO_2) may be delivered if there is equipment failure or human error. Hypoxia may be caused by switching of nitrous oxide and oxygen lines, malfunction of a nitrous oxide–oxygen proportioner, exhaustion of an oxygen cylinder or the use of a nitrous oxide–air mixture. A properly calibrated oxygen analyzer with the low alarm limit set 10% below the intended F_1O_2 helps to avoid this anesthetic catastrophe. Diffusion hypoxia, caused by the rapid washout of nitrous oxide from the blood and into the alveoli at the end of an anesthetic, can be prevented by administering 100% oxygen for several minutes after discontinuing N_2O.

Absolute shunts may be caused by **endobronchial intubation.** Even a previously well-positioned tube migrates toward the carina when the head is flexed. An oxygen saturation near 100% does not rule out tube migration if a high inspired oxygen concentration is used. An increase in inspiratory pressure is often the first sign of bronchial intubation. Pneumothorax and atelectatic collapse are also true shunts.

V/Q mismatching is increased by anesthetics, muscle relaxants, and positive pressure ventilation, as well as aspiration, pulmonary embolus (air, fat, or thrombus), bronchospasm, pneumonia, or atelectasis.

Hypoventilation may occur in spontaneously breathing patients because of anesthetic drugs, residual muscle weakness, or airway obstruction. Patients receiving mechanical ventilation may suffer hypoventilation and hypoxia if disconnection or equipment failure occurs.

Low mixed venous oxygen tension may also cause arterial hypoxemia. This is likely to occur if there is decreased oxygen delivery (anemia or low cardiac output) or increased oxygen consumption (shivering, increased temperature, or other hypermetabolic state).

Severe hypoxemia is an emergency requiring the administration of 100% oxygen. Hand ventilation allows instantaneous assessment of pulmonary compliance. Observation of symmetrical chest rise and auscultation of bilateral breath sounds suggests normal pulmonary mechanics. Milder levels of desaturation allow one to review these parameters at a less frantic pace while obtaining arterial blood gas analysis and a chest x-ray and assessing oxygen delivery and consumption.

HYPERCARBIA

The normal, nonspecific clinical signs of hypercarbia (cardiorespiratory stimulation, dysrhythmia, or vasodilation) are blunted by anesthetics. Diagnosis requires blood gas analysis. In a well-oxygenated patient, transient hypercarbia is usually benign. Treatment is directed toward discovery and correction of the underlying cause. Quantitative CO_2 monitoring of anesthetized patients should be routinely used to detect hypercarbia. CO_2 wave forms are useful for diagnosing some ventilatory problems. End-tidal CO_2 is usually lower than arterial CO_2 tension by several mm Hg, but the difference may not be constant throughout the course of anesthesia. Inspiratory CO_2 should be O mm Hg and an elevation of inspired CO_2 may be caused by rebreathing of CO_2 from increased dead space, faulty unidirectional valve, or exhausted absorbent in a circle system, or by inadequate fresh gas flow to a Mapleson-type circuit.

1. Anesthetics ordinarily decrease oxygen consumption and the rate of CO_2 formation. If a patient's minute ventilation remains constant, hypercarbia will occur if there is an increase in CO_2 production (altered RQ as with IV hyperalimenta-

tion, febrile illness, malignant hyperthermia, thyroid storm, or other hypermetabolic state).

2. More commonly, hypercarbia results from a **diminished CO_2 removal.** Since patients frequently receive supplemental oxygen perioperatively, hypoventilation and hypercarbia may occur with normal oxygen saturation. Rebreathing of exhaled CO_2 occurs if there is a defective expiratory valve, exhaustion of the soda lime canister, or (as is possible on older machines) complete bypass of the CO_2 absorber. Spontaneously breathing patients, either anesthetized or in the post-anesthesia period, may be hypercarbic from inhalational agents, sedatives, or narcotics that alter the CO_2 response curve. Inadequately reversed muscle relaxant may also impair spontaneous ventilation.

3. **Increases in dead space ventilation** result in CO_2 retention. Vd/Vt is greater if pulmonary blood flow is diminished by hypovolemia, PEEP, pulmonary emboli, or low cardiac output. If there is more than a 5 torr gradient between arterial and end-expired CO_2 levels, an increase in dead space ventilation may be suspected.

WHEEZING

Causes

Wheezing signifies an increased resistance to air flow, but even in patients with bronchospastic disease, all that wheezes is not asthma. In addition to bronchospasm, wheezing may be caused by "passive bronchoconstriction." Secretions or obstruction of the endotracheal tube (ET at carina) result in greater airflow resistance yet normal bronchial smooth muscle tone. Pulmonary edema and aspiration of gastric contents may present as wheezing.

Treatment

1. If wheezing occurs, the **depth of anesthesia should be increased** by the administration of opioids, volatile anesthetics, intravenous lidocaine, or ketamine. Next, a suction catheter should be passed the length of the tube and aspirated as the catheter is withdrawn. This verifies tube patency and removes obstructing secretions. If wheezing persists, the endo-

tracheal tube cuff should be deflated and the tube with-drawn slightly, lest cuff hyperinflation or bronchial intubation has occurred.

2. **β-Agonist administration** is the first-line pharmacologic treatment of bronchospasm. Metered doses of β-agonists may be administered down the endotracheal tube using a special adapter. Some of the dose clings to the walls of the endotracheal tube, 8–10 puffs may be required. **Ipatropium** (Atrovent), an anticholinergic agent, may also be given in this manner. **Methylprednisolone,** 120 mg, or **hydrocortisone,** 4 mg/kg IV, may be useful in severe attacks, although steroids do not exert maximal antiinflammatory effects for several hours. The role of **aminophylline** in the treatment of bronchospasm has become less clear. The efficacy of aminophylline is questionable, and tachydysrythmias frequently occur. A loading dose of 4–6 mg/kg of aminophylline may be useful if a severe attack is refractory to β-agonist and anticholinergic therapy.

3. Often patients with bronchospastic disease wheeze immediately after intubation and continue to wheeze despite therapy. Removal of the endotracheal tube may resolve the problem. Deep extubation may be indicated, but one must also consider the likelihood of gastric aspiration as well as the ease of reintubation, should it become necessary.

ASPIRATION

High-Risk Groups

Aspiration of gastric contents remains a significant anesthetic risk. The likelihood of aspiration is increased in patients with **diabetes, hiatal hernia, obesity, pregnancy, achalasia, bowel obstruction, and any emergency procedure.** Traditional teaching is that aspiration pneumonia occurs if the pH of the aspirate is less than 2.5, the volume of aspirate is greater than 25 ml, or if particulate matter is present.

Prevention (Table 7.8)

Omperazole (Prilosec) is a gastric acid pump inhibitor that may also be a useful pharmacoprophylactic agent. Most oral medications require 60–90 minutes for maximum effectiveness. So-

Table 7.8
Measures to Reduce Risk of Pulmonary Aspiration

Maintenance of NPO status
Decompression of stomach with gastric tube
Awake intubation
Rapid sequence intubation
Successful regional anesthesia and minimal sedation
H_2 blockers
  Cimetidine 300–400 mg PO
  Ranitidine 50 mg IV or 150 mg PO
  Famotidine 20 mg
Gastrokinetic agent—metoclopramide 10–20 mg
Nonparticulate antiacid—sodium citrate 30 ml PO

dium citrate is an exception; it neutralizes existing stomach acid immediately but has a duration of action less than 3 hours and may need to be repeated.

Diagnosis

Aspiration may be suspected if gastric material is visualized near the glottis during laryngoscopy or is suctioned from the endotracheal tube. Wheezing, coughing, and hypoxia are dramatic signs of aspiration.

Treatment

1. If significant aspiration has occurred, **tracheal intubation** should be performed as expeditiously as possible. The trachea should be suctioned before instituting positive pressure ventilation. Mechanical ventilation with increasing levels of positive end-expiratory pressure should be used to maintain adequate oxygenation with a goal of reducing FIO_2 to less than 0.5. Aminophylline may be used to treat bronchospasm. β-Agonist and anticholinergic aerosols may also be helpful.

2. **Antibiotic prophylaxis** is indicated only if infected material has been aspirated. Otherwise, antibiotics are reserved to treat secondary bacterial infections. The use of steroids after aspiration has occurred is controversial. Tracheal lavage with bicarbonate or saline to neutralize or dilute the acid concentration is futile and may worsen pulmonary damage.

3. Extubation, if indicated, should be undertaken only in patients with minimal A-a gradients who possess protective airway reflexes and who have had their stomachs decompressed
with a gastric tube. Acid damage to pulmonary endothelium
may lead to progressive atelectasis, pulmonary congestion,
and hypoxemia. Patients who have aspirated merit close observation and assessment of oxygenation for several hours
because pulmonary function may deteriorate.

AUTONOMIC HYPERREFLEXIA

Patients with spinal cord injuries above T6 may have autonomic
hyperreflexia characterized by hypertension, bradycardia, and
arrhythmias during surgical procedures on the lower extremities, during cystoscopy, or when the bladder or rectum is stimulated from being full. Sympathetic hyperactivity from spinal reflexes below the level of the injury are not inhibited from the
central nervous system from above and produce vasoconstriction below the lesion. This hypertension activates carotid and
aortic baroreceptors, leading to bradycardia. Autonomic hyperreflexia can be prevented by general or regional anesthesia.
The symptoms can also be controlled with direct vasodilators
like nitroprusside.

HYPOTHERMIA

General anesthetics decrease basal metabolic rate, inhibit hypo-
thalamic temperature regulation, and result in vasodilation.
The concomitant use of muscle relaxants prevents shivering as
a means of heat production. Spinal or epidural anesthetics produce motor block and vasodilation, which also leads to heat
loss. This heat loss may continue postoperatively if the block is
prolonged.

Hypothermia shifts the oxyhemoglobin dissociation curve
to the left, diminishes blood coagulability, reduces MAC, slows
the biotransformation of intravenous drugs, and potentiates
muscle relaxants. Nonetheless, body temperatures of 33–34°C
are usually well tolerated intraoperatively. As the patient
emerges from general anesthesia, shivering occurs. Shivering
raises oxygen consumption and CO_2 production fivefold at a
time when residual ventilatory depression and muscular weakness may be present. The resultant tachycardia and hyper-

tension increase myocardial oxygen demand further. This is particularly deleterious in elderly patients who lose heat more rapidly intraoperatively and rewarm more slowly after surgery.

Temperature Measurement

Core temperature is most accurately recorded from a probe placed in the distal esophagus, on the tympanic membrane, or in the tip of a pulmonary artery catheter. Rectal temperatures are frequently 0.5–1°C higher than core temperature and are slow to reflect changes. A rectal temperature probe should not be used routinely.

Prevention

The rate of heat loss is greatest during the first hour of anesthesia, so efforts to conserve heat must begin as soon as possible following induction. Hypothermia rarely occurs if the ambient temperature is above 24°C and is a certainty if the room is colder than 21°C. Radiant heat loss may be minimized by covering exposed body parts with a forced-air warming blanket. Particular attention should be paid to the head and neck. The head of an intubated patient may be wrapped in a bonnet fashioned from a folded towel and placed inside a clear plastic bag. A heated water mattress under the patient is not effective in warming patients.

Heat loss is increased by the use of cold irrigation or preparatory solutions, unheated IV fluids, and cool breezes generated by opening and closing operating room doors. Bags of IV fluids may be stored in a warmer at 40°C, eliminating the need for cumbersome in-line fluid warmers. Blood should be warmed to body temperature before infusion, using any acceptable device, but overheating blood may cause hemolysis from thermal injury to RBCs. Ventilation with dry gases results in evaporative heat losses, which may be minimized by the use of heat and moisture exchangers, active heat and humidification devices, or closed-circuit anesthesia.

Meperidine 6.25–12.5 mg IV may be used to treat postoperative shivering. Radiant heaters or forced-air heat are most useful postoperatively to help restore core temperature to normal.

MALIGNANT HYPERTHERMIA

Malignant hyperthermia (MH) is a syndrome that occurs when susceptible individuals receive triggering anesthetic drugs, specifically succinylcholine and all potent volatile agents (Table 7.9). During an MH crisis there is an abnormal increase in myoplasmic calcium, resulting in sustained muscle contractures, an increased metabolic rate, and ultimately, a rise in body temperature. MH has varied presentations and clinical courses, ranging from a gradual increase in heart rate, PCO_2 , and blood lactate over several hours, to a fulminant temperature rise (1°C every 5 minutes) immediately following induction.

Incidence and Risk Groups

The estimated incidence of MH ranges from 1:5,000 to 1:50,000 anesthetics. MH occurs more frequently in children than in adults, but this may reflect the common pediatric induction sequence of halothane by inhalation followed by succinylcholine. Until adolescence, MH occurs equally among boys and girls; after puberty there is a male preponderance. Patients with the following preexisting neuromuscular or skeletal diseases are at a greater risk for developing MH: **muscular dystrophy, myopathy, strabismus, cryptorchidism, and inguinal hernia.** There is also an incompletely understood genetic predisposition.

Table 7.9
Malignant Hyperthermia Nontriggering Drugs

Induction agents
  Barbiturates
  Benzodiazepines
  Etomidate
  Narcotics
  Propofol
Nitrous oxide
Nondepolarizing muscle relaxants
Anticholinesterases
Anticholinergics
Sympathomimetics, nitroglycerin, nitroprusside, β-blockers
Local anesthetics
Droperidol

Diagnosis

Total body rigidity is the most specific sign of MH. More commonly, however, other signs of hypermetabolism occur, including tachycardia, tachypnea, skin mottling, dark blood in the surgical field, arterial desaturation, and dysrhythmias, as well as heating and exhaustion of the CO_2 absorber. Blood gas analysis reveals a mixed respiratory and metabolic acidosis. A doubling or tripling of the end-tidal CO_2 concentration is the most sensitive indicator of MH. Despite the name of the syndrome, body temperature may remain normal during a malignant hyperthermia episode.

Treatment (Table 7.10)

Untreated, MH has an 80% mortality rate. Delay in diagnosis increases mortality, so prompt recognition and treatment of MH is essential. Initial supportive therapy includes stopping all volatile anesthetics and hyperventilation with 100% O_2 at high flow rates. If the procedure cannot be stopped, the above measures should be taken, and the anesthetic continued with nontriggering agents (Table 7.9).

Dantrolene decreases intracellular calcium concentration and is the specific therapy for MH. The initial dose is 2–3 mg/kg, which may be repeated at 20-minute intervals up to 10 mg/kg total until symptoms subside. Dantrolene is poorly soluble; reconstitution requires large volumes of sterile water for injection USP without a bacteriostatic agent. During an MH crisis, a trustworthy individual should be assigned the sole task of dantrolene preparation. Sufficient supplies of dantrolene and its diluent should be available wherever succinylcholine or volatile anesthetics are used.

Late complications of MH include hyperkalemia, rhabdomyolysis, and myoglobinuria leading to renal failure, as well as coagulopathy and recurrence of MH. Patients should be observed in an intensive care unit for at least 24 hours.

MH versus Masseter Spasm

One percent of pediatric patients receiving succinylcholine experience masseter muscle rigidity; half of these patients are determined to be MH susceptible after muscle biopsy testing. There is

Table 7.10
Emergency Therapy for Malignant Hyperthermia (Revised 1993)[a]

Acute Phase Treatment

1. Immediately discontinue all volatile inhalation anesthetics and succinyl-choline. Hyperventilate with 100% oxygen at high gas flows; at least 10 L/min. The circle system and CO_2 absorbent need not be changed.

2. Administer dantrolene sodium 2–3 mg/kg initial bolus rapidly with increments up to 10 mg/kg total. Continue to administer dantrolene until signs of MH (e.g. tachycardia, rigidity, increased end-tidal CO_2, and temperature elevation) are controlled. Occasionally, a total dose greater than 10 mg/kg may be needed. Each vial of dantrolene contains 20 mg of dantrolene and 3 grams mannitol. Each vial should be mixed with 60 mL of sterile water for injection USP without a bacteriostatic agent.

3. Administer bicarbonate to correct metabolic acidosis as guided by blood gas analysis. In the absence of blood gas analysis, 1–2 mEq/kg should be administered.

4. Simultaneous with the above, actively cool the hyperthermic patient. Use IV iced saline (not Ringer's lactate) 15 mL/kg q 15 min X 3.
   a. Lavage stomach, bladder, rectum and open cavities with iced saline as appropriate.
   b. Surface cool with ice and hypothermia blanket.
   c. Monitor closely since overvigorous treatment may lead to hypothermia.

5. Dysrhythmias will usually respond to treatment of acidosis and hyperkalemia. If they persist or are life threatening, standard anti-arrhythmic agents may be used, with the exception of calcium channel blockers (may cause hyperkalemia and CV collapse).

6. Determine and monitor end-tidal CO_2, arterial, central or femoral venous blood gases, serum potassium, calcium, clotting studies and urine output.

7. Hyperkalemia is common and should be treated with hyperventilation, bicarbonate, intravenous glucose and insulin (10 units regular insulin in 50 mL 50% glucose titrated to potassium level). Life threatening hyperkalemia may also be treated with calcium administration (e.g. 2–5 mg/kg of $CaCl_2$).

8. Ensure urine output of greater than 2 mL/kg/hr. Consider central venous or PA monitoring because of fluid shifts and hemodynamic instability that may occur.

9. Boys less than 9 years of age who experience sudden cardiac arrest after succinylcholine in the absence of hypoxemia should be treated for acute hyperkalemia first. In this situation, calcium chloride should be administered along with other means to reduce serum potassium. They should be presumed to have subclinical muscular dystrophy.

Post Acute Phase

A. Observe the patient in an ICU setting for at least 24 hours since recrudescence of MH may occur, particularly following a fulminant case resistant to treatment.

B. Administer dantrolene 1 mg/kg IV q 6 hours for 24–48 hours post episode. After that, oral dantrolene 1 mg/kg q 6 hours may be used for 24 hours as necessary.
C. Follow ABG, CK, potassium, calcium, urine and serum myoglobin, clotting studies and core body temperature until such time as they return to normal values (e.g. q 6 hours). Central temperature (e.g., rectal, esophageal) should be continuously monitored until stable.
D. Counsel the patient and family regarding MH and further precautions. Refer the patient to MHAUS. Fill out an Adverse Metabolic Reaction to Anesthesia (AMRA) report available through the North American Malignant Hyperthermia Registry (717)531-6936.
Caution: This protocol may not apply to every patient and must of necessity be altered according to specific patient needs.

Note: Names of on-call physicians available to consult in MH emergencies may be obtained 24 hours a day through: Medic Alert Foundation International (209) 634–4917. Ask for: Index Zero. For non-emergency or patient referral calls: MHAUS Post Office Box, 191 Westport, CT 06881–0191. (203) 847–0407.

---

[a]Reproduced with permission of Malignant Hyperthermia Association of the United States.

controversy regarding the management of patients who are scheduled for elective surgery and develop masseter rigidity after receiving succinylcholine. Most pediatric anesthesiologists have limited their use of succinylcholine, and one manufacturer has indicated that succinylcholine should be used only in specific circumstances (airway emergencies) in pediatric patients.

HYPERSENSITIVITY REACTIONS

Hypersensitivity reactions include immune-mediated anaphylaxis as well as nonimmunogenic anaphylactoid responses. Both involve the formation and release of mediators that evoke a spectrum of physiologic effects. In anesthetized patients, hypersensitivity most commonly presents as profound hypotension, but bronchospasm, angioneurotic edema, and urticaria also occur. The onset of a reaction may occur immediately after exposure to the allergen or be delayed as long as 2 hours. Severe reactions usually occur within minutes. Intravenous barbiturates, muscle relaxants (including succinylcholine), blood products, and β-lactam antibiotics are most frequently associated with allergic reactions. Any foreign material contacting the body, however, including latex surgical gloves, prosthetic devices, or antibacterial irrigation, may provoke a hypersensitivity response. Rapid administration of vancomycin produces hypotension and "red man syndrome" from histamine release.

Treatment

Initial treatment requires stopping exposure to the allergen and ventilating with 100% oxygen. If airway edema or compromise occurs, immediate tracheal intubation is necessary. Rapid infusion of 2–4 liters of crystalloid may be required to maintain intravascular volume.

Epinephrine is the drug of choice for severe hypersensitivity reactions because it inhibits mediator release, supports blood pressure, and relieves bronchospasm. An initial dose of 4–8 μg IV (1–2 ml of a solution containing 1.0 mg epinephrine in 250 ml dextrose solution) is used to treat hypotension, but 0.1–1.0 mg may be required if cardiovascular collapse occurs. Subsequent doses, if necessary, should be doubled at 2- to 3-minute intervals until hemodynamic stability is restored. Refractory hypotension may necessitate the use of norepinephrine infusion.

Diphenhydramine (Benadryl) 0.5–1.0 mg/kg and H_2 blockers are frequently administered in an attempt to limit the effects of histamine release. Aminophylline 5–7 mg/kg is used to treat bronchospasm. Methylprednisolone 15 mg/kg may help stabilize cell membranes.

Suggested Readings

Ellis JE, Shah MN, Briller JE, Roizen MF, Aronson S, Feinstein SB. A comparison of methods for the detection of myocardial ischemia during noncardiac surgery: automated ST-segment analysis systems, electrocardiography, and transesophageal echocardiography. Anesth Analg 1992;75:764–772.

Holzman RS. Latex allergy: an emerging operating room problem. Anesth Analg 1993;76:635–641.

Levitt RC. Prospects for the diagnosis of malignant hyperthermia susceptibility using molecular genetic approaches. Anesthesiology 1992;76:1039–1048.

Levy JH. Anaphylactic Reactions in Anesthesia and Intensive Care. 2nd ed. Stoneham, MA: Butterworth-Heinemann, 1992.

Tokics L, Hedenostiera G, et al. Lung collapse and gas exchange during general anesthesia: effects of spontaneous breathing, muscle paralysis, and positive end expiratory pressure. Anesthesiology 1987;66:157.

Chapter 8

Neurosurgical Anesthesia

Providing anesthesia for patients who undergo intracranial procedures requires special considerations.

1. The patient's position during surgery may be varied. This requires prior discussion with the surgical team so that an appropriate plan can be devised.
2. The anesthesiologist is removed from the airway once the procedure is started and this, coupled with the fact that the patient's neck is frequently flexed and/or rotated, makes the use of the reinforced endotracheal tube desirable. The depth of the tube's insertion depends upon the head's final position: in extension the tube should be inserted deeper, and in flexion it should be inserted shallower than usual.
3. Blood loss is very difficult, if not impossible, to estimate accurately. Also, a considerable amount of blood may be lost from the scalp vessels during opening and closure.
4. Craniotomies tend to be lengthy cases. Every effort should be made to prevent hypothermia, thickened secretion in the tracheobronchial tree, pressure points, and nerve injuries.
5. Postoperatively, it is essential that the patient regain consciousness as quickly as possible, since level of consciousness is an important part of the patient's overall evaluation. However, some patients may not regain consciousness quickly, including those with large brain tumors where only a biopsy was done and those in whom excessive traction was placed on the frontal lobe for procedures in the subtemporal area.

The following factors govern IV fluids management:

1. Craniotomy causes minimal third space and evaporative losses.

145

2. Changes in osmotic pressure of the plasma will affect the water movement from and into the brain across the blood-brain barrier.

3. Hyperglycemia is harmful to ischemic brain tissue.

Taking these factors into consideration, IV fluids are managed as follows:

1. Fluid restriction (1.5–2.5 ml/kg/hr)—this fluid restriction should not be to the point of causing severe hypovolemia or cardiovascular instability.

2. Solute-free solution (e.g., D5W or D5 1/2 NS) should not be used.

3. Ringer's lactate or normal saline are the fluids of choice unless blood products or colloids are needed

4. Blood glucose should be closely monitored and kept between 100 and 150 mg/100 ml.

5. Hypernatremic and chronic hyponatremic states should be corrected slowly (no faster than 1 mosm/hr).

PATIENTS WITH INTRACRANIAL HYPERTENSION

Preoperative Evaluation

1. General medical evaluation

2. Level of consciousness and orientation

3. Cranial nerve deficit and its sequelae (e.g., patient with tenth nerve palsy may have aspiration pneumonia)

4. Diagnostic studies, such as arteriography and CT scan, and their sequelae (remember, contrast material is a diuretic, and it may cause hypovolemia or electrolyte disturbances)

5. Side, site, and vascularity of the intracranial lesion

6. Electrolyte imbalance may be caused by syndrome of inappropriate antidiuretic hormone or diabetes insipidus

7. ECG—patients with intracranial lesions may have any ECG abnormality from heart disease or from the neurologic pathology

8. Hospital course since admission (e.g., a patient with a brain tumor who was admitted comatose, then improved with steroids and mannitol, most likely will be hypovolemic, may have electrolyte imbalance, and most importantly, has a narrow margin of safety as far as the intracranial pressure (ICP) is concerned)

Premedication

1. A moderate dose of hypnotic (e.g., diazepam) is generally adequate (narcotics should be avoided in patients with increased ICP).
2. Antiseizure and steroid medications should be continued.
3. Cardiac or antihypertensive drugs should be handled appropriately.

Monitoring

1. Standard monitors for general anesthesia
2. Urine output
3. Capnometer
4. Direct arterial pressure
5. The decision to insert a central venous pressure catheter or pulmonary artery catheter should depend on the patient's condition and vascularity of the intracranial lesion.

Induction and Maintenance of Anesthesia

1. Induction with pentothal and short-acting narcotics (e.g., fentanyl). Nondepolarizing muscle relaxants are preferable to succinylcholine. Moderate hyperventilation is begun. The cardiovascular responses to laryngoscopy can be minimized by the use of intravenous lidocaine, alfentanil, pentothal, or sympathetic antagonists.
2. Endotracheal tube must be *securely* fixed.
3. Positioning of the patient's head should allow surgical access but not interfere with venous drainage from the brain. Positions known to decrease venous drainage form the brain include extreme flexion and/or rotation of the cervical spine and putting the head at a level below that of the heart.
4. Anesthesia is maintained with a mixture of O_2 and N_2O, fentanyl and isoflurane (0.5–1%). This drug regimen, combined with hyperventilation, does not increase cerebral blood flow considerably.

Methods of Decreasing Intracranial Pressure

1. Diuretics, mannitol, and/or furosemide; mannitol (0.5–1 gm/kg) should be given slowly, <1 gm/min.

2. Hyperventilation—usually begun during induction, but since hyperventilation begins to lose its effectiveness after about 4 hours, *maximal* hyperventilation should be reserved until the surgeon is about to open the dura.
3. Intrathoracic pressure is kept as low as possible by proper patient positioning, clear unobstructed airway, muscle relaxants, ideal ventilator volumes and flows, and treating bronchospasm if it is present.
4. Fluid restriction.
5. Blood pressure fluctuation, especially hypertension, must be minimized.
6. CSF drainage, if needed, is usually done through a lumbar subarachnoid catheter or needle. CSF drainage should *not* start before the dura is opened.

If all of these measures fail to provide a relaxed brain and good working conditions for the surgeon, then the use of pentothal and tilting the operating table to a head-up position may be necessary.

Unexplainable brain swelling may be caused by pneumocephalus or intracranial hemorrhage away from the surgical field.

Emergence

Anesthesia should be maintained until the anesthesiologist has access to the patient's airway. Removing the patient's head from the holder and applying head dressing is very stimulating. If the patient is lightly anesthetized, there may be bucking or coughing, which may cause intracranial hemorrhage or edema. The use of IV lidocaine may be beneficial. Once the patient's head is wrapped, the muscle relaxant is reversed and the anesthetic agents are turned off. Use of a narcotic technique usually allows the patient to respond to commands within a few minutes without bucking on the ET tube. If the patient doesn't respond as expected, small doses of narcotic antagonist (e.g., 20–40 μgm of naloxone) can be given. In the absence of normal awakening, after possible anesthetic causes are excluded, the patient should be evaluated in consultation with the surgeon. CT scanning or other diagnostic tests may be needed.

INTRACRANIAL ANEURYSM

Patients with intracranial aneurysms are frequently admitted after subarachnoid hemorrhage, but since the introduction of the CT and MRI scans, more patients are diagnosed before the aneurysm ruptures.

Clinical Problems after Hemorrhage

1. Altered mental status
2. Focal CNS symptoms and signs
3. Rebleeding
4. Vasospasm
5. Hydrocephalus
6. Seizures
7. Electrolyte imbalance (secondary to syndrome of inappropriate antidiuretic hormone or diabetes insipidus)
8. ECG changes

Preoperative Medical Management

1. Sedation
2. Antihypertensive agents
3. Nimodipine to prevent vasospasm

Timing of surgery remains controversial:

1. *Early surgery* (within 2–3 days after the initial bleeding) is technically more difficult, but it permits hypertension and intravascular volume expansion to be used postoperatively to prevent vasospasm without fear of rebleeding.
2. *Late surgery* (10–14 days after the initial bleeding) is easier to perform and less likely to be followed by vasospasm but rebleeding may occur during the delay.

Management outcome is the same with either approach. There is a tendency to operate early when the patient is young and in good clinical condition.

Preoperative Evaluation

Preoperative evaluation is the same as that for the patient with increased ICP (see above).

In addition, the patient should be evaluated for

1. Presence of vasospasm
2. Number of aneurysms
3. Grade according to Hunt and Hess classification (1–5, grade 1 is asymptomatic, grade 5 is in deep coma)

Premedication

Premedication should not be too heavy, but adequate to prevent extreme apprehension. Extreme apprehension may cause the patient to be hypertensive, which increases the possibility of the aneurysm bleeding.

Invasive Monitors

1. Arterial line
2. CVP
3. Urinary bladder catheter
4. Possibly, EEG or somatosensory evoked potentials (SSEP)

Goals

Induction of anesthesia goals are to prevent a sudden increase in the ICP and, more importantly, an increase in BP. The critical times for BP increase are endotracheal intubation, application of the head-holder, and skin incision. Hypertension is minimized by having the patient deeply anesthetized and the use of rapidly acting drugs (e.g., alfentanil) before painful stimuli. Local anesthetic can be injected in the scalp before applying the head-holder or skin incision. Sympathetic antagonists (labetolol, esmolol) or vasodilators (nitroprusside) are useful in preventing or controlling hypertension.

Anesthetic Management

Anesthetic management is the same as that for patients with increased ICP, except

1. Adequate venous access for rapid fluid replacement if the aneurysm ruptures is needed.
2. Patient may be hypovolemic.
3. Side effects of nimodipine treatment (e.g., hypotension and bradycardia).

4. Efforts to decrease the ICP should be initiated slowly, since sudden decrease in the ICP may cause the aneurysm to rupture.
5. Prevent hypertension.
6. Necessity to provide controlled hypotension for aneurysm clipping or rupture.

Fluid Management (Three Phases)

1. Fluid restriction and diuresis during the craniotomy and the initial exposure
2. Normovolemia as the surgeon approaches the aneurysm and controlled hypotension is started
3. Hypervolemia (after the aneurysm is clipped) to prevent vasospasm

Controlled Hypotension

Controlled hypotension is required to diminish the risk of aneurysm rupture and to minimize blood loss if it accidentally ruptures. Our agent of choice is sodium nitroprusside and, if needed, deep isoflurane. If the patient develops tachycardia as a result of these agents, then β-blockers (esmolol, propranolol) can be used. Hypovolemia must be corrected before controlled hypotension is commenced. Controlled hypotension should be started slowly, since autoregulation requires a few minutes to adapt. One has to be sure that transducers are accurately calibrated and positioned at the level of the head. In patients with untreated hypertension, the autoregulation curve of cerebral blood flow is shifted to the right.

Aneurysm Rupture

Aneurysm rupture occurs during approximately one out of five aneurysm clippings. Management includes adequate volume replacement and controlled hypotension. Use of barbiturates should be considered to decrease cerebral metabolism.

Use of Temporary Clip

After the aneurysm ruptures or because of difficult exposure, it may be necessary to put a temporary clip on a major artery to isolate the aneurysm. The surgeon should tell this to the anesthesiologist, whose management of this situation includes

1. Hypertension with volume expansion, light anesthesia and, if necessary, vasopressors
2. Mannitol
3. Barbiturates
4. Normocarbia or mild hypocarbia

Anesthetic Management of Patient with Vasospasm

1. Maintain adequate blood volume.
2. Keep blood pressure slightly higher than normal.
3. Do not use controlled hypotension. When forced to do so (e.g., if the aneurysm ruptures), then controlled hypotension should be used as briefly as possible and not to the same degree as in patients without vasospasm. Barbiturates and mannitol should be given for brain protection.

Emergence

Prompt awakening is highly desirable. *Blood pressure* fluctuations should be minimized. Some patients may still have an unclipped aneurysm, and hypertension in those patients should be treated aggressively. *Focal CNS symptoms and signs* may be caused by improper placement of the clip; such patients may require immediate angiography. Postoperatively, the patient is maintained in a *hypervolemic state* with mild hypertension, especially if vasospasm exists.

ARTERIOVENOUS MALFORMATION

The presenting symptoms and signs of arteriovenous malformation (AVM) are somewhat similar to those of intracranial aneurysm. Anesthetic management is similar to that of aneurysm, with the following differences:

1. Vasospasm is not likely to happen with the AVM.
2. Resection of the AVM requires more time than the aneurysm clipping, and blood loss could be considerable.
3. After resection of the AVM, there is a concern about the *"breakthrough" phenomenon,* which is unique to the AVM. It is caused by redirection of the blood flow from the AVM into the surrounding areas of brain tissue whose vessels have lost

their autoregulation. This leads to hyperperfusion, which may cause brain edema and/or intracranial hemorrhage. To minimize the chances of this "breakthrough" phenomenon taking place, the patient's blood pressure is kept slightly below its preoperative level. Vasodilators (e.g., labetalol or nitroprusside) are used for this purpose and are continued for a few days. The patient's blood pressure is then allowed to increase slowly to its normal level. Obviously, hypertension on emergence and in the recovery room should be prevented very aggressively.

SITTING POSITION

Sitting position is used for procedures in the posterior fossa or on the cervical spine (Fig. 8.1).

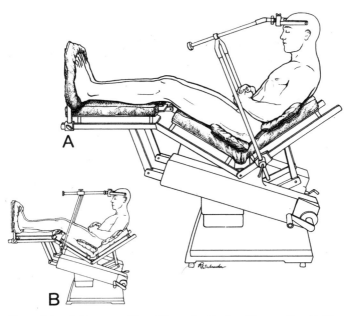

Figure 8.1.   A, Proper position of the patient in the sitting position. B, The frame position prevents lowering the patient in emergency situations. (Reproduced with permission from Martin JT. Positioning in Anesthesia and Surgery. 2nd ed. Philadelphia: WB Saunders, 1987.

Advantages

1. Good venous drainage from the surgical field leading to less venous congestion, less blood loss, and better surgical exposure
2. Easy access to the airway, face, chest, and extremities
3. Favorable respiratory compliance

Disadvantages (Table 8.1)

Hypotension

1. Causes
   a. Vasodilation secondary to the anesthetic agents
   b. Decreased venous return
   c. Myocardial depressants
2. Treatment
   a. Light anesthesia
   b. Minimal or no diuresis
   c. Liberal use of IV fluids
   d. Wrapping the lower extremities with Ace bandages
   e. Proper patient positioning
   f. Vasopressors if necessary

The patient is not only more likely to have decreased blood pressure in the sitting position but also is more vulnerable to cerebral ischemia from moderate hypotension, because the pressure perfusing the brain is less than that measured in the radial artery. The difference between the two pressures results from the vertical distance between the radial artery and the brain. To monitor the cerebral perfusion pressure accurately, the arterial pressure transducer is placed at the level of the patient's brow.

Table 8.1
Disadvantages of Sitting Position for Neurosurgery

Hypotension
Air embolism
Pneumocephalus
Quadriplegia
Endobronchial intubation
Head and neck swelling
Nerve injury

Air Embolism

Although air embolism (AE) can take place when other positions are used, the highest incidence is found in the sitting position. AE can occur when the pressure in an open vessel is subatmospheric.

1. Sources for air entry
   a. Open veins in the surgical field
   b. Holes in the scalp and skull caused by pins of the head holder
   c. Cracked or loosely connected central venous lines
2. Methods to minimize the AE
   a. Surgical vigilance
   b. Controlled ventilation
   c. High venous pressure by liberal use of IV fluids
3. Detection
   a. Precordial Doppler
   b. End-tidal CO_2: decrease
   c. End-tidal N_2: increase
   d. Pulmonary artery pressure: increase
   e. Central venous pressure: increase
   f. Frequent ABG: widened A–a DO_2, increased $PaCO_2$ in the presence of decreased ET CO_2
   g. Blood pressure changes: small AE may cause mild hypertension, but, if more air is entrained, hypotension will follow
   h. Mill-wheel murmur heard through an esophageal stethoscope indicates a large amount of intracardiac air
      i. Transesophageal echocardiography (TEE) (still not used on a large scale)
4. Treatment
   a. Discontinue the use of N_2O.
   b. Inform the surgeon.
   c. Aspirate on the CVP catheter to recover air from SVC.
   d. Apply jugular compression.
   e. Support the circulation with vasopressors if necessary.
   f. Patient may need to be put in the horizontal or left lateral decubitus position.
5. Systemic air embolism (SAE)

   Air may cross to the left side of the heart at the atrial or ventricular level and produce significant morbidity or death.

Table 8.2
Nerves at Risk for Injury in the Sitting Positions, with the Proposed Mechanism and Prevention

Nerve	Mechanism	Prevention
Ulnar	Pressure on the nerve at the elbow	Padding the elbow
Brachial plexus	Trapping the plexus between the clavicle and first rib stretching the plexus by the weight of the arm	Putting the arms in the patient's lap with some support
Sciatic	Stretching the nerve; pressure on the nerve	Padding patient's buttocks; flexion of the knees; avoid *excessive* *flexion* of the hips
Lateral, peroneal	Pressure on the nerve (below the head of the fibula) against the frame	Avoiding pressure on the nerve

The SAE risk can be minimized by preoperatively identifying patients with a patent or potentially patent foramen ovale, ASD, or VSD, by TEE. Intraoperatively, air can be visualized in the left heart by TEE.

Pneumocephalus

Due to the effect of gravity, CSF is lost through the surgical wound and is replaced by air—minimized by avoiding diuresis and marked degree of hyperventilation, and by not using N_2O.

Quadriplegia

This very rare complication is caused by extreme flexion of the cervical spine coupled with hypotension.

Endobronchial Intubation

Produced by migration of the tip of the endotracheal tube (ET) caudally when the cervical spine is flexed, endobronchial intubation is easy to prevent, detect, and correct. When the ET tube is inserted, it should be inserted about 2 cm less than usual, so that the tip will be in an ideal position when the patient is positioned with the cervical spine flexed.

Head and Neck Swelling

Produced by severe flexion of the neck and "crowding" of the pharynx with tubes and oral airway causing interference with venous and lymphatic drainage, head and neck swelling is best avoided by minimal flexion of the neck and the use of a small or shortened oral airway.

Nerve Injury (Table 8.2)

Anesthetic Management

Preoperative evaluation is the same as that for patients with increased ICP. Hydrocephalus is not uncommon in patients with infratentorial lesions. The presence of ventriculoatrial shunt is a contraindication for surgery in the sitting position. Any heart murmur should be evaluated by echocardiographic examination to detect an intracardiac shunt. Echocardiography in patients without murmurs has a high false-negative rate for diagnosing intracardiac shunt.

Special Monitors

1. Precordial Doppler
2. Continuous capnometer
3. CVP—multiple orifices, position confirmed by x-ray or ECG
4. Arterial catheter
5. PA catheter, if warranted by the patient's conditioning—a good monitoring tool for AE, but its therapeutic value for this complication is very limited
6. End-expired N_2
7. Evoked potentials (special cases)

Premedication

Premedication should not include any vasodilators.

Positioning

Figure 8.1 shows the proper position for the patient.

1. Neck not extremely flexed, with minimum of two fingers distance between the chin and chest

2. Arms in the lap, supported, and with soft cushions under the elbows
3. Cushion under the buttocks, hip joints *not excessively* flexed
4. Knees flexed, check for pressure on the peroneal nerve
5. Cushion under the feet

The operating table should be adjusted to put the knees at about the level of the heart, to improve venous return.

Anesthetic Agents

$O_2 \pm N_2O$
Inhalational agents in low concentration
Narcotics
Muscle relaxants

Ventilation is controlled. Attention should be paid to changes in cardiac rhythm and blood pressure and the surgeon should be notified.

Event	Cause
Bradycardia, usually with hypotension	Brain stem compression or vagus nerve stimulation
Tachycardia, usually with hypertension	Brain stem compression or trigeminal nerve stimulation
Extrasystoles	Brain compression

Occasionally, the surgeon may seek the anesthesiologist's help in localizing some cranial nerves (5th, 7th, 11th, 12th). If the patient is completely paralyzed, a small dose of reversal drug will be required before the cranial nerve is stimulated.

Emergence and Postoperative Period

1. Before extubation, the patient should be breathing adequately and awake enough to protect the airway. Swelling in the lips, tongue, submandibular area, or neck should raise suspicion about edema of the pharynx and larynx. The ET should be left in place until the swelling subsides.
2. Posterior fossa surgery is likely to cause nausea and vomiting.
3. Assess for possible injury to lower (7th, 9th, 10th, and 12th) cranial nerves.
4. Sequelae of air embolism (venous or systemic) may present at this stage.

Table 8.3
Glasgow Coma Scale

Eye opening	
Spontaneous	4
To speech	3
To pain	2
None	1
Verbal response	
Oriented	5
Confused conversation	4
Incomprehensible words	3
Incomprehensible sounds	2
Nil	1
Best motor response	
Obeys	6
Localizes	5
Withdraws	4
Abnormal flexion	3
Extensor	2
Nil	1

5. It is not uncommon for signs of hypervolemia to manifest on emergence. This results from return of vascular tone, change in the ventilatory pattern, and mobilization of fluids that were sequestered in the lower extremities and trunk.

HEAD INJURY

Goals of Therapy

1. Prevent hypoxia and hypercarbia
2. Protect the airway
3. Stabilize the cervical spine by avoiding flexion, rotation, or extreme extension
4. Stabilize the cardiovascular system

Possible Associated Conditions

1. A patient with head injury should be assumed to have cervical spine injury until proven otherwise.
2. 50% of patients with head injury have detectable blood alcohol.
3. Except in small children, head injury by itself does not cause hypotension. If hypotension is present in an adult patient, a

cause should be identified. The patient should be evaluated for intraabdominal or thoracic injury, bone fractures, or excessive blood loss from scalp lacerations.

4. Head injury can cause neurogenic pulmonary edema.

Patients should be evaluated for lateralizing signs and their level of consciousness graded according to the Glasgow Coma Scale (Table 8.3).

The patient may require an anesthesiologist's services for

1. Airway protection, including endotracheal intubation
2. Diagnostic procedures, such as CT scanning
3. Operative procedures for intracranial or associated injuries

Endotracheal Intubation

Endotracheal intubation is necessary if the patient's airway is obstructed or unprotected.

Use the oral route (avoid the nasal route).

Use rapid sequence intubation.

Use moderate cricoid pressure (severe pressure can displace a broken C-spine).

Have an assistant hold the head still in *moderate* extension

Muscle relaxant use is usually necessary—use a nondepolarizer if possible. (Succinylcholine is not the drug of choice, but it can be used during the immediate postinjury period if necessary).

The patient with head injury is generally in a hyperdynamic state that includes tachycardia and hypertension. One should not be overzealous in treating this hypertension, since it may be needed to maintain adequate cerebral perfusion pressure (CPP). Remember that the CPP equals mean BP minus ICP.

Once stabilized, with the airway protected and cervical spine evaluated and stabilized, the patient is usually taken for a CT scan. Head injury management will depend on the CT scan findings and the patient's condition. Craniotomy may be needed for evacuation of intracranial hematoma, elevation of depressed skull fracture, or debridement of necrotic tissue. ICP monitoring of the patient during craniotomy for head injury is similar to that of the patient with increased ICP.

Associated injuries such as bone fractures or visceral injury should be handled appropriately. Anesthetic management includes proper measures to minimize an increase in the ICP and proper fluid management for the associated injuries. Hyponatremia, hyperglycemia, and excessive decrease in serum oncotic pressure should be avoided. A patient with decreased level of consciousness preoperatively who undergo craniotomy is not expected to regain consciousness in the immediate postoperative period. This is because the patient generally has brain edema and multiple small intracranial hematomas that cannot be evacuated.

Postoperative management includes sedation, muscle relaxation, hyperventilation, head elevation, antiseizure therapy, and blood pressure control. If the patient has an ICP measuring device in place, then the ICP level is used as a guide for medical interventions. Measures to lower elevated ICP include mannitol, furosemide, and barbiturates. Use of steroids does not change the outcome in head injury patients.

TRANSSPHENOIDAL SURGERY

Pituitary tumors are accessible for resection through the transsphenoidal approach. Indications for the resection include adenomas secreting prolactin, growth hormones (GH), and adrenocorticotrophic hormone (ACTH). Nonsecreting adenomas causing pressure symptoms and signs are also resected. Preoperatively, patients are thoroughly evaluated by neurologic and endocrine studies.

Pathology

Cushing's disease	Hypertension, obesity, and diabetes mellitus
Acromegaly	Airway changes; large nose, prognathism, hypertrophied mucous membrane, cricoid narrowing, and vocal cord paralysis
	Diabetes mellitus
	Hypertension
	Cardiac; myocardial hypertrophy and fibrosis, conduction defects, and accelerated coronary artery disease

Some patients may present with panhypopituitarism, and their hormonal therapy should be included in the preoperative medication.

Anesthetic Management

Procedure is done in the supine position, with the anesthesiologist on the left side of the patient.

Airway Management

1. Consider fiberoptic intubation for acromegalic patients.
2. Use armored ETT.
3. Tube is fixed at the left side of the mouth.
4. No oral airway is inserted during the procedure.

Invasive Monitors

Invasive monitors will be dictated by the patient's condition and diagnosis. Arterial line is indicated in poor-risk patients, and in those with acromegaly or Cushing's disease. Venous air embolism is possible if the patient's head is elevated and, therefore, the use of capnometer is recommended. Episodes of hypertension during the procedure are very common. This is believed to be secondary to the surgical stimulation and the use of cocaine and epinephrine by the surgeon, for hemostasis. Because the procedure may interfere with the release of ACTH, patients are given a maintenance dose of hydrocortisone.

When the procedure is terminated and the anesthesiologist has control of the patient's airway, an oral airway is inserted so that the patient doesn't bite and occlude the endotracheal tube. Any blood in the pharynx is suctioned. Patients are extubated when they are awake enough to respond to commands. Use of narcotics in the anesthetic management and IV lidocaine at the end allows awake extubation without excessive bucking on the endotracheal tube. Postoperative care includes keeping the airway clear of blood and observing the patient for diabetes insipidus. If the latter is diagnosed, management includes pitressin and fluid replacement.

Suggested Readings

Bedford RF, Colley PS. Intracranial tumors: supratentorial and infratentorial. In: Matjaski J, Katz J, eds. Clinical Controversies in Neuroanesthesia and Neurosurgery. Orlando, FL: Grune & Stratton, 1986.

Campkin TV, Turner JM, eds. Neurosurgical Anaesthesia and Intensive Care. 2nd ed. Stoneham, MA: Butterworth, 1981.

Cottrell JE, Turndorf H, eds. Anesthesia and Neurosurgery. 2nd ed. St Louis: CV Mosby, 1986.

Cucchiara RF, Michenfelder JD, eds. Clinical Neuroanesthesia. 1st ed. New York: Churchill Livingstone, 1990.

Harvey M. Shapiro and John C. Drummond. Neurosurgical anesthesia and intracranial hypertension. Chap 54 in Miller RD, ed. Anesthesia. 3rd ed. New York: Churchill Livingston, 1990.

Horwitz NH, Rizzoli HV. Postoperative Complications of Intracranial Neurological Surgery. Baltimore: Williams & Wilkins, 1982.

Martin JT. The head-elevated positions: anesthesiologic considerations. In: Martin JT, ed. Positioning in Anesthesia and Surgery. 2nd ed. Philadelphia: WB Saunders, 1987.

Michenfelder JD. Anesthesia and the Brain. New York: Churchill Livingston, 1988.

Sperry RJ, Stirt JA, Stone DJ, eds. Manual of Neuroanesthesia. Philadelphia: BC Decker, 1989.

Walters FJM, Willatts SM. Anaesthesia and Intensive Care for the Neurosurgical Patient. Boston: Blackwell Scientific Publications, 1986.

Chapter 9

Ophthalmologic Anesthesia

Because of the delicate nature of ophthalmologic surgery, proper anesthetic management can contribute greatly to the successful outcome, just as improper management can have disastrous outcomes including loss of sight and death. Mortality rates from 0.1% to 0.015% have been reported for patients having eye surgery. The type of anesthetic provided has little effect, except in the elderly cataract patient who has had a previous myocardial infarction, in which case the myocardial reinfarction rate is lower following local anesthesia (0.3%) than following general anesthesia (6.1%) (1). There is a higher incidence of nausea and vomiting and unexpected hospital admissions after general anesthesia for outpatient cataract surgery (2). The special requirements for ophthalmologic surgery are outlined in Table 9.1.

OCULAR ANATOMY

Orbit

1. Dimensions: 40 mm wide × 35 mm high × 40–45 mm deep
2. Volume: 30 ml
3. Cone apex structures
   a. Optic foramen transmits optic nerve (CN II) and ophthalmic artery
   b. Superior orbital fissure transmits CNs III, IV, and the ophthalmic division of V

Eye (Fig. 9.1)

1. Sclera and cornea—tough protective outer layer that maintains the eye's shape

Table 9.1
Special Requirements for Ophthalmologic Surgery

Akinesia of the globe during surgery
Control of factors that reduce ocular bleeding
Avoidance or obtundation of oculocardiac reflex
Normalization of intraocular pressure (IOP)
Knowledge of anesthetic implications of ophthalmologic medications
Smooth intraoperative course and controlled emergence from general anes-
  thesia, to control IOP and maintain hemostasis
Limit N_2O with intraocular gas injection
Airway control despite proximity to operative field

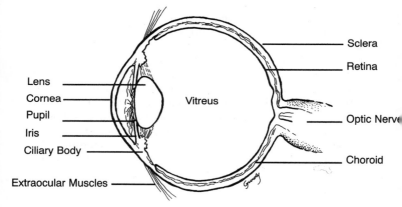

Figure 9.1. The eye with major structures.

2. Uveal tract (iris, ciliary body, and choroid)—vascular layers,
   separated from the sclera by the suprachoroidal space
   a. Iris made up of 3 sets of muscles:
      Iris dilator—sympathetically innervated
      Iris sphincter—parasympathetically innervated
      Ciliary muscle—parasympathetically innervated
   b. Ciliary body produces aqueous humor and contains the
      ciliary muscles that adjust lens curvature
3. Retina—neurosensory membrane that converts light into
   neural impulses
   a. Blood supply—the central retinal artery (an end artery)
   b. Innervation—optic nerve (CN II)

4. Vitreous—a gelatinous substance forming 4/5 of the globe
5. Lens refracts light to focus on the retina; the highly myopic patient with a long eye globe has a greater risk of eye perforation with a blocking needle

Extraocular Muscles

1. Four rectus muscles (superior, interior, medial, and lateral) anchor posteriorly into the annulus of Zinn surrounding the optic nerve
   a. Innervation of superior, inferior, and medial rectus muscles—CN III
   b. Innervation of lateral rectus muscle—CN VI
2. Superior oblique muscle innervated by trochlear nerve (CN IV)
3. Inferior oblique muscle innervated by CN III

Lacrimal System

The lacrimal system supplies tears, which are drained via the lacrimal duct into the nasal cavity below the inferior turbinate.

OCULAR PHYSIOLOGY

Intraocular Pressure (IOP)

1. Normal pressure: 15–20 mm Hg
2. Maintenance of IOP is by balance of
   a. Production of aqueous humor by the ciliary body
   b. Free circulation of aqueous humor around the iris into the anterior chamber
   c. Drainage of aqueous humor via the canal of Schlemm into the episcleral venous system
3. Complications of sudden changes in IOP include
   a. Retinal detachment
   b. Intraocular bleeding
   c. Wound dehiscence
   d. Loss of vitreal contents
4. Factors influencing IOP are listed in Table 9.2.

Oculocardiac Reflex (OCR)

1. A trigeminal-vagal reflex
   a. Afferent path—long and short ciliary nerves (CN V) to

Table 9.2
Factors Affecting Intraocular Pressure

Increase	Decrease
Endotracheal intubation*	Decreased venous pressure
Cough, strain, and bucking* (30–40 torr increase)	Decreased arterial pressure
Succinylcholine* (transient increase in IOP of 10 mm Hg lasting about 5 minutes)	Hyperventilation
Transtracheal injection	Decreased temperature (secondary to vasoconstriction causing decreased aqueous production)
Retrobulbar block	Open eye
Resistance to aqueous humor outflow	Osmotically active substances (mannitol, urea, sorbitol, dextran)
Increased choroidal volume (enlargement of lens secondary to age, intraocular tumors, edema of vitreous)	Inhalation anesthetic agents
	Intravenous barbiturates
Increased aqueous production	Benzodiazepines
Significant hypoventilation with increased PCO_2	Nondepolarizing muscle relaxants
Increased arterial blood pressure beyond the normal range of autoregulation	Actezolamide
Nitrous oxide (in the presence of intraocular gas injection)	Narcotics
Ketamine	

*Most severe

the Gasserian ganglion via the ciliary ganglion and trigeminal nerve
   b. Efferent path from the nucleus of the vagus (CN X) to the cardiac depressor nerve (2)
   c. Exhibits vagal escape and fatigues easily
2. Incidence
   a. 32–90% (more often in children because of increased parasympathetic tone)
   b. Similar for general anesthesia and local anesthesia
   c. Less common in elderly (3)
   d. Hypoxemia and hypercarbia may increase the occurrence (3, 4)
3. Manifestations
   a. Bradycardia (most common)
   b. Serious ventricular arrhythmias such as ventricular fibrillation and/or asystole (3, 4)

    c. Supraventricular arrhythmias such as multifocal atrial tachycardia and sinus arrest (3, 4)

4. Causes (4)
    a. Traction on the extraocular muscles, especially medial rectus
    b. Pressure on the globe
    c. Intraorbital hematomas or hemorrhage
    d. Ocular trauma
    e. Eye pain
    f. Retrobulbar injection (by putting pressure on the eye)
5. Treatment—see Table 9.3

IMPORTANT EFFECTS OF OPHTHALMOLOGIC DRUGS DURING ANESTHESIA

Although the eyes represent only a small portion of the total body weight, the rich vasculature and large surface area of the conjunctiva and nasolacrimal duct mucosa provide a rich absorption site for locally applied drugs.

Parasympathomimetic Drugs (Miotics)

1. Used topically to treat glaucoma by producing miosis
2. Mimic the effects of acetylcholine on parasympathetic postganglionic nerve endings
3. Categories
    a. Direct-acting agents (cholinergics)
        i. Carbachol
        ii. Pilocarpine hydrochloride
    b. Indirect-acting agents (anticholinesterases)
        i. Physostigmine sulfate: relatively short-acting
        ii. Echothiophate iodide: longer duration of action

Table 9.3
Treatment of Oculocardiac Reflex

Immediate cessation of manipulation of the eye or extraocular muscle
Hyperventilate the patient
IV atropine (0.02 mg/kg, maximum 0.6 mg) or glycopyrrolate (0.01 mg/kg, maximum 0.3 mg) for persistent bradyarrhythmia
Local lidocaine infiltration in specific eye muscles
Retrobulbar block (may also cause reflex)
Ensure patient is well-oxygenated

4. Systemic effects of miotics
   a. General effects—muscle weakness after succinylcholine, hypersalivation, sweating, nausea and vomiting, abdominal pain, urinary incontinence, diarrhea, bradycardia, severe hypotension, and bronchial spasm
   b. Central nervous system (CNS) effects—ataxia, confusion, convulsion, coma, muscular paresis; (death can result from respiratory failure)
   c. Adverse effects can occur in patients with bronchial asthma, bradycardia or hypotension.
   d. Patients who have had lacrimal surgery with lacrimal drainage tubes may have increased drug absorption
   e. Long-acting anticholinesterase miotics can significantly depress plasma cholinesterase levels. They should be discontinued 2–4 weeks before giving succinylcholine.
   f. Anticholinesterase miotics should be given carefully to patients receiving systemic anticholinesterase therapy (e.g., patients with myasthenia gravis).

Sympathomimetic Drugs (Mydriatics)

1. Ophthalmic uses
   a. To dilate the pupil to examine the fundus or to allow extraction of a cataract without damaging the iris
   b. To reduce the incidence of posterior synechiae in uveitis
   c. In open angle glaucoma, to decrease production of aqueous humor by local vasoconstrictor action

2. Categories
   a. Direct-acting (e.g., epinephrine bitartrate)
   b. Indirect-acting (e.g., phenylephrine hydrochloride)
3. Systemic effects of sympathomimetics
   a. Cardiovascular effects
      i. Tachycardia, hypertension (especially with 10% phenylephrine hydrochloride), ventricular arrhythmias, angina, myocardial infarct, cardiac arrest
      ii. Use cautiously in patients with recent infarct or cardiac arrhythmias.
      iii. Halogenated agents, such as halothane, may sensitize the heart to catecholamines, especially after repeated use of a strong ephedrine solution.

b. CNS and other effects—Subarachnoid hemorrhage and hyperhidrosis, blanching, tremor, agitation, and confusion.

c. Cyclopentolate hydrochloride (Cyclogyl), commonly used for funduscopy; can cause ataxia, hallucinations, grand mal seizures, vomiting, abdominal distention and pain, disorientation, and psychosis, especially in children and elderly patients

Anticholinergic Agents (e.g., Atropine and Scopolamine)

1. Ophthalmic uses—mydriatics and cycloplegics
2. Cardiovascular effects—tachycardia and cardiac arrhythmias
3. CNS and other effects
   a. Fever, dry mouth, flushing
   b. Confusion often seen in children
   c. Hallucination and disorientation more often with scopolamine

Adrenergic Antagonists (e.g., Timolol and Betaxolol)

1. Blockade of β-adrenergic receptors in ciliary body lowers IOP by decreasing aqueous humor secretion; may be readily absorbed systemically
2. Cardiovascular effects
   a. Bradycardia (most common), hypotension, congestive heart failure
   b. Use cautiously in patients with congestive heart failure and AV conduction disturbances
   c. Effects may be additive with other β-blocking agents or calcium channel blockers
3. CNS and other effects
   a. Fatigue, lethargy, depression, anxiety, psychosis, disassociation, confusion, and hallucinations
   b. GI side effects—anorexia, nausea, and dyspepsia
   c. Respiratory system effects—decreased forced expiratory volume in patients with COPD; bronchospasm, especially in asthmatics
   d. Hypoglycemic episodes in diabetic patients on insulin
   e. May aggravate symptoms of myasthenia gravis

Table 9.4
Factors Influencing Anesthetic Choice

Patient anesthetic preference
Type and length of procedure
Abnormalities in coagulation status
Ability of the patient to communicate and cooperate
Ability of the patient to remain immobile (lie flat) for an extended time

Hyperosmotic Agents (e.g., Glycerin, Urea, Mannitol)

1. Decrease IOP by decreasing intraocular volume through a blood-ocular osmotic gradient
2. Acute expansion of the extracellular fluid volume with large IV dose may cause cardiac decompensation in a marginal patient.

Carbonic Anhydrase Inhibitors (e.g., Acetazolamide)

1. Inhibits carbonic anhydrase, which catalyzes the formation of bicarbonate in various tissues, and decreases aqueous humor secretion and IOP
2. Systemic effects—metabolic acidosis, diuresis, drowsiness and paresthesias, hypersensitivity reactions (rare), calculus formation, and ureteral colic
3. Patients with hepatic cirrhosis may have episodes of disorientation.

TYPES OF ANESTHESIA FOR OPHTHALMOLOGIC SURGERY: GENERAL VERSUS REGIONAL

The choice of anesthetic may be influenced by factors listed in Table 9.4. The surgeon, anesthesiologist, and most especially, the patient should be comfortable with the type of anesthetic selected.

General Anesthetic for Ophthalmologic Surgery

Acceptable Induction Agents

All induction agents, with the possible exception of ketamine, decrease IOP and may be used successfully. The choice will depend on the patient's other medical conditions.

Maintenance Agents

1. Acceptable anesthetics all decrease IOP in the deeply anesthetized patient.
   a. Nitrous oxide—if sulfur hexafluoride gas (SF_6) is injected into the vitreous by the surgeon, nitrous oxide should be discontinued 15–20 minutes before gas injection
   b. Halogenated agents—enflurane, isoflurane, halothane, desflurane are acceptable
2. Neuromuscular blocking agents
   a. Nondepolarizing muscle relaxants (pancuronium, vecuronium, atracurium, and d-tubocurarine) may all be used safely.
   b. Depolarizing muscle relaxants (e.g. succinylcholine) are usually not used for general anesthesia for ophthalmology procedures, especially in penetrating eye injuries or wound dehiscence. However, in an emergency situation with a rapid sequence induction in the patient with a full stomach, succinylcholine has been used safely (5).

Complications of General Anesthesia

1. Systemic complications
   a. Mortality and morbidity rates for patients undergoing eye surgery approximate those for patients of similar health undergoing other surgical procedures. Mortality in young patients undergoing eye surgery is usually related to a congenital problem; in the elderly, it is usually due to chronic disease, (e.g., diabetes, hypertension, coronary disease).
   b. Ocular cardiac reflex (see above)
   c. Ocular gastric reflex is commonly seen after surgery on the eye muscles (e.g., strabismus surgery).
      i. Symptoms—postoperative nausea and vomiting (occasionally seen intraoperatively)
      ii. Treatment—0.075 mg/kg droperidol IV before eye muscle manipulation can reduce incidence from 85% to 10%; patients may experience increased drowsiness
2. Coughing and bucking—if these occur under a light general anesthetic, IOP will increase and may cause wound de-

hiscence and expulsion of vitreous humor in the penetrated eye injury; choroidal vascular bleeding may occur in the hypertensive patient with an open eye; smooth induction, smooth maintenance, and smooth emergence help maintain a good IOP

Regional Anesthesia for Ophthalmologic Surgery

In elderly patients with multiple concurrent medical problems that may pose an increased risk for general anesthesia, local anesthesia with either peribulbar or retrobulbar blocks may be preferable, although most studies comparing general anesthesia and monitored anesthesia care (MAC) find no statistical increase in relative risks. For pediatric patients, most procedures are performed under general anesthesia.

Monitoring, Positioning, and Other Considerations

1. Monitors—Blood pressure cuff, pulse oximeter, monitor for ventilation (precordial stethoscope or end-tidal CO_2 monitor), ECG
2. Positive pressure ventilation and full resuscitative equipment should be available.
3. Support the surgical drapes above patient's nose and mouth.
4. Oxygen should be provided with or without air admixture via face shield at rapid flow (8 liters/min) to prevent CO_2 buildup under drapes (2).
5. Careful positioning of patient, with special attention to arthritic backs, hips, and knees, to prevent uncomfortable fidgeting during surgery

Intravenous Sedation

Titrate carefully to decrease the stress of the eye block. Oversedation may cause airway obstruction and hypoventilation

Drugs commonly used include

Midazolam (0.5–2.0 mg)
Fentanyl (25–50 μg)
Thiopental (25–75 mg)
Methohexital (10–30 mg)
Propofol (10–30 mg)

Techniques for Local Anesthesia for the Eye

1. Local anesthetics
   a. 0.75% bupivacaine (plain) with or without 0.1–1.0 ml hyaluronidase (150 USP/ml) added to 10 ml to facilitate anesthetic diffusion
   b. 1–2% lidocaine with or without 1:100,000 epinephrine added to the bupivacaine mixture to shorten onset time
   c. 9:1 BSS/1% lidocaine mixture injected in the skin with a 0.5-inch 27–30 gauge needle at the site of blocking needle entry
   d. Local anesthetic eye drops (proparacaine) to anesthetize the conjunctiva for transconjunctival blocks through the retracted lower lid in lieu of blocks through the exterior lid
2. Needles—"blunted" type 22–25 gauge, 1.25 inch (31 mm) or less in length used to avoid penetration of globe, optic nerve, or optic foramen
3. Retrobulbar block (RB) technique (see Fig. 9.2)
   a. Fingertip on external lid under the globe to elevate it out of advancing needle path

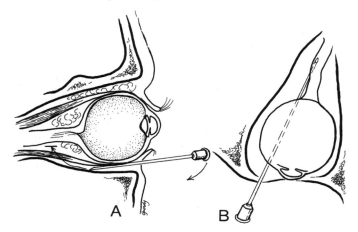

Figure 9.2. Retrobulbar block, showing the needle motion and position in (A) horizontal view and (B) superior view. (*Note:* Final needle position is below the optic nerve.)

Table 9.5
Complications of Retrobulbar Blockade

Contralateral amaurosis
Cardiac arrest
Ophthalmic artery laceration and retrobulbar hemorrhage
Brainstem anesthesia
Puncture of the globe causing retinal detachment, vitreous hemorrhage, and possible intraocular injection
Oculorcardiac reflex stimulation
Needle penetration of the optic nerve
Optic neuritis and/or atrophy
Occlusion of the central retinal artery
Toxic CNS and cardiovascular effects of intravascular injection of local anesthetic

   b. Needle insertion at junction of lateral and middle thirds of external lower lid at orbital rim
   c. Needle advancement, parallel to orbital floor, medially toward optic foramen (watch eye for motion suggesting globe perforation)
   d. Needle placement—after the equator of the eye is passed, the needle tip is directed slightly superiorly to enter muscle cone
   e. Local anesthetic injection—aspirate, inject 2–3 ml slowly to avoid sudden increase in intraorbital pressure (6)
   f. Firm digital pressure or pressure applied with a Honan balloon to help distribute the anesthetic solution and lower IOP (3)
4. Complications specific for RB anesthesia (Table 9.5)
5. Peribulbar block technique (see Fig. 9.3)
   a. Needle insertion and finger position (see "3a" and "3b")
   b. Needle advancement—with bevel facing the globe, the needle is advanced along the bony orbital floor in a position further from the globe, more laterally and less superiorly than with RB; deposit 2–3 ml of anesthetic at or anterior to the globe equator
   c. Needle placement—outside and slightly lateral to muscle cone
   d. Local anesthetic injection—aspirate, inject 4–7 ml of local anesthetic slowly until the superior lid fold disappears

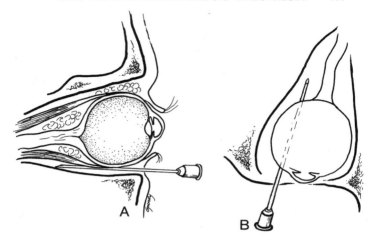

Figure 9.3. Peribulbar block, showing final needle position in (A) horizontal view and (B) superior view.

    e. Apply light digital pressure or pressure with Honan balloon
    f. Superior and medial rectus block—deposit 1–2 ml of local anesthetic at the eye equator from the orbital rim between the supraorbital notch and trochlea, parallel to orbital roof (7)
    g. Glaucoma patients—deposit anesthetic in graded doses of 2–3 ml to avoid increasing the IOP
    h. Peribulbar block advantages and disadvantages in Table 9.6

Complications of Regional Anesthesia

1. Globe perforation—immediate ocular pain and restlessness follow; hypotony, retrobulbar hemorrhage, or vitreous hemorrhage with poor red reflex may be seen
2. Retrobulbar hemorrhage, the most common complication, may occur in up to 1–2% of retrobulbar injections. Signs of retrobulbar hemorrhage include increasing proptosis and/or chemosis with possible subconjunctival blood (if anterior extension of the hemorrhage occurs). The OCR may be stimulated. External pressure of the hemorrhage on the globe may elevate IOP.

Table 9.6
Peribulbar Block

Advantages	Disadvantages
Extraocular muscles avoided	Chemosis with subconjunctival hemorrhage may occur
Sclera avoided	Orbit compression device essential
Optic nerve contact avoided	Higher supplementation rate
Visual acuity often preserved	Slower onset
Dural sheaths and optic foramen avoided	Larger volume of local anesthetic required
Less pain on injection	
Superior orbicularis akinesia	

3. Optic atrophy and retinal vascular occlusion
   Optic atrophy with permanent loss of vision may occur because of retrobulbar hemorrhage, direct nerve injury from intraneural injection or compression from intraneural sheath hemorrhage, or after a seemingly uneventful retrobulbar block.
4. Allergic reactions
5. Systemic toxicity of local anesthetics usually results from either accidental intravascular injection or administration of an excessive dose.
6. Brainstem anesthesia is believed to be caused by penetration of the optic nerve sheath with direct injection of the local anesthetic into the subdural or subarachnoid space. Symptoms usually appear between 2 and 10 minutes after injection and progress to a maximum over a 10-minute interval (3). Symptoms suggesting central spread of local anesthetic include mental confusion or unconsciousness, convulsive shivering, nausea or vomiting, hypotension, bradycardia, respiratory depression, paresis of the contralateral eye, and cardiac arrest (8). Full cardiopulmonary resuscitation equipment should be readily available wherever these blocks are performed. Treatment of this complication involves the respiratory and cardiac support usual in any resuscitation. Total recovery usually occurs in 20–60 minutes.

POSTOPERATIVE CARE OF THE OPHTHALMOLOGIC PATIENT

1. Avoid accidental pressure on the operated eye during recovery from anesthesia.

2. Appropriately treat the causes of restlessness, such as hypoxia, hypercarbia, pain, bladder distension, or delirium from perioperative medications.
3. Ophthalmic patients who have had surgery on their *only functioning* eye may become anxious or may hallucinate because of lack of visual orientation. Give frequent verbal reassurance and orientation and assistance in the bathroom, etc.

PEDIATRIC OPHTHALMOLOGIC PATIENT

The pediatric patient may present for ophthalmologic surgery for many reasons ranging from eye-muscle surgery, examination under anesthesia, chalazion removal, corneal transplants, and traumatic injury, including an open eye.

Anesthetic Plan for Pediatric Open Eye

1. Regional anesthesia usually contraindicated
   a. Poorly tolerated by younger patients
   b. Local anesthesia volume in smaller orbit may increase IOP
2. General anesthesia techniques in the pediatric patient
   a. Avoid crying and increased IOP in open eye.
      i. Gentle inhalation induction with parents present to avoid trauma of separation
      ii. Rectal methohexital (20–30 mg/kg) for sedation
      iii. Intranasal midazolam may be used for premedication (4)
   b. Minimize positive pressure ventilation.
   c. Avoid pressure of mask on open globe (4).
   d. Intravenous lidocaine (1.5 mg/kg) on induction and before extubation will decrease airway reactivity.
   e. Avoid dramatic increases in IOP produced by coughing and bucking.

Oculocardiac Reflex

The incidence of OCR has been studied most frequently during strabismus surgery. An incidence of 90% is reported in infants and children without prophylactic administration of an anticholinergic drug such as atropine or glycopyrrolate. Manipulation of the medial rectus may produce the highest frequency of

OCR; however, it is also the extraocular muscle most often manipulated during strabismus surgery. Many pediatric anesthesiologists advocate giving prophylactic intravenous atropine or glycopyrrolate immediately before induction of anesthesia.

GERIATRIC OPHTHALMOLOGIC PATIENT

Physiology of Aging and Anesthetic Considerations

Evidence suggests that elderly patients have an improved prognosis if their surgical procedure is performed with local rather than general anesthesia or major regional anesthesia (9). The most common surgical procedure on the elderly patient is cataract removal. With trends away from inpatient hospitalization toward ambulatory care, more elderly patients with severe systemic disease will be undergoing these surgeries on an outpatient basis. Table 9.7 lists some physiologic changes of aging that affect drug pharmacokinetics. These changes prolong the half-life of lipid-soluble drugs because of slower metabolism and excretion.

Preoperative Preparation

1. Medication history—types of medication can give indication of presence of systemic disease
   a. Hypertensive patients on diuretics may have serious hypokalemia.
   b. If given on the day of surgery, diuretics may cause an uncomfortably full bladder in the patient for regional anesthesia.

Table 9.7
Physiologic Changes of Age Affecting Drug Pharmacokinetics

Decreased liver drug metabolism
Decreased renal clearance of drugs
Decreased cardiac output and cardiac index
Decreased pulmonary function because of diminished vital capacity and decreased maximal breathing capacity
Body composition changes including decreased total body water, decreased lean body mass, and increased fat
Increased drug effect caused by decreased plasma protein binding of drugs
Decreased physiologic function of the CNS, producing a higher incidence of dementia

c. Continue β-blocking drugs, calcium channel blockers, and ACE inhibitors.

d. Patients with uncontrolled hypertension may have decreased blood volume causing severe hypotension on induction of general anesthesia.

e. For patients on cardiac and pulmonary medications see chapter on preoperative evaluation.

2. Physical examination—cardiac, pulmonary, and airway examination

3. Objective tests

   a. ECG less than 1 year old (sooner if patient has had symptoms suggesting a cardiac event)

   b. Potassium levels, especially in patients on diuretics or digoxin

   c. Glucose level

   d. Hemoglobin and/or hematocrit

4. Ensure that patients know what to expect and what is expected of them (e.g., procedure for local or general anesthesia, NPO, medication regimen)

5. Ensure that elderly outpatients have a physically and mentally competent adult available to stay with them for the 24-hour postoperative period, in case help is needed.

Choice of Anesthesia

General Anesthesia

Factors in the selection of general anesthesia in the elderly eye patient include increased risk of morbidity and possibly mortality, more frequent unanticipated hospital admission, increased chance of postoperative nausea and vomiting, long-lasting disorientation and dementia caused by slower drug metabolism, increased risk for aspiration because of decreased tracheal reflexes, increased risk of hypoxia during recovery, and increased risk for problems during intubation such as fragile dental work and arthritic changes in the airway and neck.

Regional Anesthesia

Factors in the consideration for regional anesthesia in these patients include the severity of coexisting pulmonary and cardiac disease, the mental capacity and ability of the patient to hear and follow instructions and to lie immobile during the procedure, disorientation after sedation because of lack of visual orientation under the surgical drapes, problems maintaining ventilation under the surgical drapes if oversedation occurs, and claustrophobia caused by drapes too close to nose and mouth.

Recovery

1. Determine adequacy of ventilation and oxygenation and give supplemental oxygen as needed.
2. Orient patients frequently to their environment.
3. Restless patients should be checked for hypoxia, full bladder, etc. before sedatives and narcotics are given.
4. Ensure that the elderly outpatient and family have and understand written postoperative instructions before discharge.
5. Return these patients as soon as is safely possible to their own familiar environment (9).

ANESTHETIC MANAGEMENT OF SPECIFIC OPHTHALMOLOGIC PROCEDURES

Emergency "Open Eye–Full Stomach" Patient

This situation presents the anesthesiologist with the dilemma of possible extrusion of ocular contents versus the risk of aspiration. If time permits H_2 receptor antagonists can be given to increase gastric fluid pH and reduce gastric acid production and metaclopromide may be given to increase gastric emptying.

Rapid Sequence Induction

Pretreat the patient with a nondepolarizing muscle relaxant (e.g., *d*-tubocurarine 0.06 mg/kg), then induce with thiopental (4 mg/kg) or other suitable induction agent. With this management, succinylcholine produces only small increases in IOP and there have been no reports of loss of intraocular contents (10).

Strabismus Surgery

Strabismus surgery is the most common pediatric ocular operation in the United States. Factors to consider in the care of these patients are an increased risk of malignant hyperpyrexia and a high incidence of nausea and vomiting, which may delay discharge and cause postoperative dehydration—75 μg/kg of droperidol given IV on induction, retrobulbar anesthesia, and/ or 0.15 mg/kg metaclopromide on arrival in the PACU help to decrease the incidence of this complication (4).

Intraocular Surgery

1. Strict control of IOP is mandatory (see Table 9.2).
2. Maximal pupillary dilation is essential to prevent damage to the iris.

Retinal Detachment Surgery

An anesthetic consideration in retinal detachment surgery is intravitreal air or sulfur hexafluoride (SF_6) injection. These substances together with nitrous oxide can cause a dramatic increase in IOP, reaching a peak within 20 minutes. The recommendation is to stop nitrous oxide administration 15 minutes before intravitreous gas injection.

Note: Subsequent anesthetics should avoid nitrous oxide for 5 days following air injection and 10 days following SF_6 injection (10).

References

1. Backer CL, Tinker JH, Robertson DM. Myocardial reinfarction following local anesthesia for ophthalmic surgery. Anesth Analg 1980;59:257–262.
2. Zahl K. Preoperative evaluation and choice of anesthesia for ophthalmic surgery. In: Zahl K, Meltzer MA, eds. Regional Anesthesia for Intraocular Surgery: Ophthalmology Clinics of North America. Philadelphia: WB Saunders, 1990:1–11.
3. Feitl ME, Krupin T. Retrobulbar anesthesia. In: Zahl K, Meltzer MA, eds. Regional Anesthesia for Intraocular Surgery: Ophthalmology Clinics of North America. Philadelphia: WB Saunders, 1990:83–91.
4. Larson CE. Anesthesia for pediatric ophthalmic surgery. In: Zahl K, Meltzer MA, eds. Regional Anesthesia for Intraocular Surgery: Ophthalmology Clinics of North America. Philadelphia: WB Saunders, 1990:57–69.
5. Libonati MM, Leahy JJ, Ellison N. The use of succinylcholine in open eye surgery. Anesthesiology 1985;62:637.
6. Galindo A, Keilson LR, Mondshine RB, Sawelson HI. Retro-peribulbar anesthesia. In: Zahl K, Meltzer MA, eds. Regional Anesthesia for Intraocular Surgery: Ophthalmology Clinics of North America. Philadelphia: WB Saunders, 1990:83–91

7. Davis DB, Mandel MR. Peribulbar anesthesia: a review of technique and complications. In: Zahl K, Meltzer MA, eds. Regional Anesthesia for Intraocular Surgery: Ophthalmology Clinics of North America. Philadelphia: WB Saunders, 1990:101–110.

8. Hamilton RC, Gimbel HV, Javitt JC. The prevention of complications of regional anesthesia for ophthalmology. In: Zahl K, Meltzer MA, eds. Regional Anesthesia for Intraocular Surgery: Ophthalmology Clinics of North America. Philadelphia: WB Saunders, 1990:111–125

9. McLeskey CH. Anesthesia for the geriatric patient. In: Barash PG, Cullen BF, Stoelting RK, eds. Clinical Anesthesia. Philadelphia, JB Lippincott, 1992:1353.

10. McGoldrick KE. Anesthesia and the eye. In: Barash PG, Cullen BF, Stoelting RK, eds. Clinical Anesthesia. Philadelphia: JB Lippincott, 1992:1095.

Chapter 10

Anesthetic Considerations for Ear, Nose, and Throat Procedures

The administration of anesthetics for ENT procedures presents the anesthesiologist with a unique group of challenges and requirements. Frequently, the patient's airway is either inaccessible or shared with the surgeon. This makes particular attention to airway monitoring and close communication with the surgeon mandatory. Preoperative evaluation of airway pathology is especially important in planning anesthetic management of these cases. A knowledge of airway anatomy, including both motor and sensory innervation is important for a safe and successful anesthetic outcome. Patients of all ages have ENT procedures and they may be compromised by chronic medical conditions or hypovolemia. ENT procedures are usually elective but can be emergent and require not only skillful but expeditious management. Finally, the use of lasers and unconventional forms of ventilation places anesthesia for ENT procedures at the forefront of medical technology.

AIRWAY ANATOMY

Nose

1. Formed by ethmoid, vomer, and maxillary bones; cartilage; and fatty tissue
2. Nasal cavity divided by cartilaginous septum, opens anteriorly via nares and posteriorly via choanae, and contains three turbinates projecting from the lateral aspect of the eth-

moid over openings for paranasal sinuses and nasolacrimal duct

3. Sensory innervation via anterior ethmoidal nerve of ophthalmic division and branches of the maxillary division of V (which can be blocked to prepare for nasal intubation)

Oral Cavity

1. Bounded anteriorly by the lips and posteriorly by the palatal arches and tonsils
2. Contains gums, teeth, and tongue
3. Tongue and tonsils are very important; they are highly vascular and can cause airway obstruction
4. **Sensory supply** to the tongue originates from four nerves:
   a. Lingual nerve—anterior two thirds of the tongue
   b. Glossopharyngeal nerve (IX)—posterior one third of the tongue
   c. Superior laryngeal nerve—base of the tongue
   d. Chorda tympani nerve (branch of VIII)—taste to anterior two thirds of the tongue

5. **Motor supply** to tongue comes from hypoglossal nerve (XII)

Pharynx

The pharynx is the area posterior to the palatal folds and choanae, and superior to the glottis and larynx. Its walls are formed by striated muscles (the superior, middle, and inferior constrictors) as well as soft tissue. The pharyngeal muscles propel food toward the esophagus and prevent regurgitation into the larynx and trachea. The motor and sensory supply of the pharynx arises from the glossopharyngeal nerve (IX) and the vagus nerve (X).

Divisions:

1. **Nasopharynx**—area posterior to choanae and superior to soft palate; contains nasopharyngeal tonsils and openings of eustachian tubes below inferior turbinates (may give rise to complications with nasal intubation).
2. **Oropharynx**—area inferior to soft palate, posterior to tongue and superior to epiglottis; anterior portion contains tonsils, tonsillar pillars; walls of oropharynx are nonrigid and

may collapse under negative pressure, causing airway obstruction.

3. **Hypopharynx**—area lateral and inferior to epiglottis, extending from superior tip of epiglottis to the inferior edge of cricoid cartilage. This includes recesses lateral to the larynx: the pyriform sinuses. Sensory innervation of this area is from internal laryngeal branch of vagus nerve (X).

Larynx

The larynx controls access to the trachea and is responsible for phonation. It is suspended from the hyoid bone, which in turn is suspended from structures higher in the neck by muscles and the stylohyoid ligament. The larynx moves superiorly during swallowing, causing the epiglottis to oppose the tongue and soft tissue of the oropharynx, preventing aspiration. Closure of the glottis is a reflex, via intrinsic adductor muscles. Laryngospasm occurs when closure persists beyond the initiating stimulus and may be caused by mucus, blood, or other foreign matter irritating the vocal cords or by airway manipulation under insufficient anesthesia.

Treatment:

1. Head in "sniff position"
2. Jaw thrust
3. Positive pressure by face mask with 100% O_2

If the above is ineffective, use reintubation facilitated with rapidly acting muscle relaxant.

Cartilages of the Larynx

(See Figs. 10.1–10.3.)

1. **Epiglottis:** Leaf-shaped, connected inferiorly to the hyoid bone and to the base of the tongue by the glossoepiglottic folds. Recesses between the folds are called valleculae. Placement of laryngoscope blade in this location and extension of neck will usually expose glottis for intubation.
2. **Thyroid cartilage:** Two plates of cartilage fused to form a shield-like structure. Posteriorly, the thyroid cartilage has projections or "horns" both superiorly and inferiorly.
3. **Cricoid cartilage:** This is circular "signet ring" shape, sits immediately inferior to the thyroid cartilage, and is suspended

from it by the cricothyroid membrane. This is an easily identified area for rapid surgical access to the airway. Its inferior border is at C-6. Anterior pressure on the cricoid occludes the esophagus—"Sellick's maneuver."

4. **Arytenoid cartilages (2):** Pyramidal, situated on the posterior aspect of the cricoid cartilages, serve as posterior attachments for the vocal cords; folds of tissue above the vocal cords between the thyroid and arytenoid, known as "false" vocal cords.

5. **Corniculate cartilages (2):** Smaller cartilages that rest on the arytenoids.

6. **Cuneiform cartilages (2):** Small cartilages embedded in the aryepiglottic folds which may assist in recoil of adducted cartilages.

Muscles of Larynx

Intrinsic Group

The intrinsic muscles have origins and insertions within the larynx and are striated and voluntary. All except the cricothyroid are innervated by the **recurrent laryngeal nerve.**

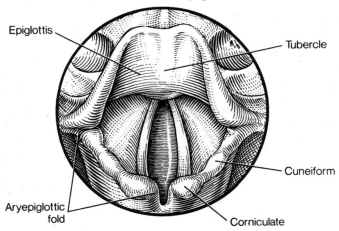

Epiglottis

Tubercle

Cuneiform

Aryepiglottic fold

Corniculate

Figure 10.1. Glottic opening as viewed via direct laryngoscopy. (Reprinted from Finucane BT, Santora AH, eds. Principles of Airway Management. Philadelphia: FA Davis, with permission.)

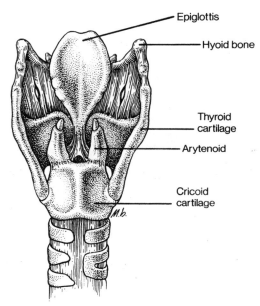

Figure 10.2. Larynx, posterior view. (Reprinted from Finucane BT, Santora AH, eds. Principles of Airway Management. Philadelphia: FA Davis, with permission.)

Posterior cricoarytenoids (2)—abduct vocal folds.
Lateral cricoarytenoids (2)—abduct vocal folds.
Transverse and oblique arytenoid (2 each) adduct vocal folds.
Aryepiglottic (2)—adduct vocal folds.
Thyroarytenoids (2)—relaxes vocal folds.
Vocalis (2)—alter vocal folds during speech.
Cricothyroid—lengthens, tenses, adducts vocal folds.

Extrinsic Group

Extrinsic muscles originate outside of the larynx, cause the larynx to move up and down in the neck, and alter the shape of the aryepiglottic folds. They are further subdivided into two groups:

The *suprahyoid group* originates on the tongue, mandible,

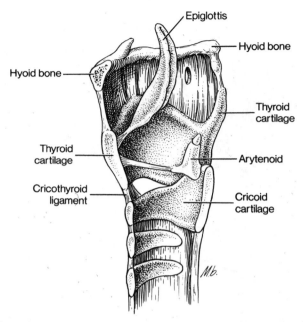

Figure 10.3. Larynx, sagittal section. (Reprinted from Finucane BT, Santora AH, eds. Principles of Airway Management. Philadelphia: FA Davis, with permission.)

and styloid process and inserts on the hyoid. This includes the digastrics, myohyoids, stylohyoids, and geniohyoids.

The *infrahyoid group* originates on the hyoid and inserts on various laryngeal structures. They generally lower the larynx. They consist of sternohyoids, sternothyroid, thyrohyoid, and omohoid.

Sensory Innervation of the Larynx

1. Internal branch of the superior laryngeal nerve—a branch of the vagus nerve (X)
   a. Supplies sensation to the mucous membrane of the larynx, hypopharynx and base of the tongue.

  b. May be blocked at two points with local anesthetics:
     i. Exteriorly at point between the lateral tip of hyoid and superior cornu of the thyroid.
     ii. From inside the pharynx in the pyriform fossae using pledgets and curved Krause forceps.
2. Recurrent laryngeal nerve—also a branch of the vagus—supplies sensation to the mucous membranes of the larynx, *below* the vocal cords.
3. The motor supply of the larynx is derived from the recurrent laryngeal nerve *except* for the tensor of the vocal cords, the cricothyroid muscle, which is supplied by the external laryngeal branch of the superior laryngeal nerve.

LASERS AND ENT PROCEDURES

Lasers are being used more frequently in the operating room, and their use in ENT procedures is common.

Laser Characteristics

Laser characteristics are generally determined by the lasing medium used, i.e., gas (CO_2), liquid, or crystalline solid (Nd-YAG).

1. CO_2 Laser
   a. Most commonly used.
   b. Beam is infrared and invisible.
   c. Highly absorbed by water-containing tissues.
   d. Beam energy is almost completely absorbed in the first 200 μm of the tissue surface.
   e. Usually used in continuous (as opposed to pulsed) mode.
   f. Cannot be transmitted down a fiberoptic bundle.
   g. Used to excise airway tumors including carcinomas, cysts, hemangiomas, and papillomas.
2. Nd-YAG (neodymium-yttrium-aluminum-garnet) lasers
   a. Beam is invisible.
   b. Usually used in pulsed mode.
   c. May be transmitted down fiberoptic bundle.
   d. Beam is strongly absorbed by pigmented lesions—depth of penetration may be somewhat unpredictable. Late tissue effects may not be seen for days.
   e. Usually used to remove pigmented lesions and larger airway tumors.

Safety Precautions

Safety precautions are aimed at avoiding airway fires, which may occur in up to 1.5% of laser airway cases.

1. Use the lowest possible FIO_2.
2. Use no N_2O (supports combustion); volatile agents are all right.
3. O_2/air may be mixed with helium—retards combustion and may improve conditions.
4. All currently available ET tubes are reported to ignite under certain conditions.
   a. "Red rubber" tubes ignite at low FIO_2.
   b. Polyvinyl chloride tubes release hydrochloric acid when ignited.
   c. Wrapping the tube with metallic tape is helpful, but tapes can also ignite, and edges on tape can cause trauma (recommended tapes: 3M #425 or Venturi copper foil).
   d. Use ET tubes specifically designed for laser surgery—stainless steel Mallinckrodt Laser Flex tube for CO_2 laser. Others have been shown to be combustible.
   e. Fill cuffs of tube with sterile saline, pack pharynx with saline-soaked gauze.

Airway Fire

Should an airway fire occur:

1. All anesthetic gases, including oxygen, should be discontinued.
2. The endotracheal tube should be removed. An extra breathing circuit should be available because the original may be damaged.
3. Syringes of saline should be available to extinguish flames.
4. Ventilate patient by mask, using 100% O_2, until reintubation or surgical control of airway is achieved.
5. Airway should be carefully evaluated for trauma or debris using endoscopy as necessary.
6. Surgery may proceed if burns are minor. Otherwise, prolonged mechanical ventilation may be necessary.

Other Precautions

1. Warning signs indicating laser use should be placed at the entrances to the OR.
2. All OR personnel should have appropriate eye protection. Plastic lenses are all right for CO_2 laser. Other lasers require specific types of lenses. Glasses should have side shields. The patient's eyes may be protected with saline-soaked sponges and/or appropriate lenses.
3. Instruments in the laser field should be nonreflective.
4. Most OR drapes are flammable. Areas adjacent to the fields may be draped with moist towels.
5. Adequate room ventilation is necessary. Carbon monoxide can be produced by tumor combustion.
6. A fire extinguisher should be available in the OR suite.

Airway Techniques Not Involving Conventional ET Tubes

Airway techniques not involving conventional ET tubes are preferred by some practitioners.

Advantages

a. Improved visualization
b. Lower incidence of airway fires

Commonly Used Techniques

Spontaneous ventilation with insufflation is usually done via nasal catheters using N_2O, O_2, and an inhalational agent. Problems include difficulty adjusting depth of anesthesia, inadequate scavenging of waste gases, movement of vocal cords, and lungs unprotected from blood, mucus, and secretions.

Venturi jet ventilation, first described by Sanders in 1967, can be performed via a catheter connected to 50 psi O_2 source and bronchoscope/laryngoscope. Because of air entrainment, O_2 is used as the high-flow gas to ensure an adequate FIO_2. The surgeon can control the timing of the jet to minimize movement of the operative field. Anesthesia is maintained with IV agents. Problems include pneumothorax, pneumomediastinum, gastric distension if jet improperly aimed (kids at particular risk), postprocedure laryngospasm, and desiccation of tissues from high flow of dry gases.

MAJOR HEAD AND NECK SURGERY

Major head and neck surgery for resection of neoplasms includes laryngectomy, radical neck dissection, glossectomy, pharyngectomy, and hemimandibulectomy, all with possible tracheostomy.

Preoperative Evaluation

1. Determine plan for establishing the airway initially and maintaining it postoperatively. These patients usually have some airway compromise secondary to tumor, edema, inflammation, or fibrosis from radiation.
2. In addition to thorough airway examination, head and neck CT scans, chest x-ray (CXR), and surgeon's indirect laryngoscopic examination may be helpful.
3. Head and neck tumors frequently occur in patients with history of tobacco or ethanol abuse.
4. Coexisting medical conditions such as hypertension, diabetes, and coronary disease should be thoroughly evaluated and optimized.
5. Possibility of awake control of airway should be discussed with the patient, if appropriate.
6. Preoperative sedation should be minimal (diphenhydramine 25–50 mg p.o. and/or glycopyrrolate 0.2–0.4 mg IM) if fiberoptic intubation is planned. Supplemental oxygen should be provided for transport and before induction.

Monitoring

Preoperative findings help determine whether specialized monitoring is required. CVP or pulmonary artery catheter may be indicated by the patient's physical status. Internal jugular access may be limited during neck procedures, and antecubital or subclavian sites should be used. A CXR should be checked for pneumothorax before induction if the subclavian approach is used. Arterial line should be used in patients with compromised cardiovascular status or when repeated blood gas, glucose, or hematocrit sampling is necessary. Lines should be placed before induction because access to many sites may be limited by surgical positioning. Processed EEG monitoring may be appropriate if carotid artery resection is contemplated.

Induction of Anesthesia and Maintenance of Airway

1. Frequently, the safest way to secure the airway is awake intubation with the patient breathing spontaneously.
   a. Fiberoptic laryngoscopy (oral or nasal)
   b. Blind nasal intubation may be traumatic and cause hemorrhage if tumor is friable.
2. Awake tracheostomy may be preferable in patients with large laryngeal tumors or pharyngeal masses.
3. Anesthesia may be maintained with a balanced technique—narcotics, N_2O, inhalational agents, and muscle relaxants. Halogenated agents may be useful because they produce bronchodilation and muscle relaxation.
4. Controlled hypotension can be used in some patients to reduce blood loss but should be avoided with coronary or cerebral vascular disease.

Intraoperative Management

1. Access to the airway may be limited by the surgical positioning, so airway patency (breath sounds, chest rise, CO_2 wave form, tidal volume, peak inspiratory pressure) must be carefully monitored. An armored ET tube may help prevent kinks.
2. Blood loss may be significant and difficult to quantitate (hidden in drapes, pooled in pharynx, etc.)
3. Sudden hemodynamic changes may be produced by hypovolemia, air embolus secondary to open neck veins (consider slight head-down position, discontinuation of N_2O), and bradycardia or sinus arrest secondary to carotid sinus manipulation. Treatment for carotid-induced bradycardia includes
   a. Informing the surgeon and asking to stop manipulation,
   b. Infiltrating the carotid sinus with local anesthetic, or
   c. Administering atropine 0.2–0.4 mg IV (adult) or pressor as indicated.
4. Radical neck dissection can lead to prolonged QT interval, malignant tachyarrythmias (torsade des pointes), or cardiac arrest. Therapy includes restoring ventricular rate with atropine or isoproterenol, cardiac pacing, or CPR if necessary. Avoid hypokalemia—it may worsen QT prolongation. Prolonged QT may be ameliorated by left stellate ganglion block.

Emergence and Postoperative Considerations

After resection, the surgeon and anesthesiologist should plan postoperative airway protection.

1. If a tracheostomy is performed, the edge of the tracheal stoma should be secured with sutures, and ET tube changed to a cuffed tracheal tube to permit positive pressure ventilation. The pharynx and trachea superior to the tracheal site should be suctioned before changing the tube.
2. If the trachea has been left intact, the patient may be extubated using the usual criteria. If the original intubation was difficult, the patient should be fully awake before extubation. Glottic edema may worsen for several days postoperatively, and postoperative intubation may be prudent in this situation. After procedures involving significant recurrent laryngeal nerve manipulation, vocal cord function may have to be evaluated. Patients with compromised pulmonary function secondary to COPD may also require postoperative ventilation.
3. Postoperative considerations should focus on the possibility of airway compromise.
   a. patients with a fresh tracheostomy should be admitted to ICU.
   b. Postoperative CXR should be checked for tube placement, lung expansion, pneumothorax.
   c. 15dg head-up position helps to decrease edema.
   d. Supplemental O_2, narcotics, and gentle suctioning are valuable if used judiciously.
   e. Topical, aerosolized, or IV lidocaine 1.5 mg/kg may be helpful in treating coughing in patients with new tracheostomies.
   f. Postoperative hypertension may be a problem secondary to carotid sinus receptor denervation, pain, or anxiety. It may resolve in 24 hours or require therapy with vasodilators. β-Blockers should be used cautiously in the presence of bronchospastic airway disease.

TRACHEOSTOMY

Tracheostomy is usually performed electively for patients who require long-term airway protection and/or ventilatory assistance. Elective tracheostomy should not be performed on hemodynamically unstable patients or those requiring high PEEP. Indications for emergency tracheostomy are limited.

General Anesthesia

Awake intubation with topicalization of the airway is the safest way to secure the airway before induction of anesthesia. In some situations, a mask induction with inhalational agents can be performed. Muscle relaxants should be used with extreme caution in patients with compromised airways. Some practitioners prefer to have the patient breathe spontaneously with high FIO_2 during the procedure. Inhalational agents can be used for amnesia and analgesia. The ET tube cuff should be deflated before the surgeon enters the trachea, to avoid cuff rupture. An anesthesia circuit is passed over the drapes to attach to the tracheostomy tube, and breath sounds are verified by auscultation and end-tidal CO_2.

Awake Tracheostomy

Awake tracheostomy can be performed under local anesthesia (local infiltration with 1% lidocaine by surgeon) in patients breathing spontaneously with a natural airway or those already intubated.

1. Give 100% O_2 by face mask, reassure patient, monitor vital signs, manually assist ventilation (if necessary).
2. Patient should be warned about coughing and loss of speaking ability as the trachea is entered.
3. After establishing an adequate airway by the tracheostomy, there may be cardiovascular collapse from rapid reversal of sympathetic stimulation produced from prior hypoxia, hypercarbia, and anxiety.
4. Postoperative care is as per major head and neck surgery.

Complications

1. Immediate
   a. Pneumothorax
   b. Subcutaneous emphysema
   c. Mucous plug
   d. Tube displacement
   e. Hemorrhage

2. Long-term
   a. Infection
   b. Tracheomalacia
   c. Tracheal stenosis

EAR SURGERY—GENERAL ANESTHESIA

There is wide variation in the complexity of procedures, ranging from myringotomy and PE tubes to microsurgical hearing restoration and tumor resection. Brief procedures may be performed in adults under local anesthesia (topical). Pediatric patients usually require general anesthesia.

Anesthetic Goals

Anesthetic goals for complex ear surgery (i.e., tympanoplasty, mastoidectomy, ossicular reconstruction, labyrinthectomy, facial nerve decompression, middle ear tumor resections) are given below.

Minimize Blood Loss

1. Patient positioned "head up"
   a. May increase risk of venous air embolus.
   b. When combined with deliberate hypotension may cause cerebral hypoperfusion. If an arterial line is used, the transducer should be placed at the level of the brain to measure pressure there.
2. Infiltration of field with lidocaine mixed with epinephrine; epinephrine-soaked pledgets applied to field topically.
   a. Solutions prepared in OR must be double-checked with regard to epinephrine concentration.
   b. Local anesthetic use must not exceed toxic dose.
3. Deliberate hypotension
   a. Systolic blood pressure reduced to 60–70 mm Hg using anesthetic or vasodilator.
   b. Many patients are young and healthy, but A-line, EEG monitoring, and capnography may be necessary to ensure adequate organ perfusion. Cardiac and CNS ischemic complications are possible.
   c. No correlation exists between the degree of hypotension and the surgeon's assessment of operative field.

Maintenance of Motionless Field

1. A motionless field is generally maintained by using nondepolarizing muscle relaxants.
2. Use of muscle relaxants should be discussed with the surgeon if surgeon plans intraoperative stimulation of the facial nerve for preservation.
3. A differential sensitivity to muscle relaxants exists between facial musculature and muscles of the hand; 10–20% twitch response maintained in the hand will allow facial muscle stimulation.

Use of N_2O

Use of N_2O is controversial during middle ear surgery.

1. In high concentrations, N_2O can enter air-filled cavities more rapidly than nitrogen can leave, because blood gas solubility 34:1.
2. If eustachian tubes are obstructed, N_2O can quickly increase middle ear pressure to 300–400 cm H_2O.
3. After N_2O is discontinued, reversal of the concentration gradient can cause N_2O to be rapidly reabsorbed, creating a negative middle ear pressure. This can result in graft rupture, serious otitis media, hemotympanum, osseous structure disruption.
4. N_2O has been implicated as causing hearing loss in patients with a history of middle ear surgery.
5. The middle ear cavity has been packed with gel foam and/or flushed with air to avoid complications.
6. N_2O should be avoided in middle ear surgery, or if used, discontinued 15 minutes before tympanic membrane closure.

NASAL AND SINUS SURGERY

Many considerations are the same as those for middle ear surgery. Modified hypotension, head-up tilt, and topical vasoconstrictors may be used to reduce intraoperative blood loss.

General Anesthesia

1. Oral "RAE" tube is positioned midline and secured to chin. It may be sutured to the nostril.

2. If a posterior pharyngeal pack has been used, it must be removed before extubation. Oral pharynx should be thoroughly suctioned and inspected for blood coming from the nose or sinuses.

3. Patients must be awake enough to support their own respirations because mask ventilation may disrupt surgical repair.

4. Patients should be extubated slightly head down and with the head turned to the side to prevent blood from entering the trachea.

5. Discomfort of nasal packing and necessity of mouth breathing should be discussed with patient preoperatively.

Local Anesthesia with Sedation

1. Some cosmetic and reconstructive surgery can be performed with this technique.

2. Careful patient selection is important (cooperation and motivation necessary).

3. Specific techniques of local anesthesia
   a. Infraorbital and external nasal nerves may be blocked by local anesthetic injection.
   b. Sphenopalatine ganglion may be anesthetized by inserting anesthetic-soaked pledgets (4% cocaine or 2% lidocaine with epinephrine) along inferior and middle turbinates.
   c. Total doses as well as effects of all agents should be carefully monitored.

4. **Cocaine** is a frequently used anesthetic agent in nasal surgery.
   a. Rapidly absorbed from the mucosa.
   b. Plasma concentration peaks at 1 hour, analgesia and vasoconstriction in 10 minutes.
   c. Metabolized by plasma cholinesterase, maximum dose 3 mg/kg or approximately 5 ml of a 4% solution in a 70-kg adult.
   d. Toxic reactions include restlessness, tachycardia, hypertension, delirium and seizures.
   e. Cocaine acts by blocking reuptake of norepinephrine or uptake of epinephrine. This makes addition of epinephrine to cocaine solutions unnecessary and potentially dangerous.

    f. Use of cocaine in patients on MAO inhibitors is contraindicated.

Nasal Surgery to Control Epistaxis

1. Emergency procedure involving ligation of anterior ethmoid, internal maxillary, or external carotid artery.
2. Secondary to blood loss, patients may be hypovolemic and considered a "full stomach" because they have probably swallowed a large volume of blood.
3. Patients are generally anxious and uncomfortable, frequently from attempts to control bleeding.
4. Sedation should be minimal, patient should be rehydrated via large-bore IV, and should be given supplemental O_2 before induction.
5. Preoperative laboratory tests should include evaluation of liver function, coagulation profile, and hematocrit. Contributing factors to epistaxis include hypertension, anticoagulant therapy, coagulopathy secondary to hepatic disease, and hematologic malignancy.
6. Either rapid sequence or awake intubation is required for airway control on induction. If profuse bleeding is occurring, visualization of the glottis may be difficult. Blood for transfusion should be available.

ADENOTONSILLECTOMY

Adenotonsillectomy is a common elective procedure for recurrent tonsillar infection or hypertrophied tonsils causing partial airway obstruction. It may be combined with uvulopalatopharyngoplasty (UPPP) to treat some types of obstructive sleep apnea. It can also be part of the surgical correction of some congenital airway anomalies (Treacher-Collins, Pierre-Robin). It is usually a benign procedure done on a "day-stay" basis. Morbidity caused by a compromised airway or hypovolemia from postoperative bleeding is possible. Acute tonsillitis and current respiratory infection are contraindications to elective adenotonsillectomy.

Preoperative Evaluation

1. Hematocrit and coagulation status should be checked preoperatively. Children should be examined for loose or damaged teeth.

2. If enlarged tonsils compromise the airway, preoperative sedation should be minimal. An antisialagogue may be used as part of the premedication.
3. Tonsillar enlargement may produce difficulty with intubation. An awake intubation using topical anesthesia may be best in adults when this is the case.

Induction

1. Induction is generally done in children using N_2O/O_2/halothane by mask with spontaneous respirations.
2. In patients with potentially difficult airways, use awake intubation after topicalization. In an uncooperative child, induction may be by mask with visualization of the glottis by gentle laryngoscopy. After this, a muscle relaxant may be given for intubation. An oral "RAE" tube is usually preferred. Equipment for difficult intubation should be immediately available (stylet, variety of blades, fiberoptic scope).
3. After intubation, the surgeon inserts a mouth gag to secure the tube and expose the pharynx. This may cause the tube to obstruct or kink. (For this reason, some advocate using an anode tube.) It is very important to check breath sounds and monitor inspiratory pressures after insertion of the gag.

Maintenance of Anesthesia

1. Anesthesia may be maintained by any technique; inhalational agent in N_2O and oxygen is common for pediatric cases. Total IV anesthesia propofol/alfentanil/relaxant) is used in adults. Rapid awakening and return of protective airway reflexes at the end of the procedure are particularly important.
2. The tonsillar bed may be sprayed or injected with local anesthetic to supplement anesthetic technique and give postoperative pain relief.
3. Blood loss is frequently difficult to quantitate intraoperatively because of drainage into the stomach and posterior pharynx. Volume deficits caused by blood loss and/or NPO status should be replaced and IV maintained postoperatively until the patient can swallow fluids.

Emergence

1. At the end of resection, the surgeon loosens the mouth gag and inspects the pharynx for hemostasis.
2. Stomach, naso-, and oropharynx are suctioned gently. Be careful not to stir up bleeding in tonsillar beds.
3. Posterior packs are removed and counted.
4. Awake extubation with minimum of coughing and bucking. Lidocaine 1 mg/kg IV helps blunt tracheal responses until consciousness level is adequate for extubation.
5. The patient is transported with head slightly down and turned to the side to facilitate drainage of secretions.

Postoperative

1. The patient is carefully observed for airway patency and post-operative bleeding.
2. Most common period for rebleeding is first 4–6 hours.
3. Initial sign of hemorrhage may be patient vomiting swallowed blood. This may be preceded by tachycardia, restlessness, or hypoxia.
4. If surgery has been to correct sleep apnea, ICU monitoring overnight is advised because a central component to the apnea may still be present. There may also be significant upper airway edema, which may be reduced by IV steroids (dexamethasone 4 mg IV) or nebulized racemic epinephrine (3 ml 2.5% solution in 3 ml saline).

"The Bleeding Tonsil"

1. Hematocrit and coagulation factors should be rechecked.
2. Volume losses should be corrected before reoperation (this may include transfusion).
3. Patients should be considered "full-stomachs" and hypovolemic. Induction should be via rapid sequence after preoxygenation. Ketamine (1–2 mg/kg) or etomidate (0.2–0.4 mg/kg) should be used if urine output is low or volume status is unclear. For potentially difficult airway patients, an awake intubation may be necessary. If no IV access is available, mask induction may be attempted, with cricoid pressure added as the patient loses consciousness. Of course this will

not prevent blood in the pharynx from entering the lungs, but it will offer some protection from passive gastric aspiration. When anesthetic depth is appropriate, the oropharynx should be suctioned and the airway secured with an endotracheal tube. Afterward, an orogastric tube may be passed to empty the stomach of blood.

ACUTE EPIGLOTTIS (SUPRAGLOTTITIS)

Epiglottitis is an infrequent but potentially life-threatening infection seen most commonly in children (ages 1–7), though it can occur in adulthood. It does not involve the subglottic structures and is sometimes referred to as "supraglottitis." The causative agent is usually *Haemophilus influenzae.*

Diagnosis

1. 4 "Ds"—drooling, dysphagia, dysphonia, dyspnea
2. Patient will be febrile, have tachycardia.
3. Lateral neck films may help rule out a foreign body, but negative films do not rule out epiglottis.
4. Blood work should be kept to a minimum (if any) because painful stimuli may cause acute airway obstruction.

Management

1. Airway obstruction may ensue within 6–12 hours, so expeditious management is important.
2. The OR should be prepared for bronchoscopy, laryngoscopy, cricothyrotomy, and tracheostomy. The ENT surgeon should be scrubbed, gowned, and gloved during induction. The airway should not be instrumented for examination in the emergency room because obstruction can occur.
3. Anesthesia airway tray should include multiple blades, tubes, and nasal and oral airways. Intubation is usually carried out with a styleted endotracheal tube a size smaller than normal.
4. Some centers allow the parents to accompany the child to the OR and hold the child during mask induction to minimize crying and agitation. Mask induction should occur with the child in the sitting position.

5. After induction, IV access should be established and appropriate antibiotics and fluids given. In children, atropine 0.02 mg/kg should be given to prevent bradycardia with laryngoscopy.

6. With the patient breathing spontaneously but at a deep level of anesthesia (eyes centered, rectus abdominus muscles flaccid), laryngoscopy should be performed and the glottis, epiglottis and periglottic structures carefully examined. Should these be normal, then bronchoscopy will be necessary.

7. If erythema and edema indicative of epiglottis are present, the trachea should be intubated if possible. The use of muscle relaxants is discouraged.

8. If intubation is not possible, the airway should be secured surgically via either tracheostomy or cricothyrotomy.

9. On emergence, the child should be sedated with a narcotic and an anxiolytic and admitted to an ICU. The child should remain intubated for the next 36–48 hours. Before extubation, laryngoscopy may be necessary to determine the degree of resolution of edema.

10. Epiglottis in adults is much more unusual, and management is more controversial. Some authors have suggested that in the absence of airway compromise, observation in an ICU setting with appropriate medical therapy is acceptable.

ANESTHESIA FOR ENT TRAUMA

Maxillary Trauma

1. First studied systematically by Rene LeFort in 1900 by striking blows to the skulls of cadavers.

2. Maxillary fractures are classified into 3 groups:
    a. LeFort I—horizontal fractures with the upper teeth, palate portions of the pterygoid process, and wall of the maxillary sinus included in fracture segment.
    b. LeFort II—fracture line running through lacrimal bones and inferior rims of the orbits and extending beneath the malar bone to the pterygomaxillary fossa.
    c. LeFort III—complete separation of the maxilla, nasal bones, and zygoma from the cranial attachments.

3. Maxillary fractures are one third as common as mandibular fractures; can be associated with CNS trauma and airway compromise.
4. All facial trauma patients should be evaluated for
   a. Intracranial trauma (25% incidence of CSF leak with Le-Fort II and III fractures)
   b. C-Spine instability
5. Airway may be occluded initially, secondary to fracture segment pressing on posterior pharynx or tongue.
   a. Ask the patient to lean forward if possible or apply gentle forward traction on maxilla.
   b. If CSF leak is absent and nasal damage is not too extensive, a well-lubricated nasal airway may be passed.
6. Nasogastric tube should not be inserted except under special circumstances because its course may be disrupted by the altered anatomy.

Mandibular Fractures

1. Frequently complicated by trismus and edema, which limit mouth opening.
2. Degree of temporomandibular joint dysfunction should be ascertained by reviewing films with surgeon.
3. For patients with poor mouth opening, airway control options include
   a. **Awake nasal fiberoptic intubation** after appropriate topicalization and antisialagogue.
   b. **Awake blind nasal intubation** also after appropriate topicalization.
   c. **Awake tracheostomy** in patients who have concomitant severe maxillary trauma.
   d. **Awake oral intubation** may be considered if the surgeon agrees. In this case, the tube may be wired in the space behind one of the posterior molars if the mouth is to be wired closed.
4. **Before emergence,** the patient should be given an antiemetic (droperidol 0.625 mg IV or ondansetron) and an antisialagogue (glycopyrrolate 0.2 mg). The pharynx and nasogastric tube should be thoroughly suctioned.
5. **Before extubation,** the patient should be alert and able to maintain airway and control sections. **Wire clippers** should

be immediately available to cut the wires securing the mandible fixation should airway difficulty arise.

Acute Laryngeal Trauma

Laryngeal trauma should be suspected in all victims of major trauma—especially motor vehicle accidents, assault, or sporting injury.

Diagnosis

1. Can be particularly insidious, **few external signs (subcutaneous emphysema and/or mild erythema), gradual loss of airway.**
2. Complaints may include dysphagia, hoarseness, or local pain.

Therapy

1. Conservative—humidified oxygen, steroids, prophylactic antibiotics may help.
2. Awake tracheostomy or, for the uncooperative patient, tracheostomy under general anesthesia with inhalational agent by mask in 100% O_2.
3. Endotracheal intubation may be hazardous:
   a. Occult C-spine injury
   b. Excessive blood, debris, mucus from trauma
   c. Supraglottic laryngeal fracture causing edema and difficulty raising the epiglottis on laryngoscopy
   d. Subcutaneous emphysema may make neck extension difficult and may be associated with air emboli and pneumothorax.
   e. In severe trauma, cricotracheal separation may, with administration of muscle relaxants, cause relaxation of splinting musculature making endotracheal intubation impossible.
   f. Blind nasal intubation and/or temporizing are not recommended in management.
   g. Fiberoptic intubation may be attempted, depending on the extent of trauma, but may be impossible if blood or excretions are present.

Suggested Readings

Casey WF, Drake-Lee AB. Nitrous oxide and middle ear pressure: a study of induction methods in children. Anaesthesia 1982;37:896–900.

Crosby E, Reid D. Acute epiglottitis in the adult: is intubation mandatory? Can J Anaesth 1991;38:914–918.

Edgerton MT Jr., Kenney JG. Fractures of the maxillae. In: Zuidema GD, Rutherford RB, Ballinger WF, eds. The Management of Trauma. Philadelphia: WB Saunders, 1985:321–322.

Flood LM, Astely B. Anaesthetic management of acute laryngeal trauma. Br J Anaesth 1982;54;1339–1342.

France W, Beste D. Anesthesia for pediatric ear, nose and throat surgery. In: Gregory G, ed. Pediatric Anesthesia. New York: Churchill Livingstone, 1989:1130–1133.

Ovassapian A. Anatomy of the Airway in Fiberoptic Airway Endoscopy in Anesthesia and Critical Care. New York: Raven Press 1990:15–22.

Owens WD, Gusave F, Selaroff A. Tympanic membrane rupture with nitrous oxide anesthesia. Anesth Analg 1978;57:283–286.

Piotrowski JJ, Moore EJ. Emergency department tracheostomy in airway management and anesthesia. Emerg Med Clin North Am 1988;6:737–744.

Rampil IJ. Anesthetic considerations for laser surgery. Anesth Analg 1992;74:424–435.

Roberts JT. Functional anatomy of the larynx. Int Anesth Clin 1990;28:101–105.

Sosis M. Anesthesia for laser surgery. Int Anesth Clin 1990;28:119–131.

Todres J, Berde C. Pediatric Emergencies in A Practice of Anesthesia for Infants and Children. Philadelphia: WB Saunders, 1986:1130–1133.

Chapter 11

Pulmonary Considerations in Anesthesia[1]

The leading cause of morbidity and mortality in surgical patients is postoperative pulmonary complications. Major risks for postoperative pulmonary complications include preexisting pulmonary disease, smoking, and obesity. Type of surgery and duration of anesthesia also affect outcome. Satisfactory postoperative analgesia is important for reducing postoperative pulmonary problems for many types of surgery. Pulmonary assessment, planning, and management are essential to good outcome.

PREOPERATIVE PULMONARY EVALUATION

Purpose of Evaluation

Preoperative pulmonary evaluation serves three purposes: *(a)* planning for anesthesia, including preoperative, intraoperative, and postoperative management; *(b)* assessment and minimization of risks; *(c)* optimizing utilization of resources (time, people, equipment, money). There are no "routine" pulmonary laboratory measurements or "routine" pulmonary function tests. Tests and measurements should depend upon each patient's disease and proposed surgery. Every patient should receive a good pulmonary history and physical examination, the

---

[1] Symbols and terminology used in this chapter are defined in a list at the end of the chapter.

two most useful sources of data for pulmonary evaluation. Orders for additional tests, measurements, and x-rays should be based upon findings in the history and physical examination. Patients warranting closer scrutiny include those with congenital pulmonary disease, occupational hazards, prolonged tobacco abuse, and known or suspected pulmonary disease.

Consultations

Anesthesiology consultation should focus on five issues.

Identification: Are there acute or chronic pulmonary diseases that place the patient at increased risk? What information is needed to define these risks?

Baseline information: What baseline information is needed to assess intraoperative and postoperative pulmonary changes?

Prediction of outcome: Will outcome for the cardiorespiratory system be changed by the planned anesthesia and surgery? What information is needed to predict outcome?

Preparation: Can pulmonary disease processes be altered preoperatively to reduce risks?

Planning: Should the anesthetic plan be moderated by existing acute or chronic pulmonary disease? Should postoperative planning be modified?

The written preoperative consultation should include documentation of pertinent normal conditions and disease. Risks should be identified, documented, and included in a discussion with the patient and family. The reasons for additional tests, measurements, and radiologic studies should be evident in your consultation. Anesthetic plan for preoperative, intraoperative, and postoperative management should be documented.

Pulmonary consultation should be requested when (a) one or more specific diagnostic or therapeutic questions need to be answered prior to anesthesia and surgery; (b) assistance is desired for preoperative pulmonary preparation or postoperative support; (c) another expert opinion needs to be incorporated into the anesthesiologist's overall assessment, documentation, and management of risks.

History and Physical Examination

See Table 11.1

Table 11.1
Pulmonary Evaluation

History
  Occupation and avocation
  Exercise tolerance
  Dyspnea (activity-related and positional)
  Cough—frequency, duration, productivity, recent changes
  Sputum—volume, color, odor, viscosity, recent changes
  Hemoptysis—onset, amount, character
  Cardiothoracic pain
  Emergency room visits, hospitalizations, ICU admissions for pulmonary
    disease
  Previous intubation/ventilation for pulmonary reasons (what? when?)
  Pulmonary medications
  Previous CXR (when? why?)
  Previous pulmonary function test (when? what? why?)
  Previous cardiothoracic surgery (when? what? why?)
Physical examination
  Color (cyanosis, plethora)
  Patient habitus
  Respiratory rate
  Breathing pattern—thoracoabdominal synchronicity
  Retractions (suprasternal, intercostal, subcostal)
  Accessory support of respiration (pursed-lip breathing, use of accessory
    muscles of neck and/or abdomen)
  Auscultation of all lung fields
  Percussion to determine hyperresonance and fluid levels

General Laboratory Measurements

Review or obtain when indicated:
  Hematocrit (rule out polycythemia)
  WBC with differential count (rule out infection)

Chest Roentgenography (chest x-ray [CXR])

Although still obtained routinely in some institutions, the
CXR's usefulness as a preoperative screening tool is questionable. Patients who smoke or have signs or symptoms of pulmonary disease should receive a preoperative CXR (PA and lateral), which you personally review.

Arterial Blood Gas (ABG)

Arterial oxygen tension (P_aO_2)
  Normal: $(104 - 0.27 \cdot AGE_{YEARS})$ mm Hg (sea level; $F_IO_2 = 0.21$)
Arterial carbon dioxide tension (P_aCO_2)
  Normal: 35–45 mm Hg. Gravid normal: 32 mm Hg.
Arterial pH (pH_a)
  Normal: 7.36–7.44
Arterial oxyhemoglobin saturation (S_aHbO_2)
  Normal: 95% (sea level; $F_IO_2 = 0.21$)
Arterial carboxyhemoglobin saturation (S_aHbCO)
  Nonsmoker normal: 0–1.5%; smoker normal: 0–10%; also elevated in urban dwellers.
Note: Elevated carboxyhemoglobin levels cannot be detected by pulse oximetry.
Cooximetric measurement is mandatory in victims of carbon monoxide poisoning.
Arterial methemoglobin saturation (S_aHbmet)
  Normal: 0–1.5%. Methemoglobinemia occurs in certain nitrate and nitrite poisonings. In these cases, S_aHbmet is the definitive measurement for diagnosis and for assessment of therapy.
Hemoglobin concentration [Hb]

Assessment of Oxygenation

Measure fractional inspired concentration of oxygen (F_IO_2) and calculate alveolar oxygen tension:

$$P_AO_2 = [(P_{bar} - P_{H2O}) \cdot F_IO_2] - \{[F_IO_2 + (1 - F_IO_2)/R] \cdot P_aCO_2\}$$

State of Oxygenation

Measure P_aO_2 and S_aHbO_2. Hypoxemia occurs when S_aHbO_2 falls below 90%.

Cardiopulmonary Oxygenating Ability

Calculate alveolar-arterial oxygen tension difference ($P_{(A-a)}O_2$); dependent on age and F_IO_2; do **not** use when $F_IO_2 > 0.3$. Room-air normal $\approx$ 5 torr/decade.

Calculate arterial/alveolar oxygen tension ratio $(P_{(a/A)}O_2)$. This is independent of age and F_IO_2. Normal: 0.75 or greater.

Assessment of Alveolar Ventilation

Measure P_aCO_2. Normal: 36–44 torr. Gravid normal: 32 torr.

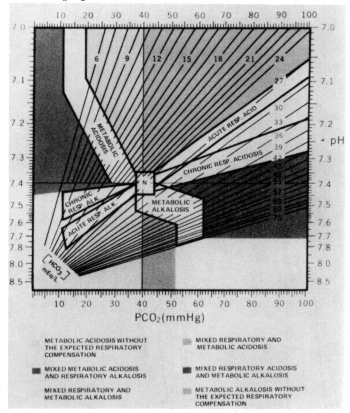

Figure 11.1. Goldberg acid-base diagram. Determine patient's acid-base condition by locating intersection of lines for pH_a and P_aCO_2, y-axis and x-axis, respectively. (From Goldberg M, Green SB, Moss ML, Marbach CB, Garfinkel D. Computer-based instruction and diagnosis of acid-base disorders. JAMA 1973;223:269–275, with permission. Copyright 1973, American Medical Association.)

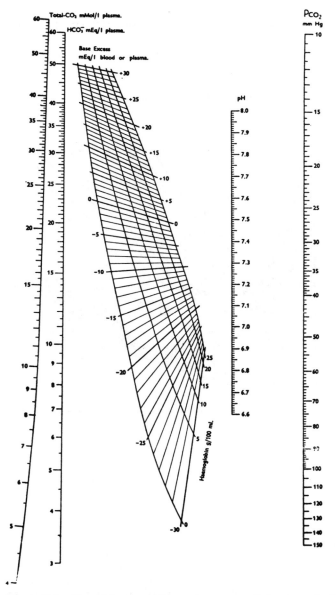

Figure 11.2. Sigaard-Anderson alignment nomogram. Determine patient's base excess, plasma bicarbonate concentration, and total plasma carbon dioxide content by aligning a straightedge on P_aCO_2 and pH_a. Note that base excess concentration depends upon hemoglobin concentration. (From Siggaard-Anderson O. Blood acid-base alignment nomogram. Scand J Clin Lab Invest 1963;15:211–217, with permission.)

Assessment of Acid-Base

Acid-base state: measure pH_a. Normal: 7.36–7.44.

Acidemia: $pH_a < 7.36$.

Alkalemia: $pH_a > 7.44$.

Acid-base condition: use Goldberg diagram (Fig. 11.1) to determine the primary condition(s)—respiratory acidosis, respiratory alkalosis, metabolic acidosis, metabolic alkalosis. Use Sigaard-Andersen alignment nomogram (Fig. 11.2) to calculate plasma bicarbonate (normal: 24 ± 2 mEq/liter) and base excess (normal: 0 ± 2.5 mEq/liter). Metabolic alkalosis is the most common acid-base disorder in hospitalized patients.

Pulmonary Function Testing

Pulmonary function tests (PFTs) can be used to *(a)* diagnose acute or chronic disease; *(b)* assess progression of disease; and *(c)* assess treatment or support of disease. Normal ranges and predicted values are affected by age, sex, race, and smoking history. The patient's results should be compared with the normal values reported for the pulmonary function laboratory in which the patient was tested. *Percent predicted* and *ratios* can be used without absolute normal values.

Flow-volume loops can be used to assess pulmonary disease and assess obstructive upper airway pathology (Figs. 11.3 and 11.4).

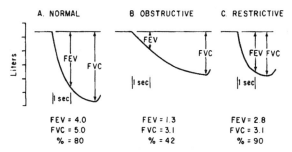

Figure 11.3. Forced vital capacity. *A,* Normal; *B,* obstructive disease; *C,* restrictive disease. Note the prolonged expiratory time and the reduced FEV_1/FVC ratio with obstructive disease. Also note the reduced vital capacity and the high FEV_1/FVC ratio with restrictive disease. (From Pulmonary Pathophysiology, 4th ed., West.)

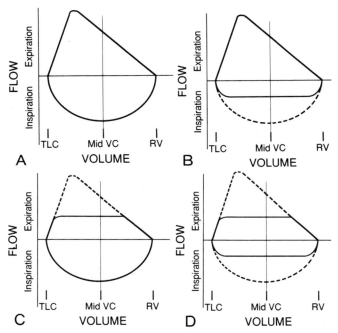

Figure 11.4. Flow-volume loops are obtained by having the patient sequentially perform inspiratory and expiratory vital capacity maneuvers. The *solid line* represents the actual flow-volume loop in **A-D**; the *dashed line* represents a normal curve for comparison in **B-D**. **A,** Normal; mid-vital capacity (mid-VC) inspiratory:expiratory (I:E) flow ratio is approximately 1. **B,** Variable extrathoracic obstruction; I:E flow ratio < 1. **C,** Variable intrathoracic obstruction; I:E flow ratio > 1. **D,** Fixed obstruction extrathoracic or intrathoracic; I:E flow ratio is approximately 1; flow-volume loop pattern is distinctly abnormal.

Lung volumes and capacities are measured either directly (spirometry) or indirectly (body plethysmography, helium dilution, nitrogen washout) (Fig. 11.5) (Table 11.2).

Mechanics Measurements

Mechanics measurements include compliance, resistance, and work.

Compliance: $\Delta V/\Delta P$, where P = pressure, V = volume.

Lung compliance: $C_L = \Delta V/\Delta P_{LUNG}$. Normal: 200 ml cmH_2O^{-1}.

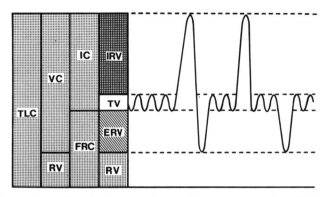

Figure 11.5. Normal spirogram. Lung volumes are mutually exclusive; lung capacities consist of two or more lung volumes or capacities. Definitions and measurements are in Table 11.2. Symbols and terminology are in Appendix I. (From Bonner JT, Hall JR. Respiratory intensive care of the adult surgical patient. St. Louis: CV Mosby, 1985, with permission.)

Thoracic compliance: $C_T = \Delta V / \Delta P_{THOR}$. Normal: 200 ml cmH$_2$O^{-1}.

Total, or lung-thorax, compliance: $C_{LT} = \Delta V / \Delta P_{AW}$. Normal: 100 ml cmH$_2$O^{-1}.

Static compliance measurements permit pressure to come to equilibrium in all airways, i.e., allow gas redistribution to occur throughout the lungs.

Dynamic compliance measurements are made with a finite respiratory rate; i.e., gas redistribution may not be complete. Compared with static measurements, pressure may be higher, and compliance lower, during dynamic measurements.

Resistance: $\Delta P / \dot{V}$, where P = pressure, $\dot{V}$ = flow.

Normal: 0.2–2.5 cmH$_2$O liter^{-1} sec^{-1}.

Gas Flow Measurements

Gas flow measurements are made both timed (forced) and nontimed and can provide an important assessment in patients with obstructive airways disease. In normal individuals, greater resistance to gas flow occurs in the larger conducting airways (generations 1–9) than in the smaller conducting airways (generations 10–17). Transition from convective (bulk) gas flow to molecular diffusion occurs at the terminal bronchioles (genera-

Table 11.2
Lung Volumes and Capacities

Total lung capacity (TLC)	Total gas volume in thorax; usually the gas volume in the lungs but will include pneumothorax, pneumomediastinum, pneumopericardium, if present	Indirect measurement
Tidal volume (V_T)	Volume of gas moved in and out of the lungs with each breath	Direct measurement
Vital capacity (VC)	Volume difference between TLC and RV; that volume of gas that a patient can maximally inspire from RV to TLC (inspiratory VC) or maximally expire from TLC to RV (expiratory VC)	Direct measurement during inspiration or expiration; rule of thumb normal: 70 ml/kg; abnormal is <80% of predicted
Inspiratory capacity (IC)	That volume of gas that a patient can maximally inspire following normal expiration; IC = V_T + IRV	Direct measurement
Functional residual capacity (FRC)	Volume remaining in the lungs at end of normal expiration; the point at which the outward recoil tendency of the chest wall is balanced by the inward recoil tendency of the lungs; the most reproducible point in the spirogram; considered the lung volume from which gas exchange occurs	Indirect measurement; abnormalcy is <80% of predicted
Inspiratory reserve volume (IRV)	The volume difference between resting tidal volume and inspiratory capacity; IRV = IC − V_T	Direct measurement
Expiratory reserve volume (ERV)	Volume difference between FRC and RV	ERV is normally 20–40% of VC
Residual volume (RV)	Volume remaining in the lungs at the end of maximal expiration	Abnormalcy: <80% or >120% of predicted

tion 17), which is the point at which the greatest increase in cross-sectional area in the lungs occurs.

Forced vital capacity (FVC) is the volume expired as rapidly and completely as possible from TLC to RV. FVC is effort dependent, and in air-trapping disease, FVC will be less than nontimed vital capacity.

Forced expiratory volume in one second (FEV_1) is the volume that is expired in the first second of an FVC. FEV_1 is effort dependent and is affected by age (peaks in third decade), sex, height, and habitus. FEV_1 may be a useful measurement in *advanced* stages of obstructive disease.

Forced expiratory flow by volume ($FEF_{200-1200\ ml}$) is the flow rate at which the initial 1000-ml volume of the FVC is exhaled. It is measured between 200 and 1200 ml to eliminate any effect of initial hesitation.

Forced expiratory flow by percentage ($FEF_{25-75\%}$), also known as maximum midexpiratory flow (MMF or MMEF), is the flow rate during the middle half by volume of the FVC. It is effort independent.

FEV_1/FVC ratio, which normally is ≥ 0.70, is useful in detecting *early* obstructive disease. Abnormalcy is less than 0.70.

Bronchodilators. Use of bronchodilators during pulmonary function testing may or may not predict the usefulness of bronchodilators in the perioperative period. *Actual efficacy is determined by the patient's response to the bronchodilators when they are needed and administered.*

Gas Distribution Measurements

Gas distribution measurements provide information about gas flow through the conducting airways.

Single-breath nitrogen test (SBNT) is initiated with an inspiratory vital-capacity breath of oxygen; then exhaled nitrogen is plotted against lung volume, producing a quadriphasic curve (Fig. 11.6).

Closing volume (CV) is the volume above RV at which gravity-dependent portions of the lung close and no longer participate in ventilation. CV is age dependent; normal value is referenced to the patient's VC: $CV_{\%VC} = 1.9 + 0.36 \times AGE_{YR}$.

Closing capacity (CC) is (CV + RV). CC is referenced to the patient's TLC.

Gas Exchange

Gas exchange occurs in the alveolar ducts, alveolar sacs, and alveoli. The matching of ventilated and perfused surface areas, as well as the gas transfer path, can affect gas exchange.

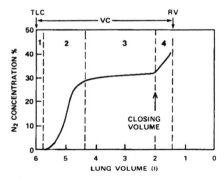

Figure 11.6. Single-breath nitrogen test. SBNT is obtained by having the patient perform a VC inspiration of 100% oxygen, followed by a VC expiration during which exhaled nitrogen concentration is measured continuously. Phase 1 contains dead space gases. Phase 2 contains a mixture of dead space and alveolar gases. Phases 1 and 2 can be used to determine anatomic dead space. Phase 3 contains alveolar gases, and its slope indicates gas distribution. Zero slope indicates even distribution; increasingly greater slopes indicate increasing maldistribution. Phase 4 indicates closure of airways in dependent portion of lungs (i.e., closing volume). (From Respiratory Physiology, 4th edition, West.)

Gas exchange units may be participating in gas exchange (alveolar ventilation) or not (alveolar dead space ventilation).

Diffusing capacity of the lung for carbon monoxide ($D_L CO$) is an indication of the surface area and transfer path for gas exchange. $D_L CO$ is affected by age, pregnancy, hemoglobin concentration, preexisting HbCO, pulmonary capillary blood volume and blood flow, lung volume, exercise, and patient position; the last two factors are controlled during PFTs. Abnormalcy is less than 75% of predicted. Diseases that involve parenchymal destruction produce low $D_L CO$.

Dead Space

Dead Space is that part of ventilation not participating in gas exchange, whether in the patient or in equipment that has bidirectional gas flow. Capnography can be used to visually assess ventilation and dead space (Figs. 11.7–11.9).

Physiologic dead space, the total dead space in the patient, is the sum of anatomic dead space and alveolar dead space. It is calculated directly from respiratory and blood gas measurements:

$$\dot{V}_D PHYSIOL = \dot{V}_E \cdot [(P_a CO_2 - P_E CO_2)/(P_a CO_2 - P_I CO_2)]$$

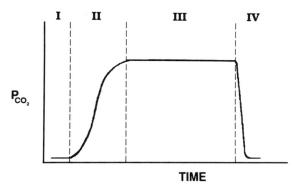

Figure 11.7. Normal capnogram. Phases I–III are expiration: I contains mechanical and anatomic dead space gases; II contains anatomic dead space gases plus initial alveolar gases; III contains gases from ventilated alveoli and alveolar dead space. Phase IV is inspiration. Value for $P_{E'}CO_2$ is obtained at the end of phase III. Slope of phase III normally is zero.

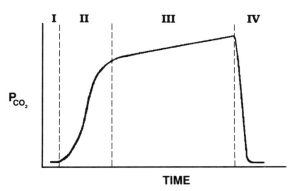

Figure 11.8. Abnormal capnogram. Increased slope of phase III is produced by uneven emptying of alveoli, caused by expiratory obstruction or parenchymal destruction.

Anatomic dead space is the volume of the conducting airways and is calculated directly from respiratory and blood gas measurements:

$$\dot{V}_{D}ANAT = \dot{V}_{E} \cdot [(P_{E'}CO_2 - P_{\bar{E}}CO_2)/(P_{E'}CO_2 - P_{I}CO_2)]$$

Approximately one-half is intrathoracic and one-half extrathoracic. Intubation eliminates extrathoracic anatomic dead space and adds physical dead space equal to the volume of

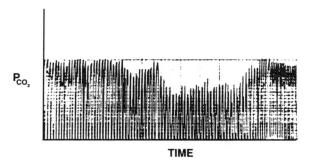

P_{CO_2}

TIME

Figure 11.9. Trend capnogram during pulmonary embolism. Decrease in $P_{E'}CO_2$ occurred over about 10 min following suspected venous air embolism.

the endotracheal tube or tracheostomy tube. Increases in anatomic dead space with bronchodilation and positive airway pressure usually are clinically insignificant.

Alveolar dead space is the volume of lung parenchyma not participating in gas exchange and is calculated indirectly from the calculations of physiologic dead space and anatomic dead space:

$$\dot{V}_D\text{ALV} = \dot{V}_D\text{PHYSIOL} - \dot{V}_D\text{ANAT}$$

Increases in alveolar dead space occur *globally* with hypotension, low perfusion states, and positive-pressure ventilation and occur *regionally* with emphysema, pulmonary embolism, and patient position. ($P_a CO_2 - P_E'CO_2$) widens as $\dot{V}_D$ALV increases. The phase III slope of the capnogram increases as $\dot{V}_D$ALV increases (Fig. 11.8).

PULMONARY DISEASES

Adult Respiratory Distress Syndrome (ARDS)

ARDS is an acute lung disease characterized by decreased lung compliance and oxygenating disability. Lung involvement may be regional or global, depending upon the etiology. There is a wide range of severity.

Diagnosis

Diagnosis of ARDS generally is made within the context of the patient's immediate history and current clinical findings. Dyspnea, tachypnea, retractions, and cyanosis occur following onset but should abate once appropriate therapy is instituted. CXR changes may occur late in the first phase of ARDS.

Perioperative Management

Maintain $F_IO_2 \leq 50\%$. Apply distending airway pressure therapy in severe cases, titrating against $\mathring{Q}_s/\mathring{Q}_t$. In moderate to severe cases, do not disconnect breathing circuit even for patient transport, since discontinuing distending airway pressure, even for 15–30 sec, can produce profound hypoxemia and cardiorespiratory instability. Transport to and from the OR with all supportive therapy and full cardiorespiratory monitoring. Use the patient's mechanical ventilator or spontaneous breathing system in OR when flow requirements for distending airway pressure or when peak inspiratory pressures exceed the capability of the anesthesia machine or anesthesia ventilator.

Airway Obstruction (Narrowing)

Airway obstruction (narrowing) can be produced over a limited length of conducting airway by tumor, cyst, lymph nodes, abscess, hematoma, enlarged thyroid, enlarged thymus. The pathophysiology, which can occur at a laryngeal, tracheal, or bronchial level, is orificial obstruction.

Assessment of moderate to severe lesions is made by history (dyspnea) and physical examination (stridor). Additional assessment tools include CT scan, MRI, and flow-volume loops.

Perioperative Management

Gas flow through a partially obstructed airway, and thereby oxygenation, can be improved by employing a gas of low density. Helium mixed with oxygen, heliox, is such a mixture.

Gas	Density
Oxygen	1.429 gm/liter
Air	1.293 gm/liter
Heliox 70:30	0.554 gm/liter
Heliox 80:20	0.429 gm/liter

Although administering a gas mixture with such a low F_IO_2 to a hypoxemic patient seems to be contraindicated, oxygenation will be enhanced by the improvement in gas flow.

Gases	Densities	Relative Flow
Oxygen vs. air	1.293/1.429	0.90
Heliox 70:30 vs. oxygen	1.429/0.554	2.58
Heliox 80:30 vs. oxygen	1.429/0.429	3.33

Heliox should be applied by tight-fitting face mask to ameliorate dyspnea and improve oxygenation preoperatively, during conventional induction of general anesthesia, to facilitate flexible fiberoptic intubation, and to provide continued support of gas flow through bronchial and tracheal lesions that are not bypassed by endotracheal intubation. F_IO_2 and S_pO_2 should always be measured when administering $He:O_2$ mixtures.

α_1-Antitrypsin Deficiency

α_1-Antitrypsin deficiency is an inherited disorder that may be moderate (heterozygous) or severe (homozygous). The underlying pathophysiology is emphysema caused by proteolytic destruction of lung parenchyma, resulting from failure to deactivate proteolytic enzymes of bacteria or leukocytes in the lung. It is seen predominantly in adults, rarely in children. Disease is exacerbated by cigarette smoking. CXR shows decreased vascular markings at lung bases, as well as bullous changes. PFTs are those of emphysema.

Perioperative Management

Prevent (treat) pulmonary infections. Other perioperative management is similar to that for emphysema.

Asthma

Asthma is an episodic COPD in which airways react to one or more stimuli. Triggers include aspirin, β-blockers, and viral URIs. Incidence is 5% of adults, 10% of children. Incidence and severity are greater in blacks. Diagnosis includes intermittent periods of dyspnea, cough, and wheezing, accompanied by hyperinflation of the lungs. Pathophysiological processes include bronchospasm, mucosal edema, and increased bronchial secretions. Intercurrent periods are free of signs and symptoms. The most severe expression of the disease, status asthmaticus, is a life-threatening emergency.

Preoperative Management

Obtain recent and remote history; assess (adjust) type and dose of current medications and give bronchodilators as part of pre-operative medications; reassure the patient; include an anxiolytic in premedication; provide good hydration. Optimally, the patient should be free of wheezing for elective surgery. Delaying surgery for active wheezing to allow intensive therapy with bronchodilators and steroids is warranted (Table 11.3).

Intraoperative Management

Monitor breath sounds and capnogram continuously; maintain good hydration; provide bronchodilators by aerosol generator or metered dose inhaler (MDI). Minimize airway stimulation. Halothane, isoflurane, enflurane, and desflurane are bronchodilators, but they should not be relied upon to the exclusion of aerosol or intravenous bronchodilators, since the bronchodilating effect of the volatile anesthetic will be lost at the end of the case. Extubate ASAP in OR or PACU. In some situations, extubation during deep anesthesia is desirable to decrease the chance of bronchospasm. Deep extubation should not be used in patients at risk for regurgitation or airways compromised by anatomy or secretions.

Postoperative Management

Monitor by inquiry and auscultation; provide humidified supplemental oxygen by aerosol face mask; continue bronchodilators (and steroid) in PACU and beyond; maintain good hydration.

Atelectasis

Atelectasis is not a disease, per se, but is the most frequent postoperative pulmonary problem. Microatelectasis is a diffuse loss of parenchymal gas volume (decreased FRC), producing $\dot{V}_A/\dot{Q}_c$ mismatching and hypoxemia. Microatelectasis is exacerbated by high F_IO_2 and by diminution or ablation of sighing, which may be due to pain or drugs. Lung compliance is decreased, which results in reduced tidal volume and tachypnea. Macroatelectasis has similar pathophysiology but also appears on CXR as radio-

Table 11.3.
Bronchodilators and Associated Drugs

Drug	Classification	Formulation	Dose	Frequency	Comments
Albuterol (salbutamol)	β_2-Agonist (saligenin)	MD: 90 μg/puff	2 puffs	q 4 hr	β_2 selective; may increase heart rate; duration hours
Aminophylline	Methylxanthine		load: 6 mg kg^{-1} (60 min)	0.4–1.0 mg kg^{-1} hr^{-1}	0.4—children, smokers; 1.0—nonsmokers, elderly, acute or chronic liver disease; effective serum concentration 10–20 μg ml^{-1}
Atropine methylnitrate	Cholinergic				Can be given by aerosal treatment
Bitolterol mesylate		MD: 370 μg/puff	2 puffs	q 4 hr	
Fenoterol	β_2-Agonist (resorcinol)				
Glycopyrrolate	Cholinergic				
Hydrocortisone	Glucocorticoid	100 ml/ml	Load: 4 mg/kg	3 mg/kg q 6 hr	Effect seen at 4–6 hr; be sure to continue in patients receiving chronic steroid therapy
Ipratropium bromide	Cholinergic	MD: 18 μg/puff	2 puffs	q 4 hr	Avoid in patients with narrow-angle glaucoma, prostatic hypertrophy, bladder-neck obstruction; more effective in COPD than in asthma
Isoethareine	Catecholamine	1%			Weak bronchodilator
Isoproterenol	β-Agonist (catecholamine)				Increases heart rate and ventricular dysrhythmias
Metaproterenol	β-Agonist (resorcinol)	MD: 650 μg/puff	2 puffs	q 4 hr	
Methylprednisolone	Steroid		125 mg	q 6 hr	Effect seen at 4–6 hr

dense lines, especially at the lung bases, and may have concurrent fever, cough, and sputum production.

Perioperative Management

Reduce occurrence by avoiding prolonged high F_IO_2 and by providing good pain therapy and incentive spirometry. If atelectasis occurs, provide humidified supplemental oxygen and incentive spirometry; rule out exacerbation of chronic bronchitis and pneumonia; treat associated pulmonary infection.

Bronchiectasis

Bronchiectasis is a COPD in which there is permanent abnormal dilation of the bronchi, produced by prolonged bronchial obstruction or infection. Hypertrophied bronchial arteries are vulnerable to rupture, resulting in hemoptysis. Diagnosis is made with bronchography. Bronchiectasis may coexist with chronic bronchitis.

Perioperative Management

Maintain good hydration; treat bronchospasm; treat respiratory infections; plan regional anesthesia whenever possible; provide postoperative chest physical therapy, including postural drainage.

Carbon Monoxide Poisoning

Carbon monoxide poisoning can occur in victims of fires and motor vehicular accidents, who may present for burn treatment or trauma surgery. It is definitively diagnosed with cooximetric measurement of S_aHbCO. CO poisoning is a medical emergency!

Treatment

Treat immediately with 100% oxygen delivered via endotracheal tube or tight-fitting mask and a nonrebreathing circuit; monitor treatment with repeat measurement of S_aHbCO.

Chemotherapies

Chemotherapies that produce pulmonary pathophysiology are listed in Table 11.4.

Table 11.4.
Chemotherapies Producing Pulmonary Pathophysiology

Drug	Pathophysiology
Aldesleukin (interleukin-2)	Respiratory distress[a]
Bleomycin	Pneumonitis; pulmonary fibrosis[a]
Busulfan	Infiltrates; pulmonary fibrosis[a]
Carmustine (BCNU)	Pulmonary fibrosis
Chlorambucil	Infiltrates; pulmonary fibrosis
Cyclophosphamide	Infiltrates; pulmonary fibrosis
Cytarabine	Acute respiratory distress; pulmonary edema
Estramustine	Infiltrates; pulmonary fibrosis
Fludarabine	Infiltrates
Lomustine (CCNU)	Pulmonary fibrosis
Melphalan	Infiltrates; pulmonary fibrosis
Methotrexate	Infiltrates; pulmonary fibrosis[a]
Mitomycin	Pulmonary fibrosis
Procarbazine	Pneumonitis

[a]May limit therapy.

Chronic Bronchitis

Chronic bronchitis is a COPD for which the diagnosis is made by history: productive cough on most days of each month for a minimum of 3 months in 2 successive years. Current clinical assessment should establish recent change in sputum (volume, color, odor, consistency); current antibiotics; fever; leukocytosis, left shift in differential.

Perioperative Management

Acute exacerbation requires antibiotics, hydration, and delay of elective surgery. Regional anesthesia should be considered for appropriate procedures.

Chronic Obstructive Pulmonary Disease (COPD)

COPD is a category of lung diseases, also known as chronic obstructive lung disease (COLD). See each separately: asthma, chronic bronchitis, emphysema, bronchiectasis, cystic fibrosis. Making a definitive diagnosis among the COPDs differs among the diseases; PFTs and laboratory measurements, although not

Table 11.5.
COPD: Laboratory and Pulmonary Function Tests

COPD	Definitive Diagnosis	Laboratory Measurements and PFTs
Asthma	History	Acute early: $\downarrow P_aO_2$, $\downarrow P_aCO_2$, $\uparrow pH_a$, resp alkalosis Acute late: $\downarrow P_aO_2$, $\uparrow P_aCO_2$, $\downarrow pH_a$, resp acidosis $\uparrow RV$, $\uparrow FRC$ $\downarrow FVC$, $\downarrow FEV_1$, $\downarrow MMFR$ NLC_LSTATIC, NLD_LCO Bronchospasm $\rightarrow\rightarrow\rightarrow$ $\uparrow V_DALV$ $\rightarrow\rightarrow\rightarrow$ $\uparrow P_{a-E'}CO_2$ & $\uparrow$ phase III slope of the capnogram
Bronchiectasis	Bronchography	$\downarrow P_aO_2$, $\downarrow S_{aHb}O_2$
Chronic bronchitis	History	$\downarrow P_aO_2$, $\uparrow P_aCO_2$, $\downarrow pH_a$, resp acidosis $\uparrow RV$, $\uparrow FRC$ $\downarrow FVC$, $\downarrow FEV_1$, $\downarrow MMFR$ NLC_LSTATIC, NL-$\downarrow D_L$CO
Cystic fibrosis	Sweat chloride	
Emphysema	Biopsy	$\downarrow P_aO_2$, LATE $\uparrow P_aCO_2$, LATE $\downarrow pH_a$, LATE resp acidosis $\uparrow\uparrow$ RV > $\uparrow$TLC $\rightarrow\rightarrow\rightarrow$ $\uparrow\uparrow$ RV/TLC ratio $\downarrow FEF_{25}$/FVC earlier than $\downarrow FEV_1$/FVC $\uparrow C_A$STATIC, $\downarrow D_L$CO Parenchymal destruction $\rightarrow\rightarrow\rightarrow$ $\uparrow V_DALV$ $\rightarrow\rightarrow\rightarrow$ $\uparrow P_{a-E'}CO_2$ & $\uparrow$ phase III slope of the capnogram

definitive, can provide useful diagnostic and monitoring information (see Table 11.5).

Chronic Restrictive Pulmonary Diseases

Chronic restrictive pulmonary diseases are those in which lung volumes and capacities are less than normal (interstitial pulmonary fibrosis, interstitial pulmonary pneumonitis, kyphoscoliosis, pleural-based diseases, pneumoconioses). Differences between chronic restrictive and chronic obstructive pulmonary diseases are listed in Table 11.6.

Table 11.6.
Obstructive versus Restrictive Lung Disease

Measurement	Obstructive	Restrictive
TLC	↑	↓
VC	NL or ↑	↓
RV	↑↑	NL or ↓
RV/TLC	↑	
FRC	↑	↓
MVV	↓ (proportional to degree of obstruction)	NL
C_L STATIC	↑	↓
R_{AW}	↑	NL
$FEF_{25-75\%}$	↓↓	NL
FEV_1/VC	↓	NL
D_LCO	NL or ↓	↓

Cor Pulmonale

Cor pulmonale is right ventricular (RV) enlargement secondary to pulmonary arterial hypertension. Cor pulmonale may be acute (e.g., RV dilation following acute pulmonary embolization) or chronic (e.g., RV hypertrophy resulting from chronic pulmonary disease). The parenchymal destruction of many pulmonary diseases results in loss of pulmonary vasculature cross-sectional area, leading to pulmonary hypertension that results in cor pulmonale. Chronic hypoxemia and the acidosis associated with chronic hypercapnia also lead to pulmonary hypertension and resulting cor pulmonale. Right ventricular failure is a serious component of cor pulmonale pathophysiology. Pulmonary vascular resistance (PVR) can be calculated from data obtained using a pulmonary artery (Swan-Ganz) catheter:

$$PVR = [(P_{\overline{PA}} - P_{\overline{PAOP}})/CO] \times 80 \ dyn \cdot cm \cdot sec^{-5}$$

Normal PVR is 50–150 dyn · sec · cm^{-5}; normal systolic pulmonary artery pressure is less than 30 mm Hg.

Perioperative Management

Optimize all aspects of underlying lung disease (viz., emphysema, chronic bronchitis, cystic fibrosis, pneumoconiosis, interstitial fibrosis). Treat new or exacerbated pulmonary infections.

Monitor pulse oximetry continuously. Avoid worsening hypoxemia or hypercapnia, which can increase pulmonary artery pressure.

Cystic Fibrosis

Cystic fibrosis is an inherited (autosomal recessive) COPD, also known as pulmonary fibrocystic disease. Incidence is $\approx 1:2500$ in whites, lower in blacks. Although the obstructive pathophysiology affects several organs, the most debilitating and ultimately life-threatening changes occur in the lung. Viscous mucus leads to airway obstruction, resulting in chronic bronchitis, recurrent infections, and bronchiectasis. Chronic air trapping and hyperinflation occur. Cor pulmonale appears in later stages. Since cystic fibrosis patients are living longer now, patients in their late 20s and 30s come for anesthesia and surgery. Pulmonary function tests show an obstructive pattern but are not really of much help in assessing risks and planning anesthesia.

Preoperative Management

Obtain recent history, chest physical examination, CBC with differential, and CXR. Preoperative evaluation and preparation should be directed to four areas for every cystic fibrosis patient (Table 11.7). Plan regional anesthesia when possible.

Table 11.7.
Preoperative Evaluation of Cystic Fibrosis Patient

Problem	Assessment	Treatment
Current infection	Temperature WBC with differential	Antibiotics Chest physical therapy
Hypoxemia	S_aHbO_2, P_aO_2 $P_{(A-a)}O_2$, $P_{(a/A)}O_2$	Supplemental humidified oxygen
Hypoventilation	P_aCO_2, pH_a	Acute ventilatory insufficiency or failure may necessitate postponing surgery, when possible
Bronchospasm	Chest physical examination	Bronchodilators

Intraoperative Management

Avoid N_2O, since bowel obstruction is a GI complication. Provide humidified inspired gases. Monitor for complications of pneumothorax, hemoptysis, worsening oxygenating disability, and ventilatory failure. Extubate ASAP in OR or PACU. Frequent suctioning via the endotracheal tube may be necessary because of secretions.

Postoperative Management

Provide humidified supplemental oxygen, chest physical therapy, and early ambulation. Work with patient's pediatrician or pulmonologist to plan postoperative care.

Drug Abuse

Cocaine

Smoking alkaloidal ("crack") cocaine produces both acute and chronic pulmonary pathophysiology. Acute findings include cough, black sputum, chest pain, and, less frequently, wheezing and hemoptysis. Chronic changes include obstructive pathology of the larger airways and impairment of gas exchange. Pulmonary function tests demonstrate decreased D_LCO and, depending upon severity, hypoxemia.

Perioperative Management

Obtain a drug-use history, including recent use. Inform the patient of increased risks (both cardiac and pulmonary) related to cocaine use. Pulmonary function testing is not helpful for either assessment or prediction. If pulmonary edema occurs, myocardial ischemia should be ruled out before hypoxemia is attributed to cocaine-related lung damage. Hypoxemic patients may benefit from application of distending airway pressure.

Heroin

Heroin along with other narcotics can produce acute pulmonary edema, which likely is due to adverse effects on the alveolocapillary membranes. Associated hypoxemia may respond to the application of distending airway pressure.

Marijuana

Regular chronic users suffer decreased VC, decreased $D_L CO$, and bronchitis. Significant pulmonary pathophysiology usually is related to concomitant cigarette smoking.

Emphysema

Emphysema is an anatomically defined COPD wherein loss of elastic tissue, septal destruction, and hyperinflation increase the parenchymal airways beyond their normal size. Pulmonary capillary networks are destroyed and cor pulmonale is a terminal component. Symptoms, physical examination findings, and laboratory and radiologic changes advance as the disease progresses. Emphysema is associated with cigarette smoking. Chronic bronchitis and bronchospasm can occur with emphysema. Emphysema and chronic bronchitis are compared in Table 11.8. Air trapping and increased alveolar dead space can significantly affect anesthesia and patient outcome.

Table 11.8.
Differentiating Chronic Bronchitis from Emphysema

	Emphysema	Chronic Bronchitis
Bronchial infection	+	+ + +
Pulmonary hypertension	+	+ + +
Cor pulmonale	Late	Early
Dyspnea	+ + +	+
Cough	Late	Early
Sputum	+ (nonpurulent)	+ + + (purulent)
P_aO_2, S_aHbO_2	↓	↓↓↓
P_aCO_2	Increases late	Increases early
pH_a	Decreases late	Decreases early
Acid-base condition	Late resp acidosis	Early resp acidosis
Hematocrit, hemoglobin	NL	↑↑
RV, TLC, RV/TLC	↑	↑
C_LSTATIC	↑	—
$D_L CO$	↓	—
$\dot{V}_D ALV$, $P_{a-E \cdot}CO_2$, phase III slope of the capnogram	↑	—

Preoperative Management

Obtain recent history, especially of associated bronchospasm, pulmonary infection, and use of home oxygen. Treat infection. Optimize bronchodilator therapy. Transport patient with usual oxygen supplement. Avoid respiratory depressants for premedication.

Intraoperative Management

For moderate to severe emphysema patients:

Monitored anesthesia care (MAC) with local anesthesia
- Supplemental oxygen
- Continuous capnography and auscultation

Regional anesthesia
- Remember that abdominal and intercostal muscles are accessory muscles of respiration and that ventilatory ability may be compromised with high levels of regional anesthesia
- Supplemental oxygen
- Continuous capnography and auscultation

General anesthesia with spontaneous respiration
- Continuous capnography and auscultation
- Do not use 100% oxygen (absorption atelectasis)
- Extubate ASAP in OR or PACU

General anesthesia with positive pressure ventilation (PPV)
- Continuous capnography and auscultation
- Do not use 100% oxygen (absorption atelectasis); N_2O should be avoided in patients with large pulmonary bullae
- Use a low inspiratory flow rate to optimize gas distribution and a long expiratory time to permit complete exhalation; overall this will result in a slow respiratory rate
- Treat bronchospasm aggressively: increased phase III slope due to bronchospasm will decrease; increased phase III slope due to parenchymal destruction will not
- PPV increases risk of pulmonary barotrauma (parenchymal destruction) and produces hemodynamic compromise (above-normal airway pressure transmission to the heart and great vessels reduces transmural filling pressures)
- Extubate ASAP in OR or PACU

Postoperative Management

- Supplemental oxygen via nasal cannula (MAC and regional anesthetics)
- Humidified supplemental oxygen (general anesthetics)
- Monitor by inquiry and auscultation
- Treat bronchospasm
- Provide early ambulation
- Provide good pain management to prevent atelectasis

Guillain-Barré Syndrome

Guillain-Barré syndrome is a neuromuscular disorder that can produce respiratory insufficiency or failure. It is characterized by increasing P_aCO_2, occurring over days to weeks as neuromuscular paralysis progresses to include the muscles of respiration. Some patients will require intubation and/or tracheostomy.

Perioperative Management

Review current history for risk of aspiration. Review CXRs for acute/chronic infiltrates. Transport with oxygen and ventilatory support. Maintain euthermia. Obtain a postoperative CXR.

Hyaline Membrane Disease (HMD)

See infant respiratory distress syndrome.

Infant Respiratory Distress Syndrome (IRDS)

IRDS, also known as hyaline membrane disease (HMD), is an acute, life-threatening lung disease of the newborn. A deficiency of surfactant results in an abnormally low lung compliance. IRDS may be treated by various means, including nasal continuous positive airway pressure (CPAP), intubation and application of distending airway pressure, and tracheal instillation of surfactant.

Perioperative Management

Maintain safe F_IO_2 to avoid retrolental fibroplasia, including during transport to/from the OR; apply distending airway pressure or reverse I:E ratio ventilation.

Interstitial Pulmonary Fibrosis

Interstitial pulmonary fibrosis is a chronic restrictive disease that can be produced by drugs (bleomycin, busulfan, nitrofurantoin), chemicals (paraquat), radiation, and collagen vascular diseases (rheumatoid arthritis, scleroderma, systemic lupus erythematosus).

Perioperative Management

Avoid high Paw_{INSP}, by using lower V_T and higher f_{RESP}. Do not use 100% oxygen (absorption atelectasis).

Interstitial Pneumonitis

Interstitial pneumonitis (allergic alveolitis, extrinsic fibrosing alveolitis) is a type 3 hypersensitivity reaction to inhaled organic dusts, affecting the lung parenchyma and producing a restrictive lung disease. Pneumonitides include bagassosis (sugar cane), birdbreeder's lung (antigens from avian feathers and excrement), farmer's lung (actinomycetes spores), maltworker's lung, and mushroom worker's lung. Pathophysiology is interstitial infiltration with lymphocytes, plasma cells, some eosinophils, and histiocytes, which can form granulomata. As the disease advances, fibrosis occurs, and the patient becomes progressively more dyspneic. CXR during acute phase shows miliary nodular infiltrate; intercurrent CXR is normal.

Perioperative Management

Avoid high Paw_{INSP}, by using lower V_T and higher f_{RESP}. Do not use 100% oxygen (absorption atelectasis).

Kyphoscoliosis

Kyphoscoliosis is a chronic restrictive disease caused by skeletal deformities of the thorax (kypho in the AP plane; scolio in the lateral plane). Infection and emphysematous changes occur as the disease progresses. Significant curvature can cause severe pulmonary compromise, which should be evaluated with PFTs before surgery.

Myasthenia Gravis

Myasthenia gravis is a neuromuscular disorder with intermittent crises, some of which produce respiratory insufficiency or failure. Some patients in crisis will present for tracheostomy. Other patients not in crisis will present for thymectomy. There is a decrease in the number of postsynaptic acetylcholine receptors at the neuromuscular junction secondary to antibodies to the receptors. Anticholinesterase drugs are used for treatment, along with steroids, immunosuppressive medications, and plasmapheresis. Patients are sensitive to nondepolarizing neuromuscular blockers and may be resistant to succinylcholine.

Perioperative Management

Review current history for risk of aspiration. Review CXRs for acute/chronic infiltrates. Maintain euthermia. Bedside PFTs include V_T, VC, VC/V_T ratio, and $P_{INSP'}$. Adequate surgical relaxation may be provided by inhalational anesthetics. Small doses of nondepolarizing relaxants can be used with neuromuscular blockade monitoring. Postoperative respiratory failure is common, so neuromuscular and respiratory function must be closely evaluated before extubation and monitored in the PACU.

Obesity

Obesity produces a chronic restrictive disease and can lead to cor pulmonale.

Preoperative Management

PFTs are not necessarily helpful. Provide preoperative teaching for incentive spirometry and for the postoperative analgesia technique.

Intraoperative Management

Use anesthetic technique that complements postoperative analgesia and will permit extubation in OR. Avoid 100% oxygen (absorption atelectasis). Apply distending airway pressure to maintain FRC and improve oxygenation.

Postoperative Management

Initiate postoperative analgesia in PACU. Provide incentive spirometry and early ambulation. There is no evidence that prolonged ventilatory support is necessary or improves outcome. Semisitting position (if tolerated) improves spontaneous ventilation.

Pleural-based Diseases

Pleural-based diseases, which may be acute or chronic, are restrictive disorders.

Pleural Effusion, Hydrothorax. May be acute or chronic. If effusion volume is sufficient to compromise FRC, drain by thoracentesis or placement of chest tube.

Fibrothorax. Inflammatory pleural disease, empyema, incompletely drained hemothorax, or continuous exposure of the pleural surface to air (viz., bronchleural fistula) can result in fibrosis of the pleural surface, a chronic restrictive disease. During positive pressure ventilation, care must be taken to prevent pulmonary barotrauma, since the unilateral presentation of fibrothorax results in distribution of airway pressure and volume to the unaffected lung. Some patients with fibrothorax will present for decortication.

Hemothorax. Hemothorax requires chest tube placement for drainage.

Pneumothorax. See Pulmonary Barotrauma.

Pneumoconioses

Pneumoconioses are chronic restrictive diseases of several etiologies, including aluminum, asbestos, beryllium, coal dust, kaolin, silica, sugar cane, talc, and other minerals. PFTs reveal ↓ VC, ↓ RV, ↓ FRC, ↓ TLC; ↓ C_LSTATIC; ↓ D_LCO; NLFEV_1/FVC. Arterial hypoxemia occurs during exercise early in disease and is a constant finding late in disease. P_aCO_2 may be normal or decreased.

Perioperative Management

Avoid high PAW_{INSP}, by using lower V_T and higher f_{RESP}. Do not use 100% oxygen (absorption atelectasis).

Pneumonia

Pneumonia is an infective lung disease; presentation depends upon the causative organism.

Elective Surgery. Delay until treated. Then reassess temperature, WBC, and differential. CXR is not a good monitor of resolution because infiltrates may not clear for 4–8 weeks.

Emergent Surgery. Begin antibiotics; provide good hydration. Use MAC with local anesthesia or regional anesthesia when possible. In cases of acute pneumonia requiring general anesthesia, immediately after intubation, sterilely obtain a sputum specimen for culture, sensitivity, and staining. Postoperative: supplemental humidified oxygen, incentive spirometry, early ambulation.

Pregnancy

Pregnancy normally has several associated respiratory changes. Progesterone increases respiratory drive, leading to $\uparrow \dot{V}_E$ and $\uparrow \dot{V}_A$ with resulting $\downarrow P_aCO_2$; ventilation reverts to normal within the first month after delivery. During the latter half of pregnancy, lung volumes change, including $\downarrow$ RV and $\downarrow$ FRC. $\downarrow$ FRC and $\uparrow \dot{V}O_2$ can lead to more rapid onset of hypoxemia, an especially important factor during induction of general anesthesia.

Pulmonary Air Embolism

Pulmonary air embolism is acute entry of air into the venous vascular system, whereupon the air travels through the heart to the lungs. Acute $\uparrow \dot{V}_D ALV$ which results in a $\downarrow P_E'CO_2$ and an $\uparrow P_aCO_2$, if the air embolus is large. The course of an air embolus effect on alveolar dead space can be seen in the trend capnogram (Figure 11.9).

Pulmonary Barotrauma

Pulmonary barotrauma is air (or another gas) under pressure entering a potential space.

Pneumomediastinum, pneumoperitoneum, pulmonary interstitial emphysema, and subcutaneous emphysema present physical examination and/or roentgenographic findings and do not require treatment.

Pneumopericardium presents auscultatory and roentgenographic findings. As pericardial pressure approaches atrial pressures, filling volume of the heart decreases, and hemodynamic collapse can result.

Pneumothorax presents percussive, auscultatory, and roentgenographic findings.

Simple pneumothorax: intrapleural pressure $\leq$ atmospheric pressure

Tension pneumothorax: intrapleural pressure $>$ atmospheric pressure; acute process requiring chest tube (CT) placement

Do not permit chest tubes to be pulled within 24 hr preceding general anesthesia. Always connect chest drainage system to vacuum in the OR (see Chest Drainage Systems).

Pulmonary Edema

Pulmonary edema is a state of abnormal increase in lung water, occurring when capillary and interstitial forces become imbalanced, lymphatic flow becomes impaired, or capillary permeability increases. Fluid moves first into the interstitium, then into alveolar spaces. Depending upon pathophysiology, CXR appearance of increased lung water may be homogenous (ARDS), central (CHF), unilateral (hilar adenopathy, lung reexpansion), or localized (aspiration pneumonitis). Overall pathophysiology: $\downarrow$ FRC leads to mismatch $\dot{V}_A/\dot{Q}_c$ leads to $\downarrow$ P_aO_2 and S_aHbO_2.

Perioperative Management

Determine and treat etiology; increase F_IO_2 (usually ≤ 0.50); apply distending pressure.

Pulmonary Thromboembolism

Pulmonary thromboembolism is an acute pulmonary vascular disease, the pathophysiologic hallmark of which is increased alveolar dead space. Large emboli will produce pulmonary hypertension and possibly RV failure. Patients with previous thromboembolism may present on coumadin therapy or be heparinized.

Perioperative Management

When pulmonary embolism is suspected intraoperatively or postoperatively: assess risk factors; measure $P_{a-E'}CO_2$; review

$P_{E'}CO_2$ trend; measure PA pressures (if indicated); pulmonary angiography, if treatment depends on definitive diagnosis; heparinization, lysis, umbrella placement—depending upon surgical risks.

Sarcoidosis

Sarcoidosis is an inflammatory process of alveoli, small bronchi, and pulmonary vasculature, resulting in restrictive pulmonary disease in 5–10% of cases. Associated findings include noncaseating granulomata and cystic changes that can rupture, producing pneumothorax. Cardiac involvement (5% of cases) includes heart block, LV dysfunction, pericarditis, CHF, and cor pulmonale (late in disease). $\mathring{V}_A/\mathring{Q}_c$ mismatch produces hypoxemia. CXR may exhibit bilateral hilar adenopathy and/or reticulonodular infiltrates. Overall incidence is 0.04%; greater in blacks. Pulmonary problems produce most of the morbidity and mortality associated with sarcoidosis.

Perioperative Management

Continue glucocorticoids; preoperative ABG, CXR; assess/monitor cardiac function.

Sleep Apnea

Sleep apnea is a cardiorespiratory disorder producing obstructive pulmonary disease. There can be central and/or obstructive components.

Preoperative Management

History and sleep studies can indicate the severity of disease. Review history, physical examination, ECG, and CXR for evidence of pulmonary hypertension and cor pulmonale. Obtain room-air pulse oximetry baseline. Sleep apnea patients should not receive sedating premedication. Administer anticholinergic preoperatively if fiberoptic intubation is anticipated.

Intraoperative Management

Some patients come to surgery for pharyngeal reconstruction to reduce obstruction. Upper airway obstruction may make intubation difficult. Patients should be extubated when awake, because a central component of sleep apnea may persist.

Small Airways Disease

Small airways disease is an obstructive disease of the peripheral airways associated with cigarette smoking, asthma, chronic pulmonary infections, viral URIs, oxidant air pollution, and chronic exposure to irritant gases. Patients may be asymptomatic; there may be no history of respiratory insufficiency; there may be no radiologic changes. PFTs reveal $\uparrow$ RV, $\uparrow$ RV/TLC; $\downarrow$ C_LDYNAMIC, NL–$\uparrow$ C_LSTATIC; ABNL SBNT; $\uparrow$ CV, $\uparrow$ CC; NLFVC, NLFEV$_1$; $\downarrow$ FEF$_{25-75\%}$; $\downarrow$ P_aO_2; $\uparrow$ $\dot{V}_D$ALV.

Tobacco Abuse

Cigarette.   Produces small airways disease in about 50% of smokers; 10% progress to chronic bronchitis or emphysema. Patients may not become symptomatic for many pack-years. Cigarette smoking reduces FEV$_1$ ($\approx$0.094 liter per decade of smoking) and increases S_aHbCO_2 (1–10%), which can interfere with D_LCO measurements. Cessation of smoking should occur 4 weeks or more before anesthesia, to avoid rebound bronchorrhea in the perioperative period. Smokers are more likely to cough extensively at the end of cases for which they have been intubated.

Pipe, Cigar.   Increases S_aHbCO_2 (1–10%), which can interfere with D_LCO measurements.

Tuberculosis

Tuberculosis, especially multiple-drug-resistant (MDR) TB, is appearing at an increasing rate, in both pulmonary and systemic forms. Patients with untreated, active tuberculosis should not undergo elective surgery.

Preoperative Management

Obtain history of known exposure, chills, fever, night sweats, hemoptysis. Review most recent CXR; classic presentation is apical infiltrates with hilar adenopathy. Review past and present treatment (drugs, dosage, duration of treatment).

Perioperative Management

Known or suspected patients should be maintained in respiratory isolation perioperatively (negative pressure relative to corridor), which requires avoiding an open holding area. Isolation masks should be worn by the patient; personnel caring for the patient should use particulate respirators. The breathing circuit of the anesthesia machine should be protected with appropriate in-line filters. Contaminated permanent equipment should be decontaminated, cleaned, and sterilized. The patient should be recovered from anesthesia in a room designated for respiratory isolation.

PULMONARY PREPARATION

Cessation of cigarette smoking should be encouraged as far ahead of anesthesia and surgery as possible. A rebound bronchorrhea may occur in the first few days following cessation of cigarette smoking and may temporarily worsen pulmonary function.

Preoperative teaching for postoperative pulmonary therapy should be provided for all patients, since postoperatively, the patient's comprehension and attention span will be affected by pain or pain therapy.

Incentive spirometry, an inspiratory, lung-expanding maneuver, is a mainstay of postoperative pulmonary therapy. Simple incentive spirometers are satisfactory for adult patients. More elaborate electronic incentive spirometers may provide additional focus and feedback for children. Blow gloves and blow bottles should never be used.

Bronchodilator therapy that has been used at home should be continued perioperatively after drugs, dosages, and administration intervals have been reviewed for appropriateness and efficacy. New bronchodilators may need to be added to the current regimen, as indicated by the patient's recent history and current physical examination. New bronchodilator therapy or changes in existing therapy should be made 24 hr or more before the planned anesthesia and surgery, to produce the desired effect and permit sufficient time to monitor adequacy of treatment. Bronchodilator drugs include β-agonists (catecholamines, resorcinols, saligenins), methylxanthines, and anticholinergics. Method of administration is MDI or aerosol generator.

Corticosteroids (glucocorticoids) reduce airway inflammation in asthma. Prior treatment should be continued, converting to IV dosage perioperatively. Dexamethasone (4 mg) or methylprednisolone (125 mg) should be added early for patients poorly responsive to bronchodilator therapy, because effects will not be seen for 6 hr or more.

INTRAOPERATIVE MANAGEMENT

Bronchodilator therapy can be continued in the operating room, using aerosol generators or MDIs. For the patient under regional anesthesia or monitored anesthesia care, conventional administration devices can be used. For the patient under general anesthesia, an in-line injection port should be placed between the circuit and the patient's endotracheal tube connector. MDI injection should be made at the beginning of large, manually administered breaths, to facilitate deposition of the agent in the patient's airways. Four to eight injections are necessary because some of the drug will be lost in the endotracheal tube and breathing circuit. Effectiveness of bronchodilator therapy should be monitored by chest auscultation and observation of the phase-three slope of the capnogram or mass spectrogram.

Chest drainage systems (Fig. 11.10), used to remove fluids or air from the pleural space, may accompany the patient to the OR or may be placed before induction of anesthesia or during surgery. For all patients, the chest drainage system should be connected to a vacuum source in the operating room to keep the lungs completely expanded and minimize the chance of developing a tension pneumothorax.

Distending airway pressure. Place PEEP valve at the anesthesia machine connection for the expiratory limb of the anesthesia circuit. Orient the valve for the direction of gas flow; maintain valve position required for function. Greater hemodynamic embarrassment from increased intrathoracic pressure will occur in anesthetized, paralyzed patients than in spontaneously breathing patients for the same level of distending airway pressure.

Heliox. $He:O_2$ is available commercially in H cylinders as a mixture of 80:20 or 70:30. Helium 100% is available for anesthesia machines equipped with appropriate compressed gas fittings, so that a mixture of helium and oxygen can be provided together with a volatile anesthetic. F_IO_2 and S_pO_2 should always

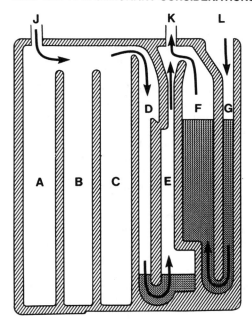

Figure 11.10. Chest drainage system. The commercial chest drainage system, Pleur-evac, contains three chambers. The first chamber provides collection of fluid drainage from the patient's chest serially into collection sections *(A, B, C)*. Air from the pleural space *(J)* moves as shown by the *arrows* through the first chamber and into the second chamber. The second chamber *(D* and *E)* serves as underwater seal. One-way valve function results from air being able to move only from section *D* into section *E*. An air leak is detected by observing bubbling in the water of section *E*. If the Pleur-evac is established as underwater seal only, this air is evacuated to the atmosphere via *K*. The third chamber *(F* and *G)* functions as a vacuum breaker. When the Pleur-evac is attached to a vacuum source via *K*, air is drawn in through vent *L* and moves through section *G*, bubbling into section *F* on its way to the vacuum source. The magnitude of negative pressure applied is a function of water depth in sections *F* and *G*. The negative pressure in the air space of section *F* is transmitted to section *E* and thereby into section *D*, and then into the air space of the collection chamber (sections *A, B, C*). (From Bonner JT, Hall JR. Respiratory intensive care of the adult surgical patient. St. Louis: CV Mosby, 1985.)

be measured when administering $He:O_2$ mixtures. Mass spectrometers should be disconnected from the breathing circuit before administering helium, to prevent loss of vacuum and instrument downtime.

High-frequency ventilation (HFV) can be applied to spontaneously breathing or apneic patients under anesthesia. In some centers, HFV is used routinely for lithotripsy, neurovascular surgery, and certain laryngoscopic and bronchoscopic procedures. For airway surgery, HFV may be provided via catheter, laryngoscope, or bronchoscope. For other surgery, the HFV ventilator should be incorporated into the conventional circuit of the anesthesia machine so that all monitors (F_IO_2, pressure, temperature) remain intact.

Supplemental oxygen during monitored anesthesia care and regional anesthesia can be provided via nasal cannula (1–4 liters/min) or simple face mask (8–12 liters/min). Capnography should be used to monitor respiratory rate and level of ventilation (Fig. 11.10).

Thoracic surgery. A major concern of lung resection—lobectomy or pneumonectomy—is that the patient not develop postoperative dyspnea or cor pulmonale. PFTs are used to identify operable candidates.

Conventional PFTs

Preoperative FEV_1 should be greater than 40% of predicted.

Split Lung Function

Percentage function for each lung can be assessed by using perfusion scanning and radiospirometry to determine relative blood flow and ventilation for each lung. Postoperative FEV_1 can be predicted. The minimum acceptable predicted FEV_1 is 800 ml.

Endobronchial intubation provides separation of right and left lungs, which is used for pneumonectomy, lobectomy, resection of thoracic aortic aneurysm, esophagogastric resection, and surgical and nonsurgical treatment of unilateral pulmonary infections. Right- and left-sided endobronchial tubes are available, although use of left-sided tubes is easier and safer. Endotracheal tubes with indwelling bronchial blocking catheters are also available. Conventional endobronchial tubes can be placed

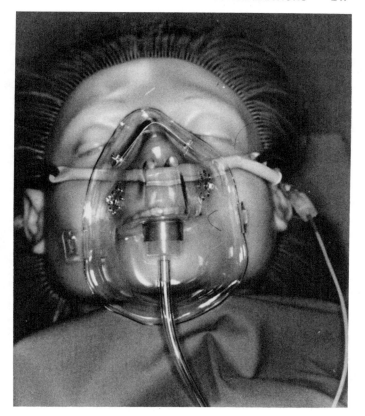

Figure 11.11. Capnography setup for the awake patient. Good fidelity in capnographic waveform can be obtained by sampling through nasal cannula while providing supplemental oxygen via simple face mask.

and tested by physical examination. Flexible fiberoptic bronchoscopes can also be used to confirm the position of conventional endobronchial tubes and are mandatory when using endotracheal tubes with bronchial blocker.

One-lung anesthesia can be provided with endobronchial tubes or endotracheal tubes with bronchial blocker. Ventilation should be provided with V_T = 8–12 ml/kg and f_{RESP} = 6–10/min, maintaining eucapnia. If possible, some inspired nitrogen (air) should be provided to promote "nitrogen splinting" and prevent microatelectasis. F_IO_2 of 0.8 usually is tolerated; S_pO_2 should be monitored continuously. Distending airway pressure can be applied to the nondependent lung to enhance oxygenation; application to the dependent lung is less efficacious.

Postoperative pain relief can be initiated during thoracotomy by performing intercostal nerve blocks or placing a pleural infusion catheter.

POSTOPERATIVE RESPIRATORY CARE

Bronchodilator Therapy

Bronchodilator therapy should be continued in the PACU. Postoperative orders for bronchodilators should be written before patient discharge from the PACU.

CXR

CXR should be obtained in the PACU for

- Suspected new acute pulmonary disease or change in chronic pulmonary disease
- Cardiothoracic surgery patients, to assess for lung expansion and pleural processes
- Assessing placement of chest tubes, NG tubes, and vascular catheters and ruling out associated complications
- Patients with a new tracheostomy to rule out pneumothorax; the most information can be obtained from an *upright* portable CXR taken in *full inspiration*; the exception is ruling out pneumothorax, for which the upright CXR should be shot in expiration

Incentive spirometry should be ordered every 2–4 hr while awake for patients at risk for atelectasis, including thoracoabdominal surgery patients, obese patients, and patients with chronic lung disease. Accompany incentive spirometry with bronchodilator therapy if appropriate. Continue a patient's supplemental oxygen during incentive spirometry using nasal cannula.

Mask CPAP can be used for awake, cooperative patients who require CPAP ≤ 15 cm H_2O. Application can be continuous or 15 min of each hour. Use a face mask with an air cushion rim or J-type seal. Patients with maxillofacial trauma or surgery of the upper aerodigestive tract are not candidates for mask CPAP. Nasogastric tube is not required but, if present, can be routed through the mask.

Supplemental oxygen is used routinely in the PACU to prevent hypoxemia, especially hypoxia due to hypoventilation, which can be seen in many patients immediately following anesthesia and surgery. Routes of delivery include aerosol face mask, face shield, or nasal cannula. Humidification should always be provided for patients who have undergone surgery of the upper airway and for patients with chronic lung disease.

SYMBOLS AND TERMINOLOGY

Lung Volumes and Capacities; Gas Flow; Pulmonary Mechanics

C_L, lung compliance
C_T, thoracic compliance
C_{LT}, total, or lung-thorax, compliance
CC, closing capacity
CV, closing volume
$D_L co$, diffusing capacity of the lung for carbon monoxide
ERV, expiratory reserve volume
$FEF_{25-75\%}$, forced expiratory flow by percentage
$FEF_{200-1200ml}$, forced expiratory flow by volume
FEV_1, forced expiratory volume in 1 sec
FRC, function residual capacity
FVC, forced vital capacity
IC, inspiratory capacity
IRV, inspiratory reserve volume
MMFR, maximal midexpiratory flow rate
R_{AW}, airway resistance
RV, residual volume
SBNT, single-breath nitrogen test
TLC, total lung capacity
TV, V_T, tidal volume
VC, vital capacity

Special Symbols and Abbreviations

• above symbol denotes *per unit time*
′ after symbol denotes end
— above symbol denotes *mixed* or *mean*

T, temperature[a]
TM, transmural[a]
MECH, mechanical[a]
PL, pleural[a]

Molecular Species

CO_2, carbon dioxide
H_2O, water
N_2, nitrogen
O_2, oxygen

Symbols for the Blood Phase (subscript to primary symbol)

a, arterial
c, capillary
PLS, plasma
t, total
v, venous
WB, whole blood
s, shunt

Symbols for the Gas Phase (subscript to primary symbol or modifier)

A, alveolar
AW, airway
BAR, barometric
D, dead space
E, expired
I, inspired
PL, pleural
T, tidal
t, total
ALV[b], alveolar
ANAT[b], anatomic
PHYSIOL[b], physiologic

[a] Subscripts.
[b] Denotes dead space compartment.

Primary Symbols

C, content or concentration in blood phase

C_aO_2, arterial oxygen content

CcO_2, carbon dioxide content (phase not stated)

F, fractional concentration

F_IO_2, fractional concentration of inspired oxygen

F_ACO_2, fractional concentration of alveolar carbon dioxide

f, frequency

f_{PT}, patient's spontaneous respiratory rate

f_{MECH}, mechanical ventilator rate

M, amount of a molecular species in the blood phase

$\dot{M}_aO_2$, systemic arterial oxygen transport

$\dot{M}_{\bar{v}}O_2$, systemic mixed venous oxygen transport

P, pressure or partial pressure

P_{H2O}, water vapor pressure (gas phase or blood phase)

P_aO_2, partial pressure of oxygen in the alveoli

$P_E{'}CO_2$, end-tidal carbon dioxide partial pressure

P_{bar}, barometric pressure

$P\bar{v}O_2$, mixed venous oxygen partial pressure

Q, amount of blood

Q_t, total blood flow, or cardiac output

S, saturation

S_aHbO_2, arterial oxyhemoglobin saturation

S_aHbCO, arterial carboxyhemoglobin saturation

S_pO_2, oxyhemoglobin saturation by pulse oximeter

V, volume of gas

V_T, tidal volume

$\dot{V}_E$, minute ventilation

$\dot{V}_A$, alveolar ventilation

$\dot{V}_{DALV}$, alveolar dead space ventilation

$\dot{V}O_2$, oxygen consumption

$\dot{V}_{DANAT}$, anatomic dead space ventilation

Other symbols

Hb, hemoglobin

[Hb], hemoglobin concentration

Hct, hematocrit

O_2UC, oxygen utilization coefficient

R   RER, respiratory exchange ratio; represents activity in the lungs

RQ, respiratory quotient; represents activity in the tissues
Under steady state condidtions, RER = RQ

Units of Measure

cm H_2O, centimeters of water; a unit of measure for pressure

mm Hg, millimeters of mercury; a relative unit of measure for pressure

torr, 1/760 of a standard atmosphere; an abolute unit of measure for pressure

vol%, volumes percent; ml of a gas per 100 ml (dl) of whole blood

Chapter 12

Anesthesia for Patients with Renal or Urinary Tract Disease

Renal function is central to fluid homeostasis and maintenance of intravascular volume in the perioperative period. An appreciation of normal renal anatomy and physiology is essential to the understanding of renal dysfunction. The anesthesiologist must be able to recognize the pathophysiology of renal disease in order to provide appropriate pre-, intra-, and postoperative anesthetic care.

ANATOMY AND PHYSIOLOGY

The kidney is very active metabolically, receiving about **25% of total cardiac output** (1250 ml/min), while comprising less than 1% of body mass. Normal glomerular filtration rate (GFR) averages 125 ml/min in the adult, with more than 99% of the filtrate reabsorbed. Approximately 60–70% of the glomerular filtrate is reabsorbed in the proximal tubule. Urine flow is about 2 liters/day. **Adequate intraoperative urine flow** is 0.5–1.0 ml/kg/min.

Glomerular Filtration

Glomerular filtration is determined by hydrostatic forces: P_{GC} (pressure in the glomerular capillary) and P_{BC} (pressure in the Bowman's capsule); oncotic pressures, π_{GC} and π_{BC}; and permeability of the glomerular membrane, K_f, glomerular filtration coefficient according the following formula:

$$GFR = K_f[(P_{GC} - P_{BC}) - (\pi_{GC} - \pi_{BC})]$$

Hypotension (by decreasing P_{GC}) and increases in plasma oncotic pressure reduce the GFR. The range of renal autoregulation is 60–160 mm Hg mean arterial pressure.

Hormones

Aldosterone—Salt transport in the distal convoluted tubule is regulated by aldosterone, which stimulates sodium and chloride reabsorption and potassium secretion.

Antidiuretic hormone (ADH) increases free water reabsorption in the distal portions of the distal convoluted tubule and in the collecting ducts. ADH is synthesized by the anterior hypothalamus and is released in response to increasing plasma osmolarity. At higher concentrations, ADH, arginine vasopressin, is a potent vasoconstrictor. When atrial stretch receptors are activated by an increase in blood volume, ADH release is inhibited.

Renin-angiotensin—The juxtaglomerular apparatus (JGA) is formed by the afferent and efferent arterioles in close proximity to a specialized portion of the distal convoluted tubule called the macula densa. The JGA releases renin in response to sympathetic nervous system stimulation, decreased renal perfusion pressure, or decreased sodium chloride delivery to the macula densa. **Renin,** a proteolytic enzyme, converts circulating **angiotensinogen** to **angiotensin I.** Angiotensin-converting enzyme in the lung then converts angiotensin I to **angiotensin II,** a vasoconstrictor that also stimulates the adrenal cortex to produce and release aldosterone.

Prostaglandins PGE_2 and PGI_2, prostacyclin, are produced in the renal medulla and act locally to modulate vasoconstrictor influences on the kidney.

Natriuretic peptides—Atrial natriuretic peptide, one of several natriuretic peptides, is secreted by the atria as they are stretched by increasing intravascular volume. The hormone relaxes vascular smooth muscle to reduce blood pressure and inhibits renin and aldosterone secretion, which promotes renal sodium loss.

Erythropoietin produced by the kidney stimulates red cell production by the bone marrow.

RENAL EFFECTS OF ANESTHESIA
Regional Anesthesia

Regional anesthesia with subarachnoid block or epidural has little effect on renal function when perfusion pressure is maintained. The renal cortex receives sympathetic input from the celiac and renal plexus with fibers originating from T4 to L1. Sympathetic block produced by major conduction anesthesia can impair renal vasoconstrictor responses to stress, helping to maintain renal blood flow.

General Anesthesia

General anesthesia is associated with a decrease in urine flow, GFR, renal blood flow (RBF), and sodium excretion. The exact mechanisms are not entirely clear but may be related to cardiovascular effects of inhalational anesthetics, changes in the sympathetic nervous system, hormonal alterations, or stress response from surgical stimulation. Circulating catecholamines, released in response to surgical stress and exacerbated by hypovolemia, increase renal vascular resistance, decreasing RBF and GFR. Aldosterone release leads to sodium retention and decreased urine output. Antidiuretic hormone, released in response to surgical stress, may reduce urine flow. Renal dysfunction persists only during the administration of anesthesia unless the patient is hypovolemic or has cardiovascular instability postoperatively.

Halothane

Halothane has been used for many of the studies on renal anesthetic effects. Halothane increases RBF in isolated kidneys and has no effect on renal autoregulation in vitro.

Methoxyflurane

Methoxyflurane may produce nephrotoxicity from a metabolite, inorganic fluoride ion (F^-). Renal damage from exposure to F^- is dose-related, with clinical nephrotoxicity noted with a serum F^- level above 50 μM/liter. **Fluoride-induced renal insufficiency** is characterized by inappropriate diuresis with hypoosmolar urine causing increased serum sodium and osmolarity.

The kidneys fail to respond to ADH or water loading, indicating both diluting and concentrating defects. Several factors predispose a patient to F^--induced nephrotoxicity, including *(a)* **enzyme induction,** as occurs with administration of isoniazid leading to increased mixed oxidase function and anesthetic metabolism (there is no direct evidence in man that barbiturates increase F^- production); *(b)* concomitant administration of other **nephrotoxic drugs** (aminoglycosides), which may exacerbate renal damage caused by the F^- ion; *(c)* **obesity;** *(d)* **age** (lower levels of F^- are produced in children); *(e)* **individual variation** in the metabolism and renal sensitivity to F^- from genetic factors; and *(f)* **preexisting renal disease.**

Enflurane

Enflurane is also metabolized to F^- although at a rate approximately 1/20th that of methoxyflurane and 1/10th that of halothane, resulting in much lower F^- levels. There have been occasional reports of fluoride nephrotoxicity after enflurane, usually in patients with risk factors as above. The low serum level of F^- after enflurane may reduce the maximum renal concentrating effect, as demonstrated by administration of exogenous ADH. Like other inhalational anesthetics, enflurane decreases RBF, GFR, and urine output.

Isoflurane

Isoflurane produces minimal effect on RBF but decreases GFR and urine output. It undergoes very little metabolism, with approximately 0.2% excreted as urinary metabolites, and has not been associated with nephrotoxicity.

Intravenous Anesthetics

Thiopental does not change RBF. Even with the hemodynamic effects at high doses, RBF is not altered because of a decrease in renal vascular resistance. In laboratory animals, thiopental reduces urine flow and GFR.

Narcotics do not reduce RBF, although fentanyl decreases GFR and urine flow.

PATHOPHYSIOLOGY OF CHRONIC RENAL FAILURE

Stages of Renal Insufficiency

Progressive renal insufficiency can be classified into several stages as noted by Weir and Chung. **Creatinine,** a product of muscle metabolism, is freely filtered by the glomerulus and is neither reabsorbed nor significantly secreted; therefore it can be used to measure glomerular filtration rate. Serum creatinine concentrations are not a sensitive measure of renal function without knowledge of baseline values because the range of normal values is quite wide (0.7–1.5 mg/dl). **Creatine clearance** (CrCl) gives the most reliable assessment of GFR. Mild dysfunction is present when CrCl is 50–80 ml/min, moderate disease with CrCl less than 25 ml/min, and when CrCl is less than 10 ml/min, the patient is functionally anephric. **Serum BUN** changes with diet, hydration states, and rate of urine flow and is not a good indicator of renal function.

1. **Decreased renal reserve** is generally asymptomatic. Laboratory data are likely within normal limits, and up to 50–60% of nephron mass may be lost without the serum creatinine concentration being elevated into an abnormal range.
2. **Renal insufficiency** is characterized by mild azotemia, hypertension, and anemia. The ability to concentrate urine is compromised, which leads to nocturia and polyuria.
3. Frank **renal failure** occurs with a GFR less than 20% of normal. There will likely be hypertension, anemia, metabolic acidosis, fluid overload, and electrolyte abnormalities (e.g., hyperkalemia, hyperphosphatemia).
4. **End-stage renal failure** with uremia is a multisystem disease requiring dialysis to remove metabolic waste products and correct fluid, electrolyte, and acid-base abnormalities. There is an inability to respond to changing sodium and water intake.

Multisystem Effects of End-Stage Renal Failure

Cardiovascular

Cardiovascular changes are common.

1. **Hypertension** develops secondary to salt and water retention or from excess renin, and often is controlled with-

out medication by intravascular volume regulation by dialysis.

2. **Left ventricular hypertrophy** may result from long-standing hypertension and lead to decreased contractility and increased susceptibility to congestive heart failure (CHF). Chronic anemia also results in a requirement for increased cardiac output to maintain oxygen delivery to tissues.
3. **Coronary atherosclerosis**
4. **Pericardial effusion or pericarditis** may be present in uremic patients or those with fluid overload. The effusion may be hemodynamically significant.
5. **Uremic cardiomyopathy** may contribute to CHF.
6. **Autonomic neuropathy** may impair sympathetic response to hypovolemia or produce orthostatic hypotension.

Respiratory

1. **Pulmonary edema or pleural effusions** may be present in patients with fluid overload or cardiomyopathy.
2. **Pulmonary infections** may be more common because of immunosuppression in renal failure.
3. **Difficult airway management**—Patients with CRF from diabetes mellitus have an increased likelihood of difficult intubation.

Nervous System

1. **Peripheral neuropathies** are often present, especially involving the common peroneal and median nerves. This can include paresthesias, weakness, and sensory deficits.
2. **Seizures** may occur secondary to uremia, hypertension, and cerebral edema.
3. **Uremic encephalopathy**

Gastrointestinal

1. **Delayed gastric emptying** leads to increased gastric volume.
2. **Nausea, vomiting, and recurrent hiccups**
3. **Gastrointestinal bleeding**

Hepatic

1. **Hepatitis B** is more common in hemodialysis patients. The prevalence of hepatitis B virus carriers is greater in hemodialysis patients than in the general population.

2. **Chronic hepatic congestion** caused by CHF.
3. **Hemosiderosis** in patients who have had multiple transfusions

Hemopoietic and Immunologic

1. Normochromic, normocytic **anemia** with usual hematocrits averaging 15–25%. Although primarily caused by a decrease in erythropoietin, decreased red cell half-life and increased membrane fragility contribute to the anemia. Compensatory responses include increased cardiac output and shift of the oxyhemoglobin dissociation curve to the right secondary to metabolic acidosis and increased 2, 3-DPG.
2. **Platelet dysfunction** is common and is characterized by decreased platelet adhesiveness, possibly leading to a prolonged template bleeding time. Platelet factor III activity may be reduced. DDAVP may be useful in correcting platelet dysfunction.
3. Hypoalbuminemia, especially in patients with loss of protein in the urine, may contribute to peripheral edema and affect intravenous drug distribution.
4. **Immunosuppression and decreased WBC phagocytosis** puts patients at risk for infection.

Endocrine System

Secondary hyperparathyroidism and uremic osteodystrophy from abnormalities in calcium metabolism. In severe cases there may be calcinosis with systemic calcium deposits. Patients with osteodystrophy are at increased risk of spontaneous bone fractures and fractures during positioning in the operating room.

Acid-Base and Electrolyte Disturbances

1. **Metabolic acidosis** is generally present when GFR is less than 25% of normal. Serum bicarbonate will be low, with a compensatory decrease in arterial Pco_2. The anion gap increases with worsening disease as sulfates and phosphates accumulate.
2. **Hyperkalemia** is rarely a problem until GFR is less than 5 ml/min but may be made worse by increased K^+ load from endogenous (trauma, infection, gastrointestinal bleeding) or exogenous (transfusion) sources.

3. **Hypermagnesemia** may develop with excess intake (e.g., Mg^{2+}-containing antacids).
4. **Serum calcium** may be elevated or abnormally low, depending on parathyroid function.
5. **Hyperphosphatemia**
6. **Hyponatremia** from inability to excrete free water.

ANESTHETIC MANAGEMENT OF PATIENTS WITH CHRONIC RENAL FAILURE

Preoperative Assessment

Preoperative assessment for the abnormalities known to occur in CRF (see above) should be part of the initial evaluation, and these conditions should be considered in optimizing the patient for surgery.

Dialysis

For patients maintained on **hemodialysis,** identify the usual schedule, the date of last dialysis, and how close they are to their "dry weight." Optimally, patients should receive dialysis within 24 hours of surgery. Hemodialysis immediately before surgery may result in a low intravascular volume if fluid is taken off and may produce hypotension on induction of anesthesia. Residual anticoagulants may prolong clotting. Laboratory values after hemodialysis should be available to ensure that electrolyte and metabolic abnormalities have been corrected. During the perioperative period, the patient's vascular access (AV graft, etc.) should be protected to prevent thrombosis from compression or low-flow states. **Percutaneous temporary vascular access devices for hemodialysis** (Vascath) should not be used for routine IV access except in a life-threatening emergency, and then it must be remembered that the catheter may contain high-dose heparin, which should be withdrawn before infusing fluids through the catheter.

Patients on **chronic peritoneal dialysis** should have their dialysis fluid drained before coming to the OR.

Premedication

Patients with advanced disease may exhibit increased sensitivity to sedative medications as well as decreased clearance of these drugs. Supplemental oxygen therapy may be indicated in patients with anemia and decreased oxygen-carrying capacity. H_2 antagonists and/or metoclopramide might be used in patients with gastroparesis.

Intraoperative Management

Monitoring

Monitoring considerations should be based on the surgery to be performed as well as the pathology in the specific patient. **Intraarterial catheterization** is useful for continuous blood pressure measurement and for frequent determination of hematocrit, acid-base, and electrolytes. Unfortunately, **IV access** and placement of A-line are often difficult in patients who have had multiple vascular access procedures in their arms. These devices, along with BP cuffs, should not be placed in an extremity used for vascular access for hemodialysis. This often means that an IV must be started in the neck or lower extremity. Measurement of **central venous pressure** may be useful for fluid management.

Positioning

1. Protect AV graft—Usually the arm should not be tucked, so that the patency can be frequently assessed.
2. Pad extremities to prevent further neural damage with neuropathy.

Fluid Management

With significant renal dysfunction, inability to excrete both free water and sodium are likely, so use of isotonic IV fluids with a sodium concentration of approximately 140 mEq/liter is best. Fluids should be given as necessary to maintain cardiovascular stability, with the realization that postoperative dialysis may be required to remove fluid after the effects of anesthesia are terminated.

Anesthetics

1. **Intravenous agents**—Most intravenous anesthetics are weak electrolytes, lipid-soluble, and readily reabsorbed from the

renal tubule. Biotransformation, most often by the liver, produces water-soluble, polar, usually inactive forms that are excreted by the kidney. For most drugs, dosage requirements are decreased in severe renal disease.

a. **Belladonna alkaloids:** Approximately 20–50% of atropine and glycopyrrolate are recovered unchanged or as active metabolites in the urine. About 10% of scopolamine is thus recovered.

b. **Thiopental** is extensively (75–85%) bound to albumin, which is decreased in uremia. Thiopental's pKa is 7.6; therefore acidosis increases the un-ionized, active form. These two factors lead to an increased free, active form, and dosage requirements may be decreased 25–50%. The blood-brain barrier may also be defective in the uremic state, allowing higher central nervous system concentrations. Metabolism is hepatic and unchanged.

c. **Narcotics:** Metabolism of narcotics occurs in the liver, and these drugs are highly protein-bound. Theoretically, duration and dose should be unchanged; however, there have been reports of prolonged respiratory depression with morphine in patients with renal failure. The duration of morphine's action may be prolonged secondary to active metabolites. Only 7% of fentanyl is excreted unchanged in the urine. Normeperidine, an active metabolite of meperidine, is renally excreted and may accumulate with repeat doses. It can cause CNS irritability, twitching, and seizure activity.

d. **Benzodiazepines** are extensively metabolized in the liver before excretion. They are less protein-bound than thiopental, and dosages need less adjustment. However, the debilitated patient with end-stage renal disease may be more sensitive to the depressant effects of benzodiazepine premedication.

e. **Ketamine** produces either no change in RBF or minimal decrease in RBF and urine output. It undergoes hepatic metabolism and renal excretion. Use with caution in patients with coexisting hypertension or cardiac disease.

2. **Inhalational agents** are useful for patients with renal insufficiency; because their elimination does not depend on renal function, they can be given with a high FIO_2, and they potentiate nondepolarizing muscle relaxants. Because of the

possibility of fluoride nephrotoxicity worsening renal function, enflurane should be avoided in patients with mild-to-moderate renal insufficiency. Myocardial depression may limit the use of these agents in patients with significant myocardial dysfunction.

3. **Regional anesthesia**—Platelet dysfunction is associated with chronic renal disease, and adequate coagulation status should be documented before undertaking regional anesthesia. Patients with recent hemodialysis may be hypovolemic and require fluid boluses before spinal or epidural anesthesia. **Brachial plexus block** is often useful for placement of vascular access for hemodialysis in the upper extremity. The duration of these blocks is likely to be reduced in patients with renal failure because of increased cardiac output and clearance of local anesthetic from tissues. Metabolic acidosis may decrease the seizure threshold associated with local anesthetics.

Muscle Relaxants

Succinylcholine is metabolized by pseudocholinesterase to succinylmonocholine, which has nondepolarizing neuromuscular blocking activity and is excreted by the kidney. Therefore, large doses of succinylcholine should be avoided with significant renal disease. A dose of 1 mg/kg normally produces a rise of 0.5–0.7 mEq/liter in serum potassium (K^+) level. The K^+ release is not exaggerated in renal failure, so when the serum K^+ is less than 5.0 mEq/liter, it is probably safe to use succinylcholine if indicated by the clinical situation. Patients exhibiting uremic neuropathy may have increased K^+ release; therefore succinylcholine should be avoided.

The dose of **nondepolarizing muscle relaxants** required may be reduced because of decreased muscle mass in many renal patients. Relaxant activity is potentiated by respiratory and metabolic acidosis as well as hypokalemia, hypermagnesemia, hypocalcemia, furosemide, and mannitol. The effects of all neuromuscular blocking agents should be monitored with a peripheral nerve stimulator, and dosages administered accordingly.

- **d-Tubocurarine:** There is not apparent increased sensitivity, but ganglion-blocking activity and vasodilation can lead to significant reduction in blood pressure. Elimination half-life is slightly increased in renal failure, as 45% is excreted in the urine.

- **Pancuronium** is metabolized to weakly active forms with 40–50% renal excretion. Elimination half-life is prolonged, and dosing should be adjusted accordingly.
- **Metocurine** activity is markedly prolonged in patients with renal dysfunction and probably is not suitable in these patients. More than 90% of **gallamine** is excreted unchanged in the urine. It is therefore contraindicated in the presence of significant renal disease.
- **Vecuronium,** a monoquaternary homologue of pancuronium, has higher biliary excretion rates, and the elimination half-life does not appear to be significantly prolonged in renal disease, although 30% is excreted in the urine. The effect and duration of the initial dose are unchanged with renal insufficiency, but subsequent doses should be reduced.
- **Atracurium** undergoes nonenzymatic Hoffman elimination and enzymatic ester hydrolysis. It does not depend on renal function for elimination, and therefore onset, duration, and elimination are unchanged with renal disease. Laudanosine, a metabolite, is renally excreted, and increased serum levels may cause CNS stimulation and seizures, although this has not been reported in clinical use.
- **Doxacurium** elimination is prolonged with renal insufficiency, and it probably should not be used.
- **Pipecuronium's** duration of action is not prolonged with renal failure, but it probably is less suitable than the intermediate-acting muscle relaxants for use in patients with renal insufficiency.

Table 12.1
Clinical Situations with Increased Risk for Acute Renal Failure

Open heart surgery
Abdominal aortic or renal artery surgery
Major abdominal surgery
Severe trauma
Severe liver failure
Sepsis, especially with multiple organ failure
Neonatal ICU admission
Aminoglycoside drug administration

Anticholinesterases

Anticholinesterases are primarily excreted by the kidneys, and elimination is prolonged with renal insufficiency. This is favorable, since it may protect against the possible prolonged effect of some nondepolarizing muscle relaxants. Adequate relaxant reversal must be confirmed by clinical signs and full return of sustained tetanus using the peripheral nerve stimulator.

PREVENTION OF ACUTE RENAL FAILURE IN THE PERIOPERATIVE PERIOD

The anesthesiologist plays a major role in the prevention of renal injury. It is important to maintain optimal hemodynamic status, cardiovascular function, and intravascular volume. Several risk categories for perioperative acute renal failure (ARF) have been identified (Table 12.1). Prevention of ARF is critical because mortality in the perioperative setting is about 50% in spite of hemodialysis and other therapies.

Diagnosis

Urine production decreases perioperatively because of angiotensin, vasopressin, and catecholamines liberated during surgery, as well as intravascular fluid shifts. The GFR is reduced during general anesthesia but returns to normal postoperatively. Oliguria, a urine output below 0.5 ml/kg/hr, may reflect

Table 12.2
Causes of Oliguria

Prerenal
    1. ↓ Cardiac output
    2. Hypotension
    3. Hypovolemia
Renal
    1. Acute tubular necrosis
    2. Nephrotoxic agents
    3. Rhabdomyolysis
    4. Transfusion reaction
Postrenal
    1. Stones
    2. Obstructed Foley catheter
    3. Bladder outlet obstruction

Table 12.3
Diagnostic Tests for Acute Renal Failure

	Prerenal	Acute Tubular Necrosis
Urine Na$^+$ (mEq/liter)	<20	>40
Urine osmolarity (mosm/liter)	>500	<350
Urine/plasma creatinine	>40	<20

these changes or represent a significant impairment of renal perfusion (Table 12.2). If oliguria is not treated, postsurgical renal failure, with its high mortality, may result. Laboratory tests to differentiate prerenal oliguria from acute renal failure caused by tubular necrosis (Table 12.3) are neither sensitive, specific, or speedy enough to be useful in the operating room, although 2-hour creatinine clearances are used in ICUs. Urine output appears to be the only reasonable monitor available to follow renal function intraoperatively.

Before aggressive means to promote diuresis are used, the proper location and function of the bladder catheter must be verified. The catheter must be inspected and irrigated.

Treatment

Common clinical signs of inadequate circulating volume may be unreliable during anesthesia. Surgical patients often have a diminished intravascular volume, so a **fluid bolus** should be given. Depending on the patient's cardiac status, 250–500 ml of crystalloid should be rapidly infused and repeated after 20 minutes. It is not uncommon to administer more than 1 liter of fluid before diuresis occurs.

If the patient is at high risk of developing pulmonary edema or if several fluid challenges have not increased the urine output, central venous or pulmonary artery catheterization is warranted to help guide further fluid therapy. Filling pressure data may dictate administration of more fluid, diuretics, or inotropic support. Dopamine, in doses of 2–5 μg/kg/min, is the inotrope of choice and may increase renal blood flow and promote a diuresis.

Diuretics do not improve outcome in renal failure and are generally not useful for treating oliguria. Exceptions include

1. Episodes of rhabdomyolysis or hemolysis (mannitol)
2. Volume overload
3. Prior to ischemic insult (i.e., aortic or renal artery cross-clamping)—(mannitol)

ANESTHESIA FOR GENITOURINARY PROCEDURES

Kidney and Ureter

Nephrectomy

Nephrectomy may be performed for tumor, infection, or hypertension from renal artery ischemia, or the kidney may be removed for transplantation into a related recipient. The patient is usually in the flank or lateral decubitus position with the kidney rest raised. This position may lead to hypotension from decreased venous return, increased venous pressure in the upper body, and ventilation-perfusion mismatching. Renal tumors may be very vascular, and adequate venous access is necessary in this situation. Also, some renal tumors may extend into the inferior vena cava and may require clamping this vessel for removal. Adequate monitoring and lines for rapid fluid administration should be used in this situation.

Renal Transplantation

The organ may come from a living related patient or cadaveric donor. Treatment of the recipient should be similar to that of patients with chronic renal failure (see above), especially with a cadaveric organ, because ARF with oliguria may occur in the immediate postoperative period.

Monitoring: Intraarterial catheterization and measurement of central venous pressure is useful for optimizing fluid volume and hemodynamics. The CVP should be maintained around 10–14 mm Hg before revascularization of the new kidney to promote renal perfusion.

Anesthesia: General or regional anesthesia is appropriate for renal transplantation. The renal vessels are usually anastamosed to the iliac artery and vein, so at least a T6 block is necessary with a regional technique. Systemic pressure should be maintained in a range that is high enough to ensure adequate perfusion of the transplanted organ but not produce vascular injury. Mannitol (0.5–1.0 g/kg) and often furosemide are given before renal reperfusion. Steroids (usually methylprednisolone) are administered early to aid with immunosuppression. Reperfusion of the kidney may produce an acute increase in serum potassium, so the K^+ concentration before this should be kept low. If the transplanted kidney begins to function after reperfusion, urine output should be adequately replaced along with other ongoing losses to ensure that cardiac preload is sufficient. For nonfunctioning organs, dopamine may be useful to increase cardiac output and perfusion pressure to optimize hemodynamics and to ensure adequate RBF.

Extracorporeal Shock Wave Lithotripsy

Extracorporeal shock wave lithotripsy (ESWL) is a procedure in which shock waves focused from a generator are used to break renal or ureteral stones into small fragments that can be passed in the urine. Contraindications to ESWL include morbid obesity, cardiac pacemaker, coagulation disorders, abdominal aortic aneurysm, and pregnancy. Anesthesia is required for the pain produced by early-generation lithotriptors that have poorly focused shock waves. Refinements in the technology have made anesthesia unnecessary with later versions of the equipment.

1. **Positioning**—With the earlier generation of lithotriptors, the patient is placed in a semi-sitting gantry and lowered into a tub of water that is used as the conducting medium for the shock waves. When in the final position, only the head, neck, and shoulders remain out of the water. After assuming the upright position, the venous return is initially reduced, possibly producing systemic hypotension, but when the patient is lowered into the water bath, the external compression by the water usually increases central blood volume and restores blood pressure. Devices contacting the patient should be waterproofed (IV site, ECG leads, etc.) to prevent contamination and ensure continued function. Electrical devices contacting the patient should be battery-powered to prevent electroshock injury.

2. **Arrhythmias**—The timing of the shock waves is synchronized by the R wave of the ECG, since arrhythmias may occur if

the shock is delivered during a vulnerable period of the cardiac cycle. Patients with pacemakers should probably not undergo ESWL because of the possibility of serious arrhythmias.

3. Anesthesia for ESWL using earlier-generation lithotriptors could be either general with endotracheal intubation or regional. Because of the variable length of the procedure, a **continuous epidural** is often used with analgesia to at least T6. The sympathectomy produced by this level of blockade may lead to hypotension when the patient is placed in the gantry before immersion, and therefore adequate hydration and temporary pharmacologic vasoconstriction are required. With regional anesthesia, awake patients can use their arms to assist with the transfer to the gantry and can help with positioning to avoid brachial plexus injuries. Some patients prefer **general anesthesia,** and in others, regional techniques are contraindicated. Although not general practice, some centers use high-frequency ventilation with general anesthesia so that the renal stone is not intermittently moved out of the focus of the shock wave by positive pressure ventilation.

Bladder

Cystoscopy may be performed for diagnostic purposes or for transurethral resection of bladder tumors. IV sedation with topical anesthetic jelly to the urethra or regional or general anesthesia can be used for diagnostic cystoscopy, but resections require regional or general. Since sensory innervation of the bladder is T9 to L2, a T9–10 analgesic level is necessary for spinal anesthesia. If retrograde pyelograms or ureteral stone extraction is performed, a sensory level of T6 is usually necessary with regional anesthesia.

    Cystectomy is a major operative procedure in which the bladder is removed for tumor and a conduit for urine (often an ileal conduit) is created. Usually general anesthesia is preferable for this long procedure. Patients are often hypovolemic preoperatively from bowel preparation and malnutrition. Intraoperatively, there may be large blood losses with the actual cystectomy, followed by major third space loss with bowel dissection. Urine output is not available as a measure of intravascular volume during the period when the bladder has been removed and the ureters are draining into the abdomen. For these reasons, invasive hemodynamic monitoring is often used.

Prostate

1. **Open prostatectomy** is indicated with larger glands (>100 gm) and can be performed via a perineal approach with the patient in the lithotomy position or retropubic approach with the patient supine. General or regional anesthesia may be appropriate for either, but with the open perineal prostatectomy, the patient is in a head-down, lithotomy position, which may compromise respiration with a regional anesthetic technique. Blood loss is usually greater with the retropubic approach, with most occurring when the prostate is removed.

2. **Transurethral prostatectomy** (TURP) is performed for bladder outlet obstruction from prostatic hypertrophy or for prostatic carcinoma. During the resection, continuous irrigation is used to allow visualization and distend the bladder. The irrigation solution is absorbed via the open venous channels created in the prostate, and therefore hypotonic preparations, which would produce hemolysis or water intoxication, are not used. Electrolyte solutions cannot be used for irrigation because they would disperse the current necessary to resect and coagulate the gland. The most commonly used irrigating solutions are nonelectrolytic and consist of sorbitol and mannitol or glycine. These are hypoosmolar and may cause symptomatic hyponatremia or fluid overload if absorbed in large volumes. This is prevented by limiting resection time (< 1 hr) and not raising the irrigation containers too high, which would increase the hydrostatic pressure of the infusion.

   a. **Anesthesia**—General or regional anesthesia can be used successfully for TURP. This procedure is usually performed in elderly men who may have coexisting pulmonary or cardiovascular disease, and anesthetic choice and monitoring techniques should be commensurate with the medical conditions. Some practitioners prefer regional anesthesia because the patient is awake and mental status can be followed to monitor for TURP syndrome, bladder perforation may be diagnosed by abdominal pain, and bleeding may be less because venous pressure is reduced and the patient will not strain or cough as may occur with general anesthesia. There have been no prospective outcome studies to confirm a benefit for any anesthetic type. If regional anesthesia is used, a T10 level of analgesia is required to prevent pain from bladder distention. Spinal anesthesia is probably better than an epidural because sacral segments will be reliably blocked, and the resection should not be prolonged, to prevent TURP syndrome.

b. **Complications**

- **TURP syndrome** may occur during or after the resection from absorption of a large volume of the irrigation solution. The patient may have symptoms secondary to fluid overload (hypertension, dyspnea, hypoxemia) or dilutional hyponatremia (restlessness, confusion, seizures). Hypoosmolarity may produce cerebral edema. This may lead to hypotension, myocardial dysfunction, and pulmonary edema. If glycine is used, there may be visual disturbances. Diagnosis of TURP syndrome can be made by measuring serum sodium concentration and cardiac filling pressures. If it occurs, surgery should be discontinued and furosemide given to begin diuresis of the absorbed fluid. For severe hyponatremia, less than 118 mEq/liter, or with CNS symptoms such as seizures, hypertonic saline (3%) solution should be administered slowly. Rapid, complete correction of hyponatremia should not be attempted. Invasive monitoring such as A-line to permit frequent blood gas and electrolyte measurements and central venous or pulmonary artery catheter to assess pressures may be warranted.
- **Bleeding** may be excessive with large, vascular glands. Since blood is drained with the irrigating solution, estimation of the blood loss is difficult, and large volumes may be lost without being visible. Bleeding may continue into the postoperative period if vessels have not been adequately cauterized. Blood for transfusion should be available for patients with large glands or if the surgeon is inexperienced. Severe bleeding may be

caused by disseminated intravascular coagulation, and appropriate tests should be performed (PT, platelets, D-dimers) if this is considered a possibility.

- **Bladder perforation** may occur from the resectoscope and is usually extraperitoneal. Awake patients may note pain in the inguinal or suprapubic region. Intraperitoneal perforation produces pain in the upper abdomen or may be referred to the shoulder. Pain may be accompanied by nausea, diaphoresis, hypotension, or hypertension. In the postoperative period, perforation should be considered if the volume of irrigation fluid used is greater than that which has drained. Surgery to correct the perforation is usually not necessary.
- **Sepsis** or bacteremia may occur with resection of an infected gland and may present as intraoperative hypotension. Prophylactic antibiotics are often used with TURP.

LAPAROSCOPIC SURGERY

Laparoscopic surgery is now being used for gynecologic procedures (tubal ligation, infertility diagnosis), urologic diagnostic purposes such as lymph node biopsy for prostate cancer staging, and upper abdominal procedures such as cholecystectomy and Nissen fundoplasty. The popularity of laparoscopic procedures is increasing because of the shortened hospital stay and recovery period, although the intraoperative time may be longer than with similar open procedures.

Intraperitoneal Gas Insufflation

Intraperitoneal gas insufflation is used to distend the abdomen to permit a scope to be percutaneously introduced and subsequently to allow visualization of structures. A trocar is inserted blindly through the abdominal wall for gas insufflation. Possible complications include puncture of bowel, an organ (bleeding), or vessel (gas embolus). Most centers use CO_2 for insufflation because it is nonflammable, absorption through the peritoneum has few adverse effects, and inadvertent gas embolus or pneumomediastinum would be rapidly reabsorbed and the CO_2 blown off through the lungs. **Absorption of CO_2** during the pneumoperitoneum requires that minute ventilation be increased to prevent hypercarbia, which may produce hypertension or tachycardia. The difference between the monitored end-tidal CO_2 and the arterial CO_2 may increase during the changes in the patient's position and with the pneumoperitoneum, so hypercarbia may exist with a normal end-tidal CO_2. The abdomen is distended to a pressure of about **15 mm Hg** through constant insufflation of gas. The increased intraabdominal pressure rarely produces hemodynamic changes but may have respiratory effects from reduction of pulmonary functional residual volume and may require an increase in peak inspiratory pressure. If the pleura is inadvertently entered, the resulting pneumothorax may have adverse hemodynamic or respiratory effects.

Position

Patients for pelvic endoscopic procedures are usually placed in Trendelenburg position, while those for upper abdominal surgery are head-up. The Trendelenburg position and the pneumoperitoneum may make ventilation difficult for spontaneously ventilating patients, so ventilation should be controlled. Cardiac preload is increased by the Trendelenburg position; head-up position has the opposite effects. Since the mediastinum is pushed cephalad with the Trendelenburg position, endobronchial intubation may result as the carina moves.

Anesthetic Management

Although some diagnostic laparoscopic procedures may be performed under local or epidural anesthesia, most require general anesthesia to provide patient comfort and ensure adequate respiration, especially when steep Trendelenburg positioning is used. Because of increased intraabdominal pressure from the pneumoperitoneum, gastric reflux is possible, and therefore endotracheal intubation is suggested. To prevent organ perforation by blind sticks, an orogastric tube should be inserted to ensure that gastric distention does not exist, and the bladder should be catheterized.

Anesthetic Agents

Many anesthetic agents have been successfully used for laparoscopic surgery. Since there is an increased incidence of postoperative nausea, use of a prophylactic antiemetic such as droperidol or ondansetron appears warranted. Some practitioners also avoid large doses of narcotics in an attempt to diminish nausea, but others feel that their use provides hemodynamic stability during the procedures. The use of N_2O is controversial because some endoscopists believe that it increases bowel distention, making the procedure more difficult, and that it increases postoperative nausea. Several studies have produced conflicting results on the role of N_2O on postoperative nausea. Propofol, a useful agent for maintenance of anesthesia, can be used at the end of the case to permit elimination of potent inhalational anesthetics for rapid awakening. Muscle relaxants should be used to facilitate controlled ventilation. A nonsteroidal antiinflammatory agent like ketorolac can be administered during the case for postoperative pain relief.

Suggested Readings

Byrick RJ, and Rose DK. Pathophysiology and prevention of acute renal failure: the role of the anaesthetist. Can J Anaesth 1990;37:457–467.

Cunningham AJ, Brull SJ. Laparoscopic cholecystectomy: anesthetic implications. Anesth Analg 1993;76:1120–1133.

Kellen M, Aronson S, Roizen MF, et al. Predictive and diagnostic tests of renal failure: a review. Anesth Analg 1994;78:134–142.

Novis RK, Roizen MF, Aronson S, Thisted RA. Association of preoperative risk factors with postoperative acute renal failure. Anesth Analg 1994;78:143–149.

Shin B, Mackenzie CF, Helrich M. Creatinine clearance for early detection of posttraumatic renal dysfunction. Anesthesiology 1986;64:605–609.

Sladen RN. Effect of anesthesia and surgery on renal function. Crit Care Clin 1987;3(2):373–393.

Weir HC, Chung FF. Anaesthesia for patients with chronic renal disease. Can Anaesth Soc J 1984;31:468–480.

Chapter 13

Endocrine Diseases

Anesthesiologists must be prepared to give perioperative care to patients with endocrine disorders. Some endocrine conditions may require postponement of elective surgery to optimize the patient, while others must be managed during surgery.

DIABETES MELLITUS

Diabetes mellitus, a common disorder in surgical patients, causes the loss of homeostatic control of blood glucose and the resulting potential risks of hyper- or hypoglycemia. It may be genetic, viral, or caused by pancreatitis or pancreatic surgery.

Classification by Insulin Requirement

1. **Type I, insulin-dependent diabetes mellitus (IDDM)**
   a. Lacks insulin secretion by the beta cells of the pancreas
   b. Often begins early in life, juvenile onset
   c. Brittle glucose control with a tendency toward ketoacidosis
   d. More likely to have associated complications
      i. **Autonomic nervous system dysfunction** from demyelination producing orthostatic hypotension, increased resting heart rate, and abnormal responses to hypovolemia
      ii. **Generalized atherosclerosis,** with twice the normal risk of stroke, myocardial infarction, and peripheral vascular disease; possible silent myocardial ischemia
      iii. **Peripheral neuropathy** with decreased sensation in the lower extremities
      iv. **Renal dysfunction** from microangiopathies leading to hypertension

     v. **Gastroparesis** (20–30% of patients) may result from autonomic dysfunction
2. **Type II, non–insulin-dependent diabetes mellitus (NIDDM)**
    a. Usually begins in adults who are obese
    b. Less severe insulin deficiency exists or there may be insulin resistance
    c. Can often be treated with diet, weight loss, or oral hypoglycemic agents

Pathophysiology

Insulin

Insulin is produced by the beta cells in the pancreas (average 40–50 units/day) and is metabolized in the liver and kidney, so patients with hepatic or renal dysfunction are at increased risk for hypoglycemia during insulin treatment. Except for the brain and liver, insulin is required for glucose movement into cells. During the **stress of surgery** with increased cortisol and catecholamine secretion, patients may have an increased insulin requirement and experience hyperglycemia. **Trauma and infection** make management of patients with IDDM more difficult, and hyperglycemia with ketoacidosis is likely.

Hypoglycemia

Hypoglycemia under anesthesia may be difficult to diagnose. Resultant catecholamine release may cause tachycardia, lacrimation, and increased blood pressure, which can easily be misinterpreted as "light" anesthesia. β-Blocking medications should be used with caution in diabetics because they mask this adrenergic response to hypoglycemia in both awake and anesthetized patients. NIDDM patients are also at risk for hypoglycemia because oral hypoglycemics can exert their effects for as long as 24–36 hours after a dose, especially with renal insufficiency.

Diabetic Ketoacidosis

Diabetic ketoacidosis (DKA) occurs most commonly in IDDM when there is insufficient endogenous or exogenously administered insulin to block the mobilization of free fatty acids that are metabolized to ketones in the liver. Trauma, concurrent illness, and stopping insulin can all precipitate DKA.

Diagnosis. In addition to **hyperglycemia and glucosuria,** the hallmark of DKA is metabolic acidosis with an **increased anion gap [(Na) − (CO$_2$ + Cl)].** The anion gap is increased when it is above 12, and acidosis is confirmed by a low pH on an arterial blood gas analysis. Other characteristics of DKA include **osmotic diuresis with a decreased intravascular volume, severely decreased total body potassium stores (with metabolic acidosis, K$^+$ shifts extracellularly so the serum [K$^+$] may be normal or even increased), nausea, and vomiting.** The glucose level is often only moderately increased (300–500 mg/dl).

Treatment

1. **Rehydration** and restoration of intravascular volume with normal saline solution and albumin.
2. Small amounts of **intravenous insulin** by continuous infusion (1–10 units/hr).
3. **Sodium bicarbonate** to treat acidosis (pH < 7.20). The dose is calculated

$$\textbf{mEq NaHCO}_3 = \textbf{wt (kg)} \times \textbf{0.3} \times \textbf{base deficit}$$
$$\textbf{(from the arterial blood gas)}$$

   Usually half of the dose is given and the pH is checked before giving additional bicarbonate.
4. As DKA resolves, K$^+$ reenters cells and severe **hypokalemia can develop.** K$^+$ repletion should take place before hypokalemia occurs, but K$^+$ should be given with caution in patients with renal failure.
5. **Decreased PO$_4$** may also occur with correction of the acidosis and may result in skeletal muscle weakness with impairment of ventilation.

Elective Surgery. Elective surgery should be delayed in patients with DKA until the condition is adequately treated. If a patient in DKA presents for **emergency surgery,** treatment should be initiated in the operating room as described above. An arterial line, Foley catheter, and CVP are indicated for monitoring, with frequent determinations of blood glucose, electrolytes, and arterial blood gases.

Hyperosmolar Hyperglycemic Nonketotic Coma (HHNK)

HHNK can occur when there is sufficient insulin present to prevent ketosis, but not enough to prevent severe hyperglycemia. The insulin prevents the mobilization and metabolism of fatty acids to acetoacetate and β-hydroxybutyrate (ketones), but the hyperglycemia produces an osmotic diuresis with significant dehydration. HHNK may be precipitated by infection or dehydration.

Diagnosis

1. Glucose >600 mg/dl and serum osmolality >330 mosm/liter
2. Decreased intravascular volume (decreased blood pressure, hemoconcentration, increased BUN, metabolic acidosis)
3. CNS dysfunction (changes in mentation, seizures, coma)

Treatment

1. Correcting hypovolemia and hyperosmolality with intravenous crystalloid until the blood pressure is stabilized
2. K^+ repletion to replace that lost via the osmotic diuresis
3. Small doses of regular insulin (10 units/hr) to gradually decrease blood glucose to approximately 300 mg/dl (rapidly decreasing blood glucose can cause cerebral edema)

Anesthetic Management

Preoperative Assessment

Preoperative assessment should include the type of diabetes (IDDM or NIDDM), the severity of the disease, the method of control of blood glucose (diet, oral hypoglycemics, or insulin regimen including exact dose/timing/type of insulin). The adequacy of control can be determined by measuring the blood glucose and electrolytes, and DKA and HHNK should not be present. History and examination should be reviewed for associated conditions such as autonomic or peripheral neuropathy, coronary artery disease (silent myocardial infarct), renal dysfunction, hypertension, or gastroparesis.

Perioperative Management

Perioperative management is facilitated with availability of rapid glucose measurements using hand held glucose meters with dipsticks. The blood glucose and K^+ should be checked preoperatively and intraoperatively (as often as every 1–2 hours if the surgery is prolonged). The perioperative goal is to maintain a mild, transient hyperglycemia (approximately 120–200 mg/dl),

prevent ketoacidosis, and prevent hypoglycemia. Oral hypoglycemics should not be given on the morning of surgery.

Insulin Regimens in Clinical Practice

1. **Give no insulin the morning of surgery. Check blood glucose
   preoperatively and every 1–2 hours intraoperatively. Give 5–
   10 units regular insulin IV for glucose levels above 250 mg/dl
   (check glucose 30 minutes after insulin dose). The maximum
   effect of IV insulin occurs at about 30 minutes.** For glucose
   levels below 100 mg/dl (there may be residual effects of previous oral hypoglycemics or long-acting insulin), begin or increase the rate of a 5% dextrose infusion. Usually at least **a
   small dose of insulin is necessary to prevent ketoacidosis** even
   though the serum glucose is in an acceptable range.
2. **Give 1/4–1/2 the usual s.c. NPH dose on the morning of
   surgery.** If the patient takes regular insulin in the morning,
   increase the NPH dose by 0.5 units for each unit of regular
   insulin. Begin a 5% dextrose infusion after the insulin dose
   (100–200 ml/hr, or 5–10 gm/hr). If glucose is not given (the
   IV infiltrates or is not started), the patient may become hypo-
   glycemic because insulin has been given s.c., and its effect may
   persist for several hours.
3. **Begin a continuous infusion of insulin on the evening before
   or the morning of surgery** (best regimen to maintain nor-
   moglycemia, but requires the use of infusion pumps) (Table
   13.1).

Table 13.1 Insulin Drip for Perioperative Management of IDDM[a]

1. $D_5$1/2 NS with 20 mEq/liter KCl at 100 ml/hr on D_{10}W at 50 ml/hr
2. Blood glucose (BG) by AccuChek q 2 h
3. When BG is >150 mg/dl, begin insulin drip at 1.0 U/hr
   Insulin drip: 125 U Regular insulin in 250 ml 0.9% saline
   (1 ml of solution = 0.5 U insulin)
4. Based on blood glucose (mg/dl), do the following:

120–180	No change
181–240	Increase insulin drip by 0.5 U/hr
>240	Increase drip by 0.5 U/hr and give 8 U Reg. insulin IV
80–119	Decrease drip by 1.0 U/hr
<80	Decrease drip by 1.0 U/hr and give 25 ml D50 IV

5. If the drip rate is reduced to zero, continue q 2 h AccuChecks; when
   blood glucose is >150, restart the insulin drip at 0.5 U/hr

[a]Based on the protocol of Endocrinology Service, Emory University Hospital.

Anesthetic Regimen. No specific anesthetic technique or agents are indicated. Patients undergoing general anesthesia may require rapid sequence induction and intubation because of the risk of aspiration with symptomatic gastroparesis. Regional anesthesia may be beneficial because it may block the stress response during surgery. It is important to check the patients' baseline neurologic status for peripheral neuropathy before performing regional anesthesia. Careful attention should be paid to positioning extremities that may already have a neural deficit. A urinary catheter is desirable in most diabetic patients to assess urinary glucose and osmotic diuresis from hyperglycemia. Patients with extremely brittle diabetes may require postoperative ICU care.

THYROID DISEASES

Thyroid diseases are often associated with inappropriate serum levels of **thyroxine (T_4)** and **triiodothyronine (T_3)**. Because these hormones are responsible for regulating cellular metabolism, thyroid diseases can result in cardiac, pulmonary, or neurologic disorders. The goal of anesthetic management of a patient with thyroid disease is to maintain a euthyroid state during the perioperative period or to blunt the physiologic responses to inappropriate levels of thyroid hormone when euthyroidism cannot be achieved.

Thyroid Function Tests

Thyroid function tests should be evaluated preoperatively in patients with known or suspected thyroid disease.

1. **Total serum T_4** is the basic test for evaluating thyroid function (increased in most hyperthyroid patients and decreased in hypothyroid). T_4 (circulating half-life of 6–7 days) is produced from iodide, and its production is inhibited by iodine. Increased **thyroid binding globulin (TBG)** (occurring with acute liver disease, pregnancy, or medications [birth control pills, opioids]) can cause an elevated T_4 in euthyroid patients.
2. Most **T_3** is produced outside the thyroid from T_4. Half-life is about 24 hr. Hyperthyroid patients may have isolated elevations of T_3. About half of hypothyroid patients have low T_3.

3. **T$_3$ resin uptake (RT$_3$U)** is an indirect measure of unbound T$_3$ (normal is 25–35%). The RT$_3$U is elevated with hyperthyroidism and decreased with hypothyroidism.
4. **Thyroid-stimulating hormone (TSH)** is produced in the anterior pituitary and is responsible for thyroid hormone secretion. TSH is increased with primary hypothyroidism, decreased with secondary hypothyroidism, and normal or decreased with hyperthyroidism.

Hyperthyroidism

Hyperthyroidism produces a hypermetabolic state from excess thyroid hormone release.

Symptoms

Symptoms include heat intolerance, hyperreflexia, weight loss, tachycardia, and dysrythmias such as atrial fibrillation. Thyroid hormone increases cardiac contractility and increases the number of β-adrenergic receptors. Excess thyroid hormone uncouples oxidative phosphorylation and causes increased heat production. Although there is no increase in catecholamine levels, hyperthyroidism results in a hyperadrenergic state.

Thyroid storm is a severe exacerbation of hyperthyroidism, often with sudden onset coincident with infection, trauma, or surgery, which results in fever, tachycardia, high-output congestive heart failure, hemodynamic collapse, dehydration, and coma. Treatment directed at correction of the underlying problem, includes fluid (cold crystalloids) and electrolyte supplementation, as well as medications to reduce thyroid hormone synthesis (propylthiouracil) and release (sodium iodide). Symptomatic treatment of cardiac effects of the thyroid hormones with β-blockers should also be undertaken. Steroid coverage may be indicated. Mortality can be high, and elective surgery should not be performed in patients with untreated hyperthyroid states. Since the intraoperative presentation of thyroid storm resembles malignant hyperthermia, the two must be differentiated so that appropriate therapy can be instituted.

Causes

Graves disease, the most frequent cause of goiter, includes exophthalmos and pretibial myxedema, and occurs most commonly in young females. Other causes include a single toxic nodule (adenoma), toxic multinodular goiter, thyroiditis, TSH-secreting pituitary adenoma, or production of hormone from remote tumors.

Treatment

1. Propylthiouracil (PTU) and methimazole inhibit the synthesis of thyroid hormone but take several weeks to make a patient euthyroid because of thyroid hormone storage within the gland. PTU also decreases the conversion of T_4 to T_3.
2. Potassium iodide, given orally, inhibits thyroid hormone release, and over about a week before surgery, it will shrink an enlarged thyroid and reduce its vascularity.
3. β-Blockers can be used to treat the cardiovascular symptoms of hyperthyroidism and also to impair the conversion of T_4 to T_3 within 1–2 weeks.
4. Radioactive iodide is used in older patients but may produce hypothyroidism in 40–60% over 10 years.
5. Surgery is an alternative to medical therapy and is used in patients with large goiters or when carcinoma is suspected.

Anesthetic Management

For elective surgery, patients should be treated until they are euthyroid to avoid the hyperadrenergic state of hyperthyroidism and to prevent thyroid storm. The primary anesthetic goal in managing hyperthyroid patients is to avoid stimulating the sympathetic nervous system by ensuring an adequate depth of anesthesia and by avoiding drugs such as ketamine and ephedrine. If a vasopressor is required, a direct agent like Neo-Synephrine is preferable. Likewise, pancuronium should be avoided because of its vagolytic effect, causing tachycardia.

The **airway** should be carefully evaluated in patients with goiters, especially if they extend into the anterior mediastinum. Review of the chest x-ray film or a preoperative CT scan of the neck helps assess tracheal compression or deviation caused by the gland. Although most patients have normal laryngeal anatomy and can be intubated after induction, those with significant tracheal deviation may be candidates for awake fiberoptic intubation. Some patients may have tracheomalacia with tracheal collapse presenting after extubation.

Routine **monitors** should suffice in euthyroid patients without other medical problems. In emergency surgery for a clinically hyperthyroid patient, an arterial line may be indicated. Since the incidence of myasthenia gravis is increased in patients with hyperthyroidism, the effect of neuromuscular blockers should be followed with a twitch monitor. Since thyroid storm may occur intraoperatively or postoperatively, temperature, heart rate, and rhythm should be monitored throughout the perioperative period.

Anesthetic. Since a nitrous-narcotic technique may not reliably inhibit the sympathetic nervous system, using an inhalational agent like isoflurane can attenuate the patient's sympathetic system without sensitizing the myocardium to catecholamines like halothane. Although MAC (minimum alveolar concentration, the dose of anesthetic effective in preventing movement in one-half of patients) is unchanged, the increased cardiac output with hyperthyroidism necessitates using a higher inspired concentration of anesthetic to reach equilibrium during induction. Drug metabolism may be increased so that isoflurane may be preferred over enflurane or halothane because it undergoes the least biotransformation. When hyperthyroidism results in hyperpyrexia, anesthetic levels must be adjusted accordingly, because for every degree Celsius above 37°, there is a 5% increase in anesthetic requirement.

For thyroidectomy under general anesthesia, most practitioners prefer to intubate the trachea, although the procedure can be performed with the patient breathing spontaneously via mask or laryngeal mask airway. The patient is placed in a beach-chair position (partial sitting) to prevent venous distention in the neck, but this results in decreased cardiac venous return and requires maintaining an adequate intravascular volume to prevent hypotension (may be worsened with inhalational anesthetics that depress myocardial contractility). Surgical dissection of the gland from the trachea may produce coughing and deep anesthesia, intravenous lidocaine, or neuromuscular blockade is required to prevent this complication.

Regional anesthesia (without epinephrine in the local anesthetic) can be used for some surgical procedures because the resultant sympathetic blockade is beneficial.

Postoperative Complications. Postoperative complications after total or subtotal thyroidectomy can lead to respiratory distress.

Tracheal compression may be the result of hematoma or tracheomalacia, and immediate reintubation may be required. Some patients with hematoma may be helped by acutely opening the incision to allow decompression. Preexisting tracheomalacia can occur as a result of a large goiter causing weakening of the tracheal cartilage.

Recurrent laryngeal nerve injury can occur during thyroid dissection but produces respiratory distress after extubation only with bilateral nerve damage. The recurrent laryngeal nerve supplies both the abductor and adductor muscles to the vocal cords, but the abductors are more sensitive to damage (e.g., bruising). Pure abductor paralysis will cause the ipsilateral vocal cord to go to midline, and with bilateral damage, the cords will approximate in the midline, and severe respiratory distress occurs. If bilateral recurrent laryngeal nerves are cut, both abductor and adductor muscles are paralyzed, the cords are stationary in the midline, but the airway is maintained. Vocal cord movement can be assessed at the end of surgery via direct or fiberoptic laryngoscopy with the patient breathing spontaneously.

Inadvertent **parathyroidectomy** during total thyroidectomy can cause symptomatic hypocalcemia (tetany) with possible stridor and laryngospasm. Since the laryngeal muscles are very sensitive to the effects of hypocalcemia, respiratory distress may be the presenting symptom of hypocalcemia. The hypocalcemia after complete parathyroidectomy usually does not occur until the first postoperative day, but it may present (perioral numbness, Chvostek and Trousseau signs) earlier when the patient is in the PACU. Routine measurements of serum total or ionized calcium are indicated. The acute treatment is calcium chloride or gluconate by intravenous infusion.

Hypothyroidism

Hypothyroidism produces a reduction in T_4 and T_3 and may result from treatment of hyperthyroidism with radioactive iodine or surgery, thyroiditis, autoimmune causes, or (rarely) decreased TSH (secondary hypothyroidism).

Symptoms

Symptoms include lethargy, cold intolerance, slowed reflexes and mental acuity, hypothermia, bradycardia and myocardial depression (cardiomyopathy), hyponatremia, hypoglycemia, and decreased ventilatory response to CO_2. Severe hypothyroidism occurs with total $T_4 < 1$ $\mu g/dl$, and moderate symptoms with total $T_4 < 3$ $\mu g/dl$. When patients with hypothyroidism are treated with thyroid replacement therapy, new onset of angina may occur with the increase in metabolic activity and increase in cardiac work.

Myxedema coma is a severe exacerbation of hypothyroidism, with a mortality of up to 50%. It may occur as a result of stress (cold, infection) or following sedative administration to a severely hypothyroid patient and presents as altered consciousness, hypothermia, CHF, hypoventilation, decreased cortisol production, and SIADH. Treatment consists of intravenous T_4 (400–500 μg) or T_3 (50–200 μg bolus) and hydrocortisone (100–300 mg).

Treatment

Anesthesia and surgery are considered safe before thyroid replacement in patients with mild-to-moderate hypothyroidism. Elective surgery should be postponed in severely hypothyroid patients until replacement can be started. Thyroid hormone should be implemented gradually because angina, dysrhythmias, and CHF may be precipitated. Thyroxine takes effect after 10 days of treatment, while T_3 begins working in 6 hours (peaks at 48–72 hours). Since patients with severe hypothyroidism are also likely to have adrenal insufficiency, steroid replacement should be given (100–200 mg/day hydrocortisone) until adrenal function can be assessed.

Anesthetic Management

Preoperative Considerations

1. With cold intolerance, peripheral vasoconstriction and cool, dry skin may be seen.

2. With lethargy and decreased ventilatory response to CO_2, preoperative narcotics should be avoided; in addition, these patients may be very sensitive to CNS-depressant medications.

3. Hypodynamic cardiovascular system may be manifested as decreased cardiac contractility (but rarely CHF), heart rate, stroke volume, and cardiac output, with cardiomegaly, pleural effusions, ascites, peripheral edema, and pericardial effusions.

4. Hyponatremia may result from impaired clearance of free water.

Other Intraoperative Considerations. **Monitoring** should be individualized to the patient and the procedure, but with the possibility of a hypodynamic cardiovascular system and decreased intravascular volume, hemodynamics should be followed closely. Careful attention should be paid to maintaining normal body temperature with a warmed operating room and forced-air warming blanket to prevent hypothermia.

Most general anesthetics can be used without any problems, and regional anesthesia is acceptable as long as appropriate intravascular volume is maintained. For induction of general anesthesia, ketamine is preferred by some, but barbiturates have been used without cardiovascular depression. Since inhalational anesthetics are cardiac depressants and vasodilators, a nitrous-narcotic technique might be used in patients with hypodynamic cardiovascular system, decreased intravascular volume, and lack of baroreceptor reflex activity. Although MAC is not changed with hypothyroidism, a decreased cardiac output results in a faster increase in alveolar concentration of anesthetic. Since drug biotransformation by the liver may be slowed, depressant drugs should be carefully titrated. For the treatment of hypotension, Neo-Synephrine increases systemic vascular resistance, which may decrease cardiac output if myocardial contractility is compromised; small doses of ephedrine may be preferred.

PARATHYROID DISEASES

Calcium Regulation

The parathyroid glands via **parathyroid hormone (PTH)** maintain the extracellular fluid Ca^{2+} concentration via a variety of mechanisms including resorption of calcium from bone and renal Ca^{2+} reabsorption. Approximately 50% of total plasma calcium is the free, ionized Ca^{2+} portion that is physiologically active (skeletal muscle contraction, coagulation, neuromuscular transmission). About 40% of total plasma calcium is protein bound, most to albumin. Therefore, in a patient with hypoalbuminemia and low total plasma calcium, the ionized Ca^{2+} concentration may be normal (change in albumin of 1 gm/dl produces a corresponding change of 0.8 mg/dl in total serum calcium).

An inverse relationship exists between serum calcium and phosphate levels. This is seen in **secondary hyperparathyroidism** associated with chronic renal failure when hypocalcemia with elevated PTH level results from hyperphosphatemia produced by decreased renal excretion of phosphate. Conversely, when a patient has hypercalcemia, hypophosphatemia can result. This becomes clinically significant at very low levels of phosphate; complications of **severe hypophosphatemia** include skeletal muscle weakness (with resultant respiratory distress), impaired cardiac contractility (possibly causing CHF), hemolysis, and platelet dysfunction.

Hyperparathyroidism

Primary Hyperparathyroidism

Some 90% of cases are due to a benign adenoma, with 10% of these being part of an multiple endocrine adenoma (MEN) type I syndrome. Hyperplasia of the four parathyroid glands may also result in primary hyperparathyroidism.

Symptoms

Symptoms include hypercalcemia (> 10.5 mg/dl or 5.5 mEq/liter), polyuria/polydipsia, depression, and psychoses (with extremely elevated calcium levels), muscle weakness, renal stones, vomiting, and peptic ulcer disease. Only a minority have significant bone demineralization. The ECG may show a shortened QT interval with hypercalcemia.

Treatment

When serum Ca^{2+} rises above 15 mg/dl, emergency treatment consists of intravascular volume expansion with intravenous normal saline solution, possibly with monitoring (e.g., central venous pressure). Furosemide is used to initiate a diuresis. Hydration dilutes serum calcium, and Na^+ diuresis causes Ca^{2+} excretion by inhibiting both Na^+ and Ca^{2+} reabsorption in the proximal renal tubule. In nonemergent situations, elevated calcium levels may be corrected with mithramycin, calcitonin, or dialysis.

Surgery may be necessary to remove an adenoma or to resect most of the hyperplastic glands. Plasma Ca^{2+} concentrations will decrease within several days secondary to rapid bone remineralization, and hypocalcemic tetany is a possible complication. Postoperative Ca^{2+} levels and clinical monitoring for hypocalcemia are indicated. Immediate postoperative complications from parathyroid surgery include vocal cord paralysis from injury of the recurrent laryngeal nerves or airway compromise from tracheal compression from hematoma.

Anesthetic Considerations

1. Adequate hydration and urine output in hypercalcemia.
2. Unpredictable response to neuromuscular blockers so that a small dose of neuromuscular blocker should be used initially and titrated according to a twitch monitor.
3. Attention to positioning and movement of patients with osteoporosis is essential to prevent fractures.

Hypoparathyroidism

Hypoparathyroidism exists when there is a deficiency of PTH or the end organs are resistant to the hormone. This results in hypocalcemia (< 8 mg/dl or 4.5 mEq/liter). Surgically induced hypoparathyroidism after thyroidectomy, parathyroidectomy, or anterior neck exploration is the most common cause of hypoparathyroidism. Chronic renal failure may produce hypocalcemia.

Hypocalcemia

Hypocalcemia with acute onset in an awake patient may present as perioral paresthesias, positive Chvostek sign (facial twitching with percussion of VII), or Trousseau sign (carpal spasm with 3 minutes of arm ischemia with a tourniquet). With chronic hypocalcemia there will be lethargy, muscle cramps, and prolongation of the Q-T interval on ECG.

Treatment

Treatment of hypocalcemia is with an infusion of calcium (chloride or gluconate), following the neuromuscular signs and serum Ca^{2+} concentrations. Thiazide diuretics may also be used chronically to increase calcium concentrations.

Anesthetic Considerations

1. Plasma Ca^{2+} concentrations should be frequently measured, indicating the need for an intraarterial catheter for sampling.
2. Q-T interval on ECG should be followed as a physiologic indication of hypocalcemia.
3. Avoid hyperventilation, which, via respiratory alkalosis, would decrease the plasma ionized Ca^{2+} concentration.
4. Hypotension or low cardiac output from decreased myocardial contractility may result from hypocalcemia and should be treated with a bolus or infusion of calcium chloride or gluconate.
5. Rapid administration of citrate-containing blood products may worsen hypocalcemia because the citrate binds ionized Ca^{2+}.
6. Nondepolarizing muscle relaxants should be cautiously titrated because their effect may be potentiated with hypocalcemia.

DISEASES OF THE ADRENAL GLAND

The two adrenal glands contain a **cortical portion** that produces glucocorticoids (regulate metabolic pathways), mineralocorticoids (regulate extracellular volume), and androgens and the **medulla,** a part of the sympathetic nervous system that synthesizes epinephrine and norepinephrine. The normal adult produces 20 mg/day of cortisol (or 12 mg/m^2 of body surface area); however, under periods of stress such as trauma, infection, or surgery, the adrenal may secrete up to 4–5 times this basal amount. (See Table 13.2 for replacement doses of exogenous steroids.) Cortisol is required for blood pressure stability (conversion of norepinephrine to epinephrine in the adrenal medulla), glucose regulation (promotes formation of glucose via protein breakdown, gluconeogenesis from amino acids, and

Table 13.2 Corticosteroid Dosages

Agent	Relative Potency	Equiv. Dose[a] (mg)	Mineralocorticoid Activity[b]
Cortisol	1	20	+
Hydrocortisone	1	20	+
Prednisone	4	5	+
Prednisolone	4	5	+
Methylprednisolone	5	4	−
Dexamethasone	25	0.75	−

[a] Doses equivalent to daily exogenous cortisol production.
[b] Mineralocorticoid activity or salt-retaining effect refers to the aldosterone-like effects of that agent (its ability to reabsorb sodium in the distal convoluted tubule of the kidney in exchange for potassium).

inhibits peripheral utilization of glucose), maintenance of intra-vascular volume (mineralocorticoid effect of Na retention and K excretion), and antiinflammatory effects (decreased capillary permeability, prevention of lysosome release). An adult normally produces 0.1 mg of aldosterone per day, with this mineralocorticoid being partially responsible for renal Na^+ reabsorption.

Hyperadrenocorticism

The chronic excess of glucocorticoids may be from either endogenous or exogenous sources. Cushing's disease is usually caused by a pituitary adenoma producing excess ACTH secretion stimulating cortisol secretion by the adrenals. Alternatively, there may be ectopic ACTH from a nonpituitary neoplasm, excess cortisol from an adrenal neoplasm, or the administration of chronic steroids.

Symptoms

Symptoms include hypertension (increased intravascular volume from renal Na^+ retention), hyperglycemia, hypokalemia, skeletal muscle weakness, osteoporosis (cortisol-induced protein loss from bone), and obesity.

Treatment

Treatment is either transsphenoidal adenomectomy or adrenal resection.

Anesthetic Considerations

Anesthetic considerations must include preoperative assessment of conditions related to obesity (airway adequacy and delayed gastric emptying), hypertension, intravascular volume (possible diuresis with potassium-sparing diuretic preoperatively), electrolytes (hypernatremia and hypokalemia may need correction), diabetes mellitus, and steroid supplementation. Because of obesity and extra fat between the scapulae, careful head positioning with extra pillows to obtain a good "sniff" position is essential.

No particular anesthetics are indicated; however, the dose of muscle relaxants should be decreased because of the possibility of skeletal muscle weakness. Regional anesthesia is an acceptable technique (if appropriate for the surgical procedure), but each patient must be evaluated for the degree of osteoporosis. Careful positioning is important to avoid injury as a result of osteopenia.

Patients for hypophysectomy (for pituitary adenomas) or bilateral adrenalectomy require supplementation with hydrocortisone (100 mg/day) to prevent postoperative adrenal insufficiency. This should be continued into the postoperative period until oral steroids can be given.

Hypoadrenocorticism

Causes

1. Addison's disease (primary adrenal insufficiency) results from destruction of the adrenal cortex (e.g., carcinoma, TB, idiopathic autoimmune destruction), and patients are deficient in both glucocorticoids and mineralocorticoids.
   a. Impaired renal sodium conservation with resultant hypotension secondary to decreased intravascular volume
   b. Hyponatremia, hypokalemia, hypoglycemia
2. With a deficiency of ACTH, patients are deficient only in glucocorticoids while aldosterone levels are normal.

3. Adrenal insufficiency secondary to prolonged exogenous administration of steroids.

Anesthetic Management

Preoperative assessment
1. Volume status (heart rate and blood pressure with patient supine and standing, skin turgor, mucous membranes).
2. Electrolytes (especially noting possible hyponatremia, hyperkalemia, and hypoglycemia).
3. Thyroid function tests may be indicated in patients with ACTH deficiency since they may also have hypothyroidism secondary to decreased TSH.

Steroid supplementation must be given to prevent an acute **adrenal crisis.** If the adrenal is unable to secrete its extra 4–5 times basal cortisol during the stress of surgery, circulatory collapse, characterized by hypotension and decreased cardiac output, can ensue. Emergency treatment consists of (*a*) 200 mg intravenous hydrocortisone followed by 100 mg every 6 hours for 48 hours, (*b*) intravenous glucose in normal saline, (*c*) colloid to restore intravascular volume, and (*d*) inotropic support, after volume repletion, with use of invasive monitoring.

Perioperative steroid replacement should take into consideration the patient's degree of adrenal suppression. The total dose of corticosteroid or duration of treatment that causes suppression of the pituitary-adrenal axis is not known. It is usually best to provide stress dose supplements in equivocal situations because an acute adrenal crisis is life-threatening and there is little risk in stress coverage. The most conservative approach is to provide stress coverage to any patient who has received daily steroids for at least 1 week within 6–12 months before surgery or to any patient currently receiving steroids. Each patient should be assessed individually regarding previous steroid dose and the type of surgery needed. Topical steroids may also suppress the pituitary-adrenal axis.

Two acceptable regimens for stress dose steroid replacement:

1. 200–300 mg hydrocortisone/70 kg in divided doses on the day of surgery (100 mg IV preoperatively, intraoperatively, and postoperatively)

Table 13.3 Clinical Features of the Multiple Endocrine Neoplasia Syndromes (MEN)

MEN I:	Hyperparathyroidism (parathyroid hyperplasia or parathyroid adenoma), pituitary adenoma, and pancreatic islet cell hyperfunction (insulin or gastrin)
MEN IIa:	Parathyroid hyperplasia, medullary Ca of thyroid, and pheochromocytoma
MEN IIb:	Medullary Ca of thyroid, multiple neuromas of oral mucosa, marfanoid habitus, and pheochromocytoma

2. Low-dose method: 25 mg hydrocortisone IV before induction of anesthesia, followed by 100 mg IV as a continuous infusion during the next 24 hours

Etomidate, an imidazole anesthetic that is often used as an induction agent, has been associated with significant adrenal suppression when used in sedative or induction dosages. This seems to have little clinical significance except an increase in mortality was noted in critically ill patients who received long-term sedation with etomidate.

Pheochromocytoma

Pheochromocytoma is a tumor of the adrenal medulla or chromaffin cells, which produces, stores, and secretes catecholamines (usually epinephrine and/or norepinephrine). Approximately 90% are solitary tumors of the adrenal medulla, 10% are extraadrenal (intraabdominal tumors of the paravertebral sympathetic ganglia) and may be associated with MEN syndromes (Table 13.3).

Symptoms

Symptoms relate to the paroxysmal release of catecholamines and include headache, palpitations, tremor, sweating, and pallor or flushing. Chronic vasoconstriction results in hypertension (chronic manifestations in 90% and paroxysmal in 40%) and a significantly decreased intravascular volume, which may manifest as orthostatic hypotension with treatment of hypertension. Catecholamine-induced cardiomyopathy, presenting as myocarditis with possible CHF and dysrhythmias, may occur. Occasionally, pheochromocytoma may present as uncontrollable hypertension and arrhythmias during the induction of anesthesia for nonrelated surgery. If pheochromocytoma is suspected, the surgery should be postponed until adequate workup can be completed, because of the morbidity associated with surgery in patients with untreated tumors.

Diagnosis

Diagnosis is made by 24-hour urine collections for catecholamines and their metabolic products, VMA (urinary metanephrines may not be predictably elevated). In addition, CT scan and MRI can be used to localize the tumor before surgery for its removal. Rarely, pheochromocytoma may be metastatic, in which case resection of the primary tumor will not completely remove the abnormal source of catecholamines.

Preoperative Preparation

Preoperative preparation is essential for prevention of severe blood pressure swings during resection of the pheochromocytoma. The goals are to reduce vasoconstriction by decreasing catecholamine synthesis or the hormones' vasconstrictor effects and to increase intravascular volume concurrently, thereby decreasing perioperative blood pressure fluctuations and heart rate changes and reducing operative mortality. Oral α-adrenergic antagonists have routinely been used as the first line of treatment to produce vasodilation.

Phenoxybenzamine, a long-acting (24–48 hour) α-adrenergic blocker, is administered at an initial oral dose of 10 mg every 8 hours and increased until blood pressure is adequately controlled (range: 80–200 mg daily). At the same time, oral and/or intravenous hydration is begun, with a decrease in hematocrit indicating that the intravascular volume is normalizing. **Prazosin,** a shorter-acting α-adrenergic blocker, is also effective in patients with a pheochromocytoma. Although the optimal preoperative treatment duration may vary, the α-blocker is usually given until the blood pressure is well controlled (some clinicians continue until there is orthostatic hypotension) and continued until the morning of surgery. Since β-adrenergic receptors are not blocked with this treatment, tachycardia and arrhythmias may occur, and a β-blocker (labetalol, propranolol) should be added. β-Adrenergic blockade should not be used before α-blockade because decreased cardiac contractility with untreated vasoconstriction may produce left ventricular failure. Also, administration of epinephrine in a patient with α-adrenergic blockade will produce β-effects, tachycardia and vasodilation.

α-**Methyl tyrosine (metyrosine),** an inhibitor of catecholamine synthesis, has also been used as a single drug (1.0–4.0 gm/day in divided doses) or in combination with α-blockers in the preoperative preparation of patients with pheochromocytoma. Metyrosine is useful for preventing postoperative hypertension in patients with metastatic pheochromocytoma who will have residual catecholamine sources.

Cardiac function should be assessed (echocardiography or MUGA scan) if history or physical examination suggests the possibility of catecholamine-induced cardiomyopathy. Also, myocardial ischemia is more likely if there is left ventricular hypertrophy.

Anesthetic Management

Perioperative invasive monitoring should include direct arterial and central venous pressures. A pulmonary artery catheter should be considered for patients with a history of cardiac disease or catecholamine-induced cardiomyopathy. These monitors are often inserted before induction of anesthesia and intubation because these events may be associated with significant hemodynamic alterations. Rapidly acting, short-duration vasodilators such as phentolamine and/or sodium nitroprusside should be available for infusions to treat hypertension, which may occur during induction and tumor manipulation. Esmolol can be used to treat tachycardia. Corticosteroids should be given to patients who require bilateral adrenalectomy.

The goal of induction and maintenance of anesthesia is to avoid techniques or drugs that stimulate the sympathetic nervous system. Patients should receive sufficient **preoperative sedation** to enable placement of their arterial and central venous lines before induction without hemodynamic response. Benzodiazepines such as diazepam or midazolam are useful because they have few hemodynamic effects. Drugs such as morphine,

curare, and atracurium, which release histamine, a sympathetic
stimulator, and vagolytics should be avoided. A variety of intravenous drugs have been used for **induction of anesthesia** without any single agent being deemed most appropriate. Droperidol should be avoided because it has produced hypertension by
an unknown mechanism in these patients. **Anesthesia is usually
maintained** with an inhalation agent because it permits rapid
changes in anesthetic depth and blunts sympathetic activity, but
narcotics have also been used. Isoflurane is probably most frequently used because of the stability in hemodynamics and minimal sensitization of the myocardium to catecholamines. **Before
intubation,** a deep level of anesthesia should be established, and
vasodilators may be given to prevent hypertension with laryngoscopy. Intravenous lidocaine (1.0–1.5 mg/kg) before intubation may blunt hypertension and prevent ventricular arrhythmias. Some practitioners avoid succinylcholine for muscle
relaxation for intubation because hypertension may result from
ganglia stimulation or from catecholamine release from the tumor with increased intraabdominal pressure with fasciculations.
Vecuronium is a good choice of muscle relaxants because it is
devoid of hemodynamic effects.

Manipulation of the tumor during surgical dissection will
release catecholamines and may result in bouts of hypertension
and tachycardia. These may be treated with intravenous nitroprusside (1–2 μg/kg) or phentolamine (1–2 mg), while tachy-
dysrthythmias may be treated with intravenous propranolol
(0.5–1 mg), labetolol, or a continuous infusion of esmolol.
Short-acting agents are preferable because the stimulus will be
intermittent, and longer-acting drugs may result in prolonged
hypotension or bradycardia. Following complete **ligation of the
tumor's venous drainage** and ablation of the source of catecholamines, profound hypotension may result if intravascular volume is inadequate. In this situation, large volumes of fluid may
be required, with the use of vasoconstrictors such as levophed
or epinephrine as necessary until adequate volume has been
restored. Some patients may require pressors into the postoperative period. Postoperative hypoglycemia may occur when insulin secretion is no longer inhibited by α-adrenergic agonists.

Plasma catecholamine levels return to normal over several
days to a week postoperatively, and approximately 75% of patients become normotensive.

Suggested Readings

Hirsch IB, McGill JB, Cryer PE, White PF. Perioperative management of surgical patients with diabetes mellitus. Anesthesiology 1991;74:346.

Murkin J. Anesthesia and hypothyroidism. Anesth Analg 1982;61:317.

Napolitano L. Guidelines for corticosteriod use in anesthetic and surgical stress. Int Anesthesiol Clin 1988;26:226.

Palleritis J. Anesthesia for phaeochromocytoma. Can J Anaesth 1988;35:526.

Weinberg AD, Brennan MD, Gorman CA, et al. Outcome of anesthesia and surgery in hypothyroid patients. Arch Intern Med 1983;143:893.

Chapter 14

Anesthesia and the Liver

To properly plan an anesthetic for the patient with liver disease, the anesthesiologist should understand the demands made on the normal liver and the consequences of an abnormal liver's inability to meet those demands.

I. Fundamental knowledge of **normal hepatic physiology and anatomy** is a prerequisite to understanding the changes that occur in a dysfunctional liver.
  A. The liver is unusual in having a **dual blood supply.**
    1. **Total hepatic blood flow is 800–1200 ml/min,** which equals 100 ml/min/100 gm of tissue.
    2. Approximately one-third of total hepatic blood flow is derived from the hepatic artery, and two-thirds from the portal vein.
    3. The portal system is supplied by the venous drainage of the alimentary canal, spleen, pancreas, and gallbladder. This blood has a relatively low oxygen content and a high nutrient content.
    4. The hepatic artery is a branch of the celiac artery and has a high oxygen content and a low nutrient content.
  B. In addition to maintaining hepatic perfusion, **the hepatic artery and the hepatic portal venous system work in concert to help maintain systemic intravascular volume** in homeostasis.
    1. The portal vein can have varying amounts of blood entering and leaving the system.
      a. Through variation in resistance of the arterioles

supplying the abdominal viscera, portal venous blood can be regulated at its source.

b. Portal blood flow can be further regulated by variations in resistance of its flow into the liver. This regulation occurs through modulation of pre- and postsinusoidal sphincters.

c. If systemic intravascular volume decreases, there is an increase in resistance to the inflow of blood into the portal system and a shift of blood from the portal system into the systemic circulation.

2. Stimulation of alpha receptors in the hepatic venous system results in a decrease in venous compliance to force blood from the hepatic to the systemic circulation.

3. **The portal and hepatic venous system can transfer as much as 500 ml of blood to the systemic circulation.**

4. The hepatic artery can alter its blood flow in response to changes in portal venous flow. The details of this **autoregulation of total hepatic blood flow and oxygenation** are still being defined.

a. If portal flow decreases there is a concomitant decrease in hepatic artery resistance and an increase in arterial flow. This allows total hepatic blood flow and oxygenation to remain constant over a range of portal blood flow.

b. In contrast, the portal vein can not increase flow in response to a decrease in hepatic artery flow.

c. Via these changes, the liver can maintain a stable oxygen supply while serving as a blood reservoir for the systemic circulation.

C. In addition to changes in intravascular volume, the sympathetic tone of the splanchnic vessels is influenced by a variety of systemic stresses.

1. A decrease in $PaCO_2$ or PaO_2 results in an increase in splanchnic vascular tone and a decrease in liver blood flow.

2. Systemic acidosis resulting from an increase in $PaCO_2$ increases hepatic arterial and portal flow. The direct vasodilation of decreased pH is balanced against a generalized increase in sympathetic vascular tone when the body becomes acidotic.

3. An increase in circulating catecholamines can affect alpha and beta receptors in the hepatic arterial system and alpha receptors in the portal venous system, resulting in a decrease in hepatic blood flow.

4. A decrease in mean arterial pressure decreases hepatic artery perfusion pressure, and therefore, hepatic blood flow is diminished concomitantly.

D. Working in parallel with the hepatic vasculature is the **bile duct system.**

1. Bile formed in the hepatocytes empties into the bile canaliculi and flows in a series of larger conduits to the hepatic duct.

2. The gallbladder is drained by the cystic duct, which joins the hepatic duct to form the common bile duct.

3. The common bile duct meets the duodenum at the sphincter of Oddi. In general, **narcotics increase the tone of the sphincter of Oddi,** which is a concern in patients with obstructive jaundice. This effect can be modulated by halothane and enflurane.

4. The same system that carries bile transports bilirubin that has been detoxified by intrahepatic conjugation with glucuronic acid. Unconjugated bilirubin is a by-product of heme breakdown.

E. The liver plays a central role in **drug metabolism, glucose and fat homeostasis, and protein synthesis and catabolism.**

1. Most drugs must be relatively lipophilic to cross cell membranes to reach their sites of action. To facilitate excretion and prevent renal tubular reabsorption following filtration, they must be converted to hydrophilic polar compounds. There are a variety of intrahepatic enzymatic systems to achieve this.

   a. The first step in the process of drug elimination is either oxidation, reduction or hydrolysis. Oxidation via the cytochrome P-450 system is the most common pathway.

   b. The second step often involves the addition of glucuronic acid. This results in a highly polarized compound that is easily eliminated by the kidneys.

2. The liver helps regulate serum glucose levels by either adding to or subtracting from its glycogen stores. Following exhaustion of hepatic glycogen after starvation of 24 hours or more, the liver can manufacture glycogen from lactate, glycerol, and certain amino acids.

3. The liver can regulate serum lipid levels by production or degradation of fatty acids.

4. **The liver serves as the body's protein factory,** producing albumin, all the procoagulants except factor VIII, plasma cholinesterase, and a variety of proteins that affect a multitude of enzyme systems. While producing protein, it disposes of unneeded amino acids by converting them to ammonia and then to urea, which is eliminated by the kidneys.

II. The care of patients with abnormal liver function requires a **proper preoperative evaluation** including a complete history, physical, and appropriate laboratory testing.

A. **Pertinent historical questions** are aimed at identifying the source and acuity of the patient's disease.

1. A careful assessment of a patient's alcohol intake includes quantity of alcohol ingested and an estimate of the duration.

2. A history of drug use, either illicit or prescribed, with specific reference to intravenous abuse, is critical information.

3. High-risk sexual behavior or a prior blood transfusion raises the possibility of viral hepatitis.

4. Recent dietary intolerance or a change in urine, sclera, or stool color points to an alteration in liver function.

5. A history of a bleeding diathesis or variceal bleeding supports a diagnosis of advanced hepatic disease.

B. The **physical examination** should include an assessment of the general appearance of the patient, in addition to a detailed search for specific stigmata of liver disease.

1. A patient who is cachectic or jaundiced or who has a protuberant abdomen from ascites probably has advanced disease.

    2. Altered mental status secondary to hepatic encepha-lopathy represents a profound depression of liver function.

    3. The abdominal examination should include palpa-tion of the liver and spleen and estimation of the quantity of ascites present.

C. **Laboratory testing** can help define whether the patient is suffering from a prehepatic, intrahepatic, or posthe-patic process. The resultant impact on liver function is of critical concern to the anesthesiologist.

    1. The relative site of hepatic disease is determined by measuring bilirubin, serum transaminases, and alka-line phosphatase.

        a. **Prehepatic disease** results in elevated unconju-gated bilirubin, normal transaminases, and nor-mal alkaline phosphatase levels. Intravascular or extravascular hemolysis fits this category.

        b. **Intrahepatic disease** is characterized by increased conjugated bilirubin, increased transaminases, and normal to moderately increased alkaline phosphatase levels.

           i. Alcoholic or viral hepatitis is a typical example of this process.

          ii. If hepatitis advances to cirrhosis, the transami-nase levels may return to normal despite ad-vanced liver damage.

        c. **Posthepatic disease** is associated with increased conjugated bilirubin, normal to moderately ele-vated transaminases, and greatly elevated alkaline phosphatase levels. An example of posthepatic disease is biliary obstruction secondary to ste-nosis.

    2. Commonly used **laboratory parameters of the syn-thetic function** of the liver are serum albumin level and the prothrombin time.

        a. **Albumin** has a relatively long half-life (3 weeks); therefore, acute deterioration of liver function will not be reflected in serum albumin levels.

           i. A decrease in the serum albumin level results in a parallel reduction in intravascular oncotic pressure and the accumulation of large volumes of extracellular fluid that is most dramatically recognized as ascites.

    ii. If extracellular fluid is greatly increased, certain drugs may have a larger than normal volume of distribution, and serum drug levels would be lower than expected (e.g., a higher dose of pancuronium is required for patients with ascites).

  b. The **procoagulants** have a short half-life (hours to days), and their concentrations will reflect acute changes in synthetic function.

    i. A prolonged prothrombin time may reflect inadequate vitamin K absorption secondary to inadequate bile salt excretion into the gut. This can be treated with parenteral vitamin K. If vitamin K does not correct the clotting abnormality, this suggests that the liver has suffered a profound insult.

    ii. Fresh frozen plasma should be available if a large surgical blood loss is expected in a patient with a bleeding diathesis secondary to abnormal procoagulant activity which is refractory to vitamin K therapy.

  3. Adequate intravenous access is essential prior to major surgery if the patient has an uncorrected bleeding diathesis.

III. Once the cause, extent, and acuity of the patient's hepatic disease are determined, consideration must be given to how the **pathology intrinsic to the liver will affect the remaining organ systems.**

  A. The diseased liver may increase resistance to portal blood flow, with the ensuing portal hypertension having several consequences.

    1. As resistance to portal flow increases, the hepatic artery must deliver a greater share of the total hepatic blood flow. Maintenance of normal mean arterial pressure is mandatory to prevent the diseased liver from becoming ischemic.

    2. A series of collateral channels will develop between the portal and systemic venous system to decom-

press the hypertensive portal circulation. These collaterals can cause catastrophic hemorrhage (e.g., ruptured esophageal varix). Surgery may be required to create an artificial shunt between the portal system and vena cava to reduce portal venous pressure.

B. The **cardiovascular system** in the patient with portal hypertension is often hyperdynamic.

1. Cardiac output is high, and systemic vascular resistance is low.

2. The etiology of this hyperdynamic state is unclear, but one contribution is the abundance of arteriovenous fistulae.

3. Liver disease secondary to ethanol abuse may be complicated by alcoholic cardiomyopathy.

C. Despite a hyperdynamic cardiovascular system, the patient with portal hypertension will often have a **lower than expected arterial oxygen saturation.** There is a multifactorial explanation for this.

1. Intrapulmonary and portal to pulmonary venous shunts allow desaturated blood to reach the systemic circulation.

2. Hypoxic pulmonary vasoconstriction is impaired in cirrhotic patients secondary to higher than normal levels of endogenous vasodilators.

3. Poor diaphragmatic excursion from ascites results in ventilation perfusion mismatch.

D. **Renal function** may be altered in the presence of liver disease. Renal blood flow may be impaired in the cirrhotic patient, and the glomerular filtration rate may be reduced. Intravascular volume must be maintained to prevent renal failure. Hepatorenal syndrome is a cause of refractory renal failure associated with severe liver disease and may be a cause of oliguria.

E. The cirrhotic patient may be encephalopathic secondary to an inability to eliminate nitrogenous waste products.

F. The cirrhotic patient is often **anemic and thrombocytopenic.**

IV. The anesthetic plan must attempt to preserve remaining liver function. Knowledge of the anesthetic and surgical effects on the liver is a prerequisite to a **well-planned operative course.**

A. The **stress response to major surgery** directly decreases liver blood flow and function, independent of the choice of anesthetics.

   1. The closer the **operative site** is to the liver, the greater the reduction in hepatic blood flow. Procedures involving the upper abdomen produce the most changes.

   2. Abdominal surgery in patients with severe hepatic disease is associated with a poor prognosis. The high morbidity in this group of patients has not changed in decades, despite improved anesthetic techniques.

B. **Both general and regional anesthesia can have a negative impact on the liver** independent of the effect of surgery.

   1. If blood pressure falls following initiation of anesthesia, hepatic perfusion will be diminished. Hepatic dysfunction may be accelerated as a result.

   2. **Various anesthetic agents can be hepatotoxic** independent of their effects on perfusion pressure.

      a. **Halothane** has been implicated as a contributor to postoperative hepatic dysfunction more often than any other drug used in anesthesia.

         i. The largest study of halothane toxicity demonstrated an incidence of fatal hepatic necrosis not attributable to other causes to be 7 per 250,000 patients.

         ii. Hepatitis secondary to halothane may occur more often than fatal hepatic necrosis, but it is often hard to distinguish postoperative halothane hepatitis from coincident viral hepatitis.

   3. **Obesity, female gender, repeated exposures,** and **middle age** are generally accepted as risk factors associated with halothane hepatitis.

      b. Studies reviewing the incidence of hepatitis following exposure to **enflurane, isoflurane,** or **nitrous oxide** fail to reliably demonstrate a clear association between these agents and postoperative hepatic dysfunction.

C. It appears that **intravenous anesthetic agents** do not cause appreciable hepatic damage that is discernible from the effect of surgery.

1. This premise holds true if the administration of the agent does not result in a dramatic reduction in hepatic perfusion pressure.

2. If the patient has cirrhosis, it is advisable to titrate intravenous anesthetic agents to effect, since pharmacokinetics may be significantly altered secondary to increased volumes of distribution, poor hepatic extraction and metabolism, and variable protein binding.

D. Consideration must be given to **operative monitoring, induction sequence,** and **maintenance agents.**

1. In addition to standard monitors, often an intraarterial catheter is used for continuous pressure monitoring and access for arterial sampling. A central venous catheter may be used for volume assessment, but a pulmonary artery catheter is indicated when the patient has pulmonary or cardiac disease.

2. Special consideration should be taken for **induction** if the patient is thought to have a full stomach. It is always a concern that an alcoholic patient has surreptitiously imbibed on the day of surgery. Succinylcholine may be used to rapidly facilitate intubation, although its action might be prolonged when there are abnormally low levels of pseudocholinesterase.

3. **Isoflurane** or **enflurane** are rational choices for potent volatile agents. Halothane is best avoided, as it may complicate the differential diagnosis if there is new postoperative hepatic dysfunction.

4. **Fentanyl** does not appear to affect hepatic oxygen supply and can be used safely.

5. **Atracurium** does not depend upon the liver for metabolism and is an ideal choice for a muscle relaxant.

V. A patient who develops **hepatic dysfunction postoperatively** must be evaluated in a fashion similar to that of the preoperative workup, including pertinent historical data, physical findings, and laboratory data. The patient's disease can then be classified as pre-, intra-, or posthepatic.

A. The most common cause of **prehepatic dysfunction** is excess bilirubin production following multiple blood transfusions. This process is self-limiting.

B. **Intrahepatic disease** may be secondary to relative hepatic ischemia during surgery, caused by periods of impaired hepatic blood flow or oxygenation. The liver will usually recover from this without sequelae. Hepatotoxicity secondary to drug exposure must be considered, and if present, repeated exposure to the offending agent should be avoided.

C. **Posthepatic dysfunction** may be caused by surgical injury of the bile duct. Secondary causes with high morbidity are pancreatitis and cholecystitis.

Suggested Readings

Gelman S. Anesthesia and the liver. In: Barash PG, Cullen BF, Stoelting RK. Clinical anesthesia. Philadelphia: JB Lippincott, 1989.

Maze M. Hepatic physiology. In: Miller RD, ed. Anesthesia. New York: Churchill Livingstone, 1990.

Maze M, Prgaer MC. Anesthesia and the liver. In: Miller RD, ed. Anesthesia. New York: Churchill Livingstone, 1990.

National Research Council (US). In: Bunker JD, Forrester WH Jr, Mosteller F, et al. National Halothane Study: A Study of the Possible Association between Halothane Anesthesia and Postoperative Hepatic Necrosis. Washington, DC: National Institute of General Medical Sciences, US Government Printing Office, 1969.

Stoelting RK, Miller RD. Hepatic disease. In: Basics of Anesthesia. New York: Churchill Livingstone, 1989; chap 21.

Chapter 15

Anesthesia for the Patient with Cardiovascular Disease

For the patient with significant cardiovascular disease, the perioperative period may be considered as perhaps the ultimate cardiac "stress test." The spectrum of patients with cardiovascular disease ranges from young to old and from vigorous to frail. Mangano's recent review highlights the magnitude of the problem of cardiovascular disease in the United States:

1. Cardiovascular disease (including hypertension and coronary atherosclerotic heart disease) affects one in four Americans.
2. Approximately 7–8 million of the 25 million patients undergoing noncardiac surgery are at risk for perioperative cardiac morbidity and mortality as a result of cardiovascular disease.
3. The prevalence and incidence of cardiovascular disease are increasing as the population ages.
4. Of all forms of cardiovascular disease, coronary atherosclerotic heart disease (CASHD) results in the highest morbidity (congestive heart failure, myocardial infarction) and mortality (541,000 deaths per year).

To provide optimal care to these patients during the perioperative period, the anesthesiologist must understand normal cardiovascular physiology, the pathophysiology of common cardiovascular diseases, and the effects of these disease processes on anesthetic pharmacology. An anesthetic plan may then be designed to minimize the potential for discomfort, morbidity, and mortality during this stressful period, whether the operative procedure is required for treatment of the cardiac condition per se or a concurrent disease process. This chapter focuses on the anesthetic management of patients with CASHD who are undergoing both cardiac and noncardiac surgical procedures, with a particular emphasis on the vascular surgery patient. The anesthetic management of patients with valvular heart disease is also discussed. The care of patients with congenital heart disease is beyond the scope of this chapter.

CARDIOVASCULAR PHYSIOLOGY

The fundamental principles involved in providing a safe anesthetic for patients with cardiac disease are based on an understanding of cardiovascular physiology.

Oxygen Delivery

The primary function of the heart is to pump enough blood to the tissues throughout the body so that oxygen-dependent metabolic processes may occur. If oxygen delivery is not adequate, homeostasis is disrupted and the tissues are forced to rely on anaerobic metabolism. If anaerobic metabolism is allowed to continue without intervention, the clinical syndrome of shock will ensue. Oxygen delivery (DO_2) depends on both cardiac output (CO) and the arterial oxygen content (CaO_2), as expressed in equation (1).

$$DO_2(\text{ml } O_2 \cdot \text{min}^{-1}) = CO(\text{liter} \cdot \text{min}^{-1}) \times CaO_2(\text{ml } O_2 \cdot \text{liters of blood}^{-1}) \tag{1}$$

In an average adult at rest, DO_2 is approximately 1000 ml $O_2 \cdot \text{min}^{-1}$. The two components of oxygen delivery, CO and CaO_2, are influenced by a number of factors, which are discussed below.

Cardiac Output

CO is a measure of the pumping function of the heart and depends on the heart rate (HR) and stroke volume (SV), as shown in equation (2). Stroke volume is simply the amount of blood ejected from the left ventricle (LV) with each contraction.

$$CO(ml \cdot min^{-1}) = HR(beats \cdot min^{-1}) \times SV(ml \cdot beat^{-1}) \quad (2)$$

To permit comparison of CO values from patients of varying body habitus, cardiac index (CI) may be calculated by dividing the CO by the body surface (BSA), as in equation (3).

$$CI(liters \cdot min^{-1} \cdot meter^{-2}) = CO/BSA \quad (3)$$

In adult patients, a normal CI ranges between 2.5 and 4.0 liters $\cdot min^{-1} \cdot meter^{-2}$. Shock may occur when the cardiac index is less than 2.0 liters $\cdot min^{-1} \cdot meter^{-2}$. Inotropic support or other hemodynamic interventions are often considered if CI falls below this value in the perioperative period.

Heart Rate. The direct relationship between changes in HR and CO is apparent from equation (2). SV may change with HR, as tachycardia shortens the time for diastolic filling of the ventricle. In children, the left ventricle is relatively noncompliant, and CO increases with heart rates to about 160 beats/min (bpm). In adults, a heart rate above 120 bpm often reduces CO by decreasing the SV. The HR is determined by intrinsic cardiac pacemakers (usually the sinoatrial node), regulated in response to the metabolic needs of the body by the autonomic nervous system. Pharmacologic (anticholinergics, sympathomimetics) and mechanical measures (electronic pacemakers) may be used to augment the HR and increase CO.

Another factor that may affect CO, although not necessarily related to heart rate, is the **heart rhythm.** With sinus rhythm, an atrial contraction precedes ventricular contraction, optimizing diastolic ventricular filling and SV. Although this mechanism is of only moderate importance in patients with adequate ventricular reserve, sinus rhythm and the associated atrial "kick" may increase CO by as much as 40% in patients requiring a high end-diastolic ventricular volume, such as those with left ventricular hypertrophy (LVH). Atrial fibrillation, atrial flutter, and ventricular tachycardia, although associated with an adequate HR, may rapidly lead to shock because of profound decreases in SV.

Stroke Volume. Concepts derived from skeletal muscle mechanics have traditionally been used to describe the determinants of SV, which include **preload, afterload,** and **contractility.** The relationship between preload and contractility affects the amount of work the ventricle can do in a given beat, while afterload determines what portion of work will be applied toward ejecting the SV.

Preload. Preload, the tension placed on a muscle before contraction, determines resting muscle length. As in skeletal muscle, cardiac muscle performance improves as preload is increased over the usual range of sarcomere length. This response is important on a beat-to-beat basis so that the ventricle can respond to changes in venous return (produced, for example, by changes in body position) and effectively pump the volume of blood it receives. This relationship between cardiac work and sarcomere length is described by ventricular function, or Frank-Starling, curves (Fig. 15.1). These curves show increasing CO with increasing preload (as measured by some indication of end-diastolic fiber length or volume) over the usual sarcomere lengths. Since left ventricular end-diastolic volume

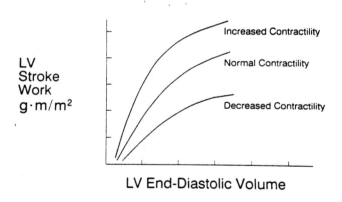

Figure 15.1. Frank-Starling curves—left ventricular (LV) stroke work vs. LV preload (expressed as end-diastolic volume). Increased contractility as produced by administration of an inotropic agent results in a shift of the curve upward and to the left. Cardiomyopathy or other causes of myocardial depression produce a shift of the curve downward and to the right. (Reproduced with permission from Reich DL, Kaplan JA. Hemodynamic monitoring. In: Kaplan JA, ed. Cardiac anesthesia. 3rd ed. Philadelphia: WB Saunders, 1993:287.)

(LVEDV) is difficult to determine, pressure measurements are used in clinical practice, but the pressure/volume relationship is usually nonlinear. Pressures that can be measured clinically to estimate the LVEDV and left ventricular preload include left atrial, pulmonary artery, and pulmonary capillary wedge pressures. Right atrial and central venous pressures are right ventricular preload estimates, and changes in these values may trend those of LV pressures in patients without significant cardiopulmonary disease.

The Frank-Starling relationship can be applied clinically to enhance the CO. Preload or venous return can be increased by expanding the intravascular volume with transfusion, use of the Trendelenburg position, or decreasing the size of the venous capacitance bed (via administration of α-agonists such as phenylephrine). Preload may be decreased by intravascular volume loss (diuresis or hemorrhage) or dilation of capacitance vessels.

Afterload. Afterload is the tension that a muscle must produce during contraction to shorten or "do work." The LV must develop sufficient wall tension during systole to generate a higher pressure than that in the aorta, so that a volume of blood (SV) is ejected. Afterload determines the portion of work that will be expended raising chamber pressure and the fraction left to eject SV. Afterload is related to several factors, including **peripheral vascular tone, compliance of the large arteries, thickness of the ventricular wall, and viscosity of the blood.** Clinically, only peripheral vascular tone changes acutely and is the focus of most discussions related to afterload. **Systemic vascular resistance (SVR)** is used to estimate vascular tone and is calculated through an equation derived from Ohm's law for electrical circuits. In this equation (4), resistance (SVR) equals the pressure difference across the systemic circulation (mean arterial pressure (MAP) minus central venous pressure (CVP)) divided by flow (CO).

$$SVR = [(MAP - CVP) \times 80 \text{ dynes} \cdot cm \cdot sec^{-5}]/CO \qquad (4)$$

SVR may be manipulated pharmacologically to alter the CO. If CO is low in the presence of high afterload (as approximated by SVR), a vasodilator may be given in an attempt to improve forward flow. This technique of afterload reduction is commonly used in the treatment of chronic congestive heart failure.

Contractility. Contractility, the final determinant of SV, is an intrinsic property possessed by the myocardial cells. Contractility can be thought of as the ability of myocardial cells to do mechanical work at any given preload. Contractility is difficult to assess with clinical monitors and may vary by region throughout the myocardium. Clinicians may alter contractility to increase or decrease CO by use of either positive or negative inotropic agents. Changes in myocardial contractility result in a shift to a new Frank-Starling function curve (Fig. 15.1).

Oxygen Content

As mentioned above, adequate oxygen delivery (DO_2) to the tissues is required for aerobic metabolism. DO_2 depends not only on an adequate cardiac output but also on the oxygen-carrying capacity of the blood. The second factor in the oxygen delivery equation (1) is the **oxygen content of arterial blood (CaO_2)**. The equation for CaO_2 (5) has several components: Hemoglobin concentration of arterial blood (Hb), oxygen saturation of arterial blood (% O_2 sat), and dissolved oxygen, which is described in the last portion of the equation.

$$CaO_2(ml\ O_2 \cdot 100\ ml\ blood^{-1}) = \qquad (5)$$
$$(Hb \times 1.39 \times \%\ O_2\ sat) + (PaO_2 \times 0.003)$$

If CaO_2 is to be maximized so that adequate oxygen is delivered to tissues, the hemoglobin must be well saturated and its concentration adequate. The amount of dissolved oxygen in blood is low and is not usually of clinical significance. The PaO_2, % O_2 sat, hemoglobin concentration, and CO can be manipulated during anesthesia to optimize oxygen delivery.

Coronary Anatomy, Physiology and Myocardial Oxygen Balance

The two main coronary arteries (left and right) branch from the aorta just distal to the cusps of the aortic valve. Each main artery divides to supply distinct portions of myocardium, (Fig. 15.2). The coronary circulation is unique in four ways:

• The heart is the only organ responsible for its own perfusion.
• The myocardium has little collateral blood supply and thus depends on the patency of the coronary arteries.

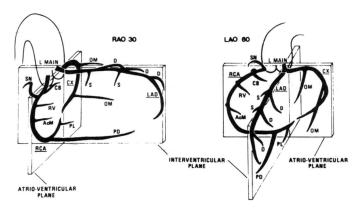

Figure 15.2. Coronary anatomy relative to the interventricular and atrioventricular valve planes as commonly viewed during cardiac catheterization. Coronary branches shown include *L MAIN,* left main (coronary artery); *LAD,* left anterior descending; *D,* diagonal; *S,* septal; *CX,* circumflex; *OM,* obtuse marginal; *RCA,* right coronary; *CB,* conus branch; *SN,* sinus node; *AcM,* acute marginal; *PD,* posterior descending; *PL,* posterolateral left ventricular branch. (Reproduced with permission from Chambers CE, Skeehan TM, Hensley FA. The cardiac catheterization laboratory: diagnostic and therapeutic procedures in the adult patient. In: Kaplan JA, ed. Cardiac anesthesia. 3rd ed. Philadelphia: WB Saunders, 1993:70.)

- Coronary oxygen extraction is near maximal at rest (8–10 ml O_2/100 gm myocardium/min), and increased demand for oxygen can be met only by increased blood flow.
- High intracavitary pressure during systole interrupts blood flow to the LV so that most LV coronary flow occurs during diastole. In contrast, the low-pressure right ventricle is perfused throughout the cardiac cycle.

The proximal portion of coronary arteries is especially prone to atherosclerotic changes that may limit myocardial blood flow. Appropriate **myocardial oxygen balance** is critical to the prevention of myocardial ischemia. This balance is determined by the relationship between the oxygen available to the myocardium (supply) and that required by the myocardium to meet the needs of the body (demand).

Myocardial Oxygen Supply

Unlike other tissues that can meet increased oxygen demand by boosting extraction from the arterial blood, the myocardium must increase coronary blood flow to meet its own needs. **Coronary blood flow** is autoregulated and is determined by the **coronary vascular resistance** and the **coronary perfusion pressure.** Coronary vascular resistance is primarily controlled by local factors such as tissue pH and oxygen levels, which are determined by local metabolic needs. The subendocardial region of the heart is particularly vulnerable to ischemia, since it is subjected to LV intracavitary pressure and is perfused only during diastole. The **coronary perfusion pressure** is calculated as the difference between the diastolic aortic pressure and the left ventricular end-diastolic pressure (LVEDP). Either a low diastolic aortic pressure or elevated LVEDP (as estimated by some measure of preload) may compromise coronary blood flow and myocardial oxygen supply.

Myocardial Oxygen Demand

The same factors that determine CO also determine the heart's requirement for oxygen: **heart rate, preload, afterload, and contractility.** Of these, HR is most significant, as it directly affects both oxygen demand and supply. Tachycardia not only increases myocardial oxygen demand but also may significantly reduce the oxygen supply by shortening the time of diastole in each cardiac cycle. Increased afterload may be favorable to the balance of myocardial oxygen supply and demand by increasing perfusion pressure or detrimental by increasing myocardial work. Increased preload and contractility both increase myocardial oxygen demand to the extent they increase CO and wall tension. All of these factors can be manipulated pharmacologically to optimize the critical balance between supply and demand.

Myocardial Metabolism

Fatty acids and lactate are the primary energy substrates used by the myocardium. During **aerobic metabolism,** most myocardial oxygen consumption goes toward oxidation of fatty acids and myocardial extraction of lactate. Under **anaerobic conditions,** glucose is the only substrate used, and lactate may accumulate in the ischemic tissues.

Heart Failure

Many disease processes may result in cardiac failure, a state in which the heart is unable to convert energy substrate into sufficient CO to maintain cellular homeostasis. Several compensatory mechanisms have evolved to cope with prolonged reductions in CO:

- Increased sympathetic tone and circulating catecholamine levels producing increased myocardial contractility
- Ventricular hypertrophy through parallel replication of contractile fibers in response to increased pressure needs
- Intravascular volume expansion by activation of the renin-angiotensin system, which increases preload and SV because of the Frank-Starling effect

These compensatory mechanisms may adversely affect other organ systems despite rectifying the patient's cardiac condition. Renal sodium retention and intravascular volume expansion may increase pulmonary venous pressures. If pulmonary capillary fluid leaks into the extravascular compartment of the lung, the increase in lung water impairs oxygen diffusion from the alveoli and produces the classic symptoms of pulmonary edema. Treatment of heart failure is directed toward relieving symptomatology as well as improving the ability of the heart to meet the metabolic needs of the body.

CARDIOVASCULAR PATHOPHYSIOLOGY

The most important cardiac disease processes in adults are CASHD and valvular heart disease.

Ischemic Heart Disease

Myocardial ischemia occurs when myocardial tissues fail to receive enough oxygen to meet their metabolic needs. The causes of ischemic heart disease (IHD) are complex, yet can be simplistically classified as CASHD and coronary vasospasm. Prinzmetal's (or variant) angina is a distinct type of symptomatology resulting from coronary vasospasm. It is important to realize that CASHD and vasospasm may both occur in the same patient.

Coronary stenosis may result from atheromatous disease, thrombus, emboli, or vasospasm and limits the usual increase in coronary blood flow (and oxygen supply) in response to stress. The spectrum of IHD includes angina, myocardial infarction, sudden death, and congestive heart failure. CASHD is the most common underlying cause of each of these syndromes, although vasospasm is occasionally responsible for some of the acute symptom exacerbations.

Angina is defined as an episode of substernal chest pain, frequently radiating to the arm or neck, that results from a demand for oxygen in a region of the myocardium in excess of the available supply. With a less critical coronary artery stenosis, an increase in oxygen demand (after eating, exercise, or exposure to stress) is required to cause ischemia. If the stenosis is sufficiently severe, angina at rest may occur.

Myocardial infarction (MI) occurs when a prolonged imbalance between myocardial oxygen supply and demand leads to necrosis. MI may range in severity from a "mild" subendocardial infarction to a life-threatening transmural MI involving the entire thickness of the myocardial wall.

The terminal event of CASHD is often **ventricular fibrillation** resulting from an ischemic myocardium. "Sudden death" is in most circumstances attributable to CASHD and may be the presenting symptom of ischemic heart disease.

Chronic congestive heart failure (CHF) may also occur secondary to CASHD. **"Ischemic cardiomyopathy"** results from loss of contractile function with chronic ischemia. This loss of contractility may be reversible, or infarction may lead to scar or aneurysm formation. Symptoms of CHF include diminished exercise tolerance, dyspnea on exertion, or paroxysmal nocturnal dyspnea.

Careful ECG monitoring of patients with CASHD has demonstrated frequent ischemic episodes without measurable changes in hemodynamic variables. The primary goals in the anesthetic management of patients with IHD are thus to avoid an imbalance between myocardial oxygen supply and demand and to minimize the detrimental hemodynamic effects of perioperative stress, especially tachycardia (Table 15.1).

Table 15.1.
Hemodynamic Management Goals in Patients with Valvular and Ischemic Heart Disease[a]

Condition	Preload	Heart Rate	Rhythm	Afterload	Contractility
Aortic stenosis	Nl to increase	Nl to decrease	Sinus is best	Increase	Usually Nl; may need increase
(Chronic) aortic insufficiency	Nl to slight increase	Nl to slight increase	Sinus is best	Decrease	Nl early; may need increase late
Mitral stenosis	Slight increase	Nl to decrease	Sinus is best; control ventricular response in atrial fibrillation	Avoid pulmonary vasoconstriction	LV Nl; RV may be decreased
Mitral regurgitation	Slight increase	Slight increase	Sinus is best; control ventricular response in atrial fibrillation	Decrease	Usually Nl

Table 15.1.
Continued

Condition	Preload	Heart Rate	Rhythm	Afterload	Contractility
Tricuspid regurgitation	Slight increase in CVP	Nl to slight increase	Sinus is best	Decrease RV afterload	Usually Nl
Hypertrophic cardiomyopathy	Increase	Nl to slight decrease	Sinus is best	Increase	Nl to decrease
Ischemic heart disease (coronary artery disease)	Optimize to maintain BP without LV distention	Nl to decrease	Sinus; keep LV response slow if atrial tachycardia is present	Nl to decrease; may need increase to maintain diastolic pressure	Nl to decrease; prevent increase
Cardiac tamponade	Increase	Increase	Sinus tachycardia OK	Nl to increase	Nl to increase

[a]Abbreviations: Nl, maintain in normal range; Increase, increase from normal range; Decrease, decrease from normal range; LV, left ventricle; RV, right ventricle; CVP, central venous pressure.

Valvular Heart Disease

Valvular heart disease leads to compensatory changes in cardiac anatomy and physiology that must be thoroughly considered in formulating an anesthetic plan. Stenotic valvular lesions lead to pressure overload, while regurgitant valvular lesions result in volume overload. Compensatory changes include increased sympathetic tone to maintain contractility and humorally mediated increases in intravascular volume to augment preload. Ventricular hypertrophy often results from chronic pressure overload, while chamber dilation occurs in response to volume overload.

Aortic Stenosis

Valvular aortic stenosis (AS) most commonly results from thickening, degeneration, and calcification of a congenitally bicuspid aortic valve but may also occur with senile degeneration of a structurally normal valve or after rheumatic fever, usually in association with rheumatic mitral valvular disease. AS usually becomes symptomatic when the aortic valve area is reduced to 1.0 cm^2 from its normal value of 3.0 cm^2. Classic **symptoms** of severe AS include syncope, angina, and late in the course of the disease, CHF.

Pathophysiologic changes occuring with AS are due to chronic pressure overload of the LV, as it must generate tremendous pressures to eject blood through the narrowed valve opening. This leads to increased LV wall tension and compensatory concentric hypertrophy, usually without a change in intracavitary size. LV hypertrophy results in deceased diastolic LV compliance, imbalances in myocardial oxygen supply and demand, especially in the subendocardial region, and eventually, deterioration of LV contractility.

CO is best maintained when the preload is normal or increased, the HR is normal or decreased, atrial contraction precedes ventricular contraction (sinus rhythm), and coronary perfusion pressure is maintained (Table 15.1). Decreased preload may be particularly detrimental because of decreased diastolic compliance from LV hypertrophy. Sudden changes from sinus rhythm may acutely diminish ventricular filling and reduce CO by up to 40%. The subsequent hypotension can be especially severe, as it may reduce coronary perfusion pressure to the thickened LV. **Ventricular fibrillation** is especially danger-ous in patients with AS, since myocardial oxygen demand is great (large mass of active muscle) while supply is nil. CPR is usually ineffective because of the valvular stenosis.

Aortic Insufficiency

Aortic insufficiency (AI) can be either **acute** from bacterial en-docarditis, connective tissue diseases such as Marfan's syn-drome, or proximal aortic dissection from trauma or atheroscle-rotic disease or **chronic,** which may be insidious in onset, from rheumatic heart disease, long-standing hypertension, or syph-ilis.

As a result of regurgitant flow, the LV must adapt to volume overload. With acute AI, the LV may rapidly decompensate in response to this additional volume. If the onset of insufficiency is slower, the LV can compensate through eccentric hypertro-phy (dilation) to maintain a nearly normal SV. Although myo-cardial oxygen requirements do not increase greatly with this form of ventricular work, this compensatory mechanism eventu-ally fails to keep pace with the increasing volume load, and con-tractility becomes impaired after a prolonged asymptomatic in-terval. LV afterload is usually reduced secondary to arteriolar dilation, manifest clinically by low diastolic pressures and a wid-ened pulse pressure. Eventually, an irreversible decrease in LV contractility ensues, and symptoms of dyspnea and diminished exercise tolerance will appear.

Factors that further increase the volume load on the LV will worsen AI, including bradycardia (more time for regurgitant flow), increased afterload (resistance to forward flow), diastolic hypertension, and myocardial depression (Table 15.1). Con-versely, modest tachycardia, adequate preload, and decreased afterload will enhance forward flow.

Mitral Stenosis

Mitral stenosis (MS) is most frequently rheumatic in origin. The onset of symptoms such as dyspnea is usually delayed for 20 to 30 years following the episode of rheumatic fever, when the mitral valve area approaches 1.0 cm^2. Patients may become symptomatic earlier if acute stresses such as pregnancy require an increased CO.

The primary pathophysiologic process in MS is pressure overload proximal to the stenotic mitral valve. Because the obstruction is "upstream" from the LV, it remains small with normal contractility, and it may be chronically underloaded. Pathophysiologic changes proximal to the stenotic valve include left atrial dilation, pulmonary arterial and venous hypertension, and if pulmonary hypertension is prolonged and severe, tricuspid regurgitation with right ventricular failure (cor pulmonale). With chronic MS, as the left atrium dilates, atrial arrhythmias (atrial fibrillation) are likely and may result in hemodynamic decompensation.

Management of a patient with MS requires that sufficient left atrial pressure be maintained to ensure adequate filling of the LV while avoiding pulmonary edema. Sinus rhythm should be maintained if possible, since atrial contraction provides a large portion of LV diastolic filling. Tachycardia should be avoided, as it decreases the diastolic time available for flow to occur across the stenotic valve, reducing LV filling and further elevating LA pressure. Any condition that increases pulmonary vascular resistance (hypercarbia, hypoxia) must be avoided, since this decreases LA filling and may worsen tricuspid regurgitation.

Mitral Regurgitation

Mitral regurgitation (MR) may develop acutely secondary to bacterial endocarditis or from a ruptured papillary muscle in the setting of acute MI. MR may be associated with chronic rheumatic heart disease or mitral valve prolapse. Although the pathophysiology of both acute and chronic MR is related to LV volume overload, the appearance of symptoms will depend on the course of the disease. There is little time for cardiac compensation with acute MR, and when a significant portion of the LV stroke volume is ejected back across the mitral valve into the LA, LA pressure rises abruptly. Acute pulmonary edema results from pulmonary venous hypertension and marked decreases in forward cardiac flow. In patients with chronic MR, compensatory mechanisms usually allow a more gradual onset of symptoms. The regurgitant fraction of the LV stroke volume is directed into the lower-pressure LA, and the LV undergoes eccentric hypertrophy (dilation) rather than the concentric hypertrophy (seen with the pressure overload of AS). LV compliance is preserved until late in the disease process. The compliant LA dilates in chronic MR, protecting the pulmonary vasculature and RV from the deleterious pressure changes that may accompany acute MR. Eventually these compensatory mechanisms may be overwhelmed, resulting in pulmonary arterial hypertension and RV failure. Over time, the dilated LV loses contractility, and overt signs and symptoms of decreased forward cardiac output are seen.

HR should be maintained at a normal or slightly elevated rate in patients with either acute or chronic MR to reduce the time available for regurgitation, decrease LV distention, and increase CO (Table 15.1). Afterload should be reduced if necessary to promote forward flow. Any factor that elevates pulmonary vascular resistance (PVR) should be avoided. Contractility and preload (normal to slightly increased) must be maintained to prevent pulmonary edema.

Tricuspid Regurgitation

Isolated tricuspid regurgitation (TR) is quite rare and is usually a complication of infective endocarditis, often secondary to intravenous drug use. TR leads to an increased volume load on the RV. This is usually well tolerated unless there is resistance to RV outflow, such as is seen in patients with elevated PVR. To manage patients with isolated TR, CVP should be maintained (or increased) to ensure an adequate RV preload. RV afterload (PVR) should be kept as low as possible by avoiding hypoxia and hypercarbia.

Other Cardiac Disease States

Hypertrophic Cardiomyopathy

Hypertrophic cardiomyopathy (HCM) or idiopathic hypertrophic subaortic stenosis (IHSS) is a heritable disease process in which asymmetric muscular development in the LV outflow tract results in a dynamic outflow obstruction, functionally similar to AS. The subaortic stenosis, usually documented by echocardiography, is produced during systole as the outflow tract is narrowed by the opposition of the hypertrophied septum and the anterior leaflet of the mitral valve.

Since the outflow obstruction is worsened by either increased LV contractility or reduced LV volume (Table 15.1), β-adrenergic or calcium channel blockers are used to reduce LV contractility and improve the outflow gradient. Volatile anesthetic agents (particularly halothane) produce similar beneficial results. Catecholamines released in response to surgical stimuli and exogenously administered inotropic agents may worsen the dynamic stenosis and reduce CO. In this unique situation, administration of positive inotropic drugs for low CO exacerbates the problem. Hypovolemia and compensatory tachycardia catastrophically reduces SV. Restoring preload while maintaining or increasing afterload minimizes LV outflow obstruction and preserves systemic pressures. With chronic outflow obstruction, LV hypertrophy increases the risk of MI.

Cardiac Tamponade and Constrictive Pericarditis

Both cardiac tamponade and constrictive pericarditis result in impairment of diastolic filling because of extracardiac compression. The severity of symptoms generally depends on the time course of the disease process. Rapid accumulation of small amounts of pericardial fluid may result in profound hemodynamic decompensation, while the chronic development of massive quantities of fluid may be well tolerated. Extracardiac compression limits systemic venous return and increases CVP. **Tamponade may be diagnosed** by the presence of hypotension, tachycardia, diminished heart tones, and jugular venous distention. Equalization of diastolic pressures is seen across all cardiac chambers.

Decreased diastolic filling limits SV, and CO becomes rate-dependent. If untreated, systemic hypotension will develop, with coronary hypoperfusion, myocardial ischemia, and a rapid downhill course. While awaiting definitive relief of the problem (drainage or resection), bradycardia must be prevented, while preload, afterload, and contractility must be maintained (Table 15.1).

ANESTHESIA FOR CARDIAC SURGERY

The anesthesiologist must have a clear understanding of potential intraoperative problems in these "high-risk" patients, so that quick, definitive action may be taken if there is a critical intraoperative event. Communication between anesthesiologists, surgeons, cardiologists, perfusionists, and intensivists is of paramount importance throughout the perioperative period.

Preoperative Evaluation

The anesthetic management of cardiac surgery patients, like all others, begins with a thorough preoperative evaluation. Consultants frequently are involved early in the preoperative process, and the anesthetic plan may be amended on the basis of their recommendations.

History

The best and least expensive tool for preoperative evaluation remains a thorough history and physical examination. The preoperative evaluation of the cardiac patient should begin with a review of the patient's medical chart, including previous anesthetic records, for information regarding hemodynamic responses at induction of anesthesia and ease of tracheal intubation.

Most patients scheduled for cardiac surgery will present with cardiac symptomatology, including unstable angina pectoris. If these cardiac complaints were part of a concurrent disease process in a patient presenting for "noncardiac" surgery, the elective surgical procedures would be postponed. In cardiac surgery cases, signs and symptoms of **congestive heart failure,** a known predictor of perioperative cardiac morbidity, are of more importance. The only symptom of impaired cardiac performance may be a diminished exercise tolerance that worsens over time as cardiac failure progresses. The presence of cerebrovascular (stroke, transient ischemic attack) or peripheral vascular disease (claudication) should be sought, as cardiac patients show a very high incidence of concomitant vascular pathology, and vice versa.

Physical Examination

Careful **auscultation of the chest** for HR, rhythm, murmurs, and gallops remains critical in cardiac patients, as heart catheterization may not reliably detect all forms of intracardiac pathology. An S3 gallop may be difficult to hear. Inspection of the jugular veins with the patient semirecumbent is useful to detect CHF. Abnormal rhythms (atrial fibrillation and ventricular extrasystoles) and impaired LV function are important adverse prognostic factors.

The lung fields should be auscultated for rales (suggestive of CHF), rhonchi, or wheezes. Having the patient perform a forced expiration may help uncover otherwise inapparent wheezing and airflow obstruction. Chronic obstructive pulmonary disease (COPD) secondary to cigarette smoking is common in patients with CASHD. Potential sites for arterial or venous cannulation should be inspected.

Preoperative Diagnostic Testing and Consultation

Baseline laboratory studies, including complete blood count, serum electrolytes, coagulation profile, and liver enzymes, are routinely obtained. A 12-lead electrocardiogram (ECG) and a chest x-ray (CXR) should be available for all patients scheduled for cardiovascular surgery. The chest radiograph is particularly helpful to the surgeon for patients undergoing reoperative cardiac surgery. ECG abnormalities (other than aberrant rhythms) have not been conclusively demonstrated to predict adverse outcome in most studies. The resting ECG is normal in 25–50% of patients with CASHD. A previous MI may predict a higher risk in cardiac surgery patients, though this decreases as time from the infarction increases.

Pulmonary function tests (PFTs) can be useful in differentiating between cardiac and pulmonary causes of dyspnea and may be helpful in identifying patients who will be difficult to wean from ventilatory support in the postoperative period. Patients with significant increases in expiratory flow obstruction because of exacerbations of chronic lung disease (COPD, asthma) frequently show improvement after administration of bronchodilators. This group may benefit from 48–72 hours of antibiotic and pulmonary hygiene therapy before elective surgery.

Along with a variety of noninvasive and laboratory studies, nearly all patients will have undergone cardiac catheterization. The cath report should contain information regarding the location and severity of coronary artery stenoses, pressures within the cardiac chambers, and if a "ventriculogram" is obtained, a gross estimate of global LV function. The LVEDP may reflect the functional status of the heart: an elevated LVEDP (above 20 mm Hg) in the absence of valvular disease suggests impaired LV function. An echocardiogram may be used to provide important (noninvasive) data regarding ventricular function and valvular pathology. Consultation with a pulmonologist may be helpful if severe pulmonary disease is present or suspected. An endocrinologist may be asked to assist with perioperative insulin management in a patient with diabetes mellitus.

Sedative Premedication

Philosophies regarding premedication of cardiac surgery patients have changed dramatically over the past few years. With economic pressures toward shorter intensive care unit (ICU) stays, heavy dose of long-acting sedative premedication are being replaced by smaller doses of short-acting agents to facilitate earlier extubation of the trachea. Sedative premedication is prescribed for anxiolysis, amnesia, analgesia (particularly important in the patient who will require placement of invasive monitoring lines), attenuation of autonomic responses to noxious stimuli, and drying of secretions. Increasing gastric pH and decreasing gastric volume may be important in patients believed to be at increased risk of regurgitation and aspiration of gastric contents.

Time-honored combinations of narcotic (e.g., 0.1 mg/kg MSO_4 IM), benzodiazepine (0.1 mg/kg of diazepam p.o.), and scopolamine (0.2–0.4 mg IM) produce a relatively calm patient, though prolonged sedation may be problematic, particularly in the elderly. Patients who are slated for "early" tracheal extubation may be better served by either titration of IV midazolam (0.5–1.0 mg increments) or lorazepam (1–4 mg p.o. or IM), with small doses of intravenous fentanyl (25–50 μg) once monitored in the preoperative holding area. Frail patients require smaller doses of all agents, including premedicants.

Prophylaxis against pulmonary aspiration should be considered in patients at risk, namely obese patients, diabetics, or those with symptomatic hiatal hernia or gastroesophageal reflux. Recent evidence suggests that a combination of metoclopramide with an H_2-blocker may be the most effective regimen.

Chronic Medications

In general, cardiac patients should receive chronic medications with a sip of water before arrival in the preoperative holding area. Studies suggest that rebound hypertension and myocardial ischemia may occur if **β-blockers** and centrally acting α_2-agonists (clonidine) are abruptly stopped before surgery. Evidence is also accumulating that myocardial ischemia may be seen with abrupt cessation of **calcium channel blocking agents.** Continuing long-acting **nitrates** has also been recommended. **Antiarrhythmics** should also be continued in the perioperative period, whether by the oral or intravenous route. While **digoxin** may be held in patients receiving it for "CHF," those taking digitalis preparations for control of supraventricular dysrhythmias should receive their morning dose before surgery. **Diuretics** are frequently withheld before surgery for the sake of patient comfort and may be given intraoperatively. **Amiodarone,** an antifibrillatory drug that has been associated with episodes of refractory, life-threatening hypotension in the presence of "depressant" anesthetics, has an extremely long half-life (weeks) and must be withheld for several months if it is to be completely cleared from the cardiac tissue before surgery. **Bronchodilators,** despite their potential interactions, are usually continued through the perioperative period in patients with reactive airway disease. A useful practice is to have the patients' bronchodilator inhalers taped to the front of their charts as they head to the operating room.

Insulin

Diabetics should be scheduled for surgery early in the day, if possible. **Oral hypoglycemics** should generally be withheld preoperatively in patients with non-insulin-dependent diabetes. (See Chapter 13 for insulin regimens.)

Special Considerations for the Patients Admitted the Morning of Surgery

The trend toward admission on the morning of operation now has expanded to include patients scheduled for cardiovascular surgery. The same, thorough preoperative evaluation must be conducted on an outpatient basis, which may be complicated by the task of obtaining preoperative consultations and study results.

Apprehensive patients may request anxiolytic therapy for either the night before or the morning of surgery. If an oral premedicant is prescribed, it should be administered before the patient's arrival at the hospital lest its effect peak too late. Incremental doses of benzodiazepines and narcotics administered in the holding area after a peripheral IV is started is generally more satisfactory. It is imperative that during the preoperative consultation, the patient be informed about the sequence of events planned in conjunction with the anesthetic, including preoperative sedation, the insertion of invasive monitoring lines, induction of anesthesia, and emergence in the ICU, and be allowed to ask questions about them.

Monitoring

Monitoring of the patient undergoing cardiac surgery has also undergone substantial changes in recent years. Although full invasive monitoring, including pulmonary artery (PA) catheterization, was the rule at many centers, the trend is now toward individualization of intraoperative monitoring to the patient's condition and planned surgical procedure.

Along with ASA standard monitors, an **intraarterial catheter** is essential for procedures involving cardiopulmonary bypass (CPB) since the nonpulsatile arterial pressure cannot be measured by cuff. The usual site chosen is the radial artery, though the femoral and axillary arteries may be used safely. **Central venous access** is truly essential for any cardiac surgical procedure. The decision to use a **PA catheter** may be more difficult, since the ability to quantify cardiac function by means of thermal dilution cardiac outputs may be helpful in the perioperative period. The appearance of "V-waves" on the PA tracing has not been shown to correlate with other determinants of myocardial ischemia in any controlled study, and no randomized studies have demonstrated improved outcome when a PA catheter has been used. PA catheterization may be reserved for the cardiovascular patient with significant LV dysfunction or severe pulmonary disease, especially when associated with pulmonary hypertension.

At an increasing number of institutions, **transesophageal echocardiography (TEE)** is being used to provide detailed information regarding cardiac function beyond that provided by a PA catheter. Regional wall motion abnormalities can be documented by TEE and are believed to represent intraoperative myocardial ischemia. Doppler technology within the TEE probe may also be used to "noninvasively" determine cardiac output. TEE requires a significant financial investment as well as considerable operator expertise. The TEE probe is not inserted until after the induction of anesthesia, and hemodynamic changes occurring during this crucial period are missed.

Sophisticated monitors of neurologic function (electroencephalography, Doppler cerebral blood flow) have not been linked to any improvement in neurologic outcome.

"Flow" of the Operation

The key to successful outcome after anesthesia may be related to the ability to anticipate surgical events and their hemodynamic consequences before they occur. A more stable anesthetic is produced by deepening the level of anesthesia before specific periods of surgical stimulation rather than merely reacting to these changes. The intraoperative "flow" of a cardiac surgery case is complicated and requires close coordination between the anesthesiologist, surgeon, and perfusionist. The typical sequence of events from arrival of the patient in the preoperative holding area through admission of the patient to the surgical ICU is summarized in Table 15.2.

Table 15.2.
Sequence of a Typical Cardiac Surgical Operation (CABG)

Preparation of the patient before induction:
1. Arrival in the preoperative holding area, verification of patient's identification
2. Query for symptomatology of angina, dyspnea; place ECG, pulse oximeter
3. Check chart for new laboratory data, consultations, etc.
4. Insertion of intravenous catheters
5. Insertion of invasive hemodynamic monitoring lines (arterial line, PA catheter, or CVP); (may occur in OR per institutional preference)
6. Transport to OR
7. Placement of "noninvasive" monitors (ECG, pulse oximeter, blood pressure cuff)

Table 15.2. Continued

8. Measurement of baseline hemodynamic values (ABGs, ACT, CO, PA pressures, etc.)

Induction:

9. Preoxygenation
10. Induction of anesthesia
11. Placement of Foley catheter, surgical preparation, and drape

Maintenance before CPB:

12. Incision (first "stimulation" since intubation)
13. Sternotomy (along with sternal retraction is very stimulating)
14. Harvesting of vein grafts and internal mammary artery (IMA) (papaverine applied to IMA may abruptly lower BP)

Preparation for CPB:

15. Heparinization, confirmation of anticoagulation (i.e., ACT >400 sec)
16. Aortic cannulation (systolic BP should be <110 mm Hg)
17. Venous cannulation, placement of retrograde cardioplegia cannula (loss of volume, dysrhythmias common during these manipulations)

Anesthetic management during CPB:

18. Initiation of CPB
19. Coronary artery bypass grafting

Preparation for separation from CPB:

20. Zero transducers
21. Confirm ventilation of lungs
22. Adequate heart rate and rhythm
23. Choice of inotropes?
24. Discontinuation of CPB

Hemostasis:

25. Reversal of heparin with protamine (ACT, thromboelastograph, and/or coagulation studies as indicated)
26. Surgical hemostasis obtained
27. Chest closure

Transport to the ICU:

28. Transfer patient to ICU bed and transport monitor
29. Transport patient to postcardiac surgical ICU (report to nurse and transfer care)

Preparation of the Patient before Induction

Preoperative orders for the cardiac surgery patient should include NPO, cardiovascular medications for the morning of surgery, sedative premedication, and supplemental oxygen to be started when sedatives or opiates are first given.

After the patient is delivered to the preoperative holding area and "checked-in" by the nursing staff, placement of intravenous and invasive monitoring lines may begin. The patient should be monitored with continuous electrocardiography and pulse oximetry and questioned at regular intervals about the presence of angina or dyspnea. One or two large-bore peripheral intravenous lines are started, and a radial arterial line is placed in the preoperative holding area. Central venous or PA catheters are usually inserted via the right internal jugular (IJ) approach. Should peripheral venous access appear inadequate, a "double-stick" technique may be used to place a double-lumen central venous line alongside the PA catheter. Most intravenous infusions (inotropes, nitrates) are best continued through the induction of anesthesia. Some practitioners will discontinue IV heparin infusions, preferring to give small (1000 unit) boluses until CPB is initiated. To be most effective, prophylactic antibiotics must be infused before the surgical incision. After baseline hemodynamic measurements are taken, the patient should be ready for the induction of anesthesia.

Induction

Agents for induction and maintenance of anesthesia are chosen with the hope of reducing the risk of perioperative cardiac morbidity and mortality. Outcome studies have shown that the choice of anesthetic technique makes much less difference than its skillful application. Many centers have used a technique relying on high-dose opiates to preserve cardiac function, maintain favorable myocardial O_2 supply/demand ratios, and produce extremely smooth intraoperative hemodynamics, although prolonged respiratory depression is often a problem. Many anesthesiologists have modified their practice to use less long-acting narcotic and more rapidly reversible anesthetic agents.

A balanced combination of sedatives, narcotic analgesics, and inhaled anesthetic agents is used in most contemporary cardiac anesthesia practices. In the patient with **normal LV function,** lower doses of narcotic analgesics and reliance on potent inhalational agents may allow earlier extubation and discharge from the ICU. The patient with **poor LV function** may be less tolerant of inhalational anesthetics, thus higher doses of narcotics and intravenous amnestic agents may be required. For example, an induction regimen for a patient undergoing myocardial revascularization with "normal" LV function might include

- Fentanyl 10–15 μg/kg
- Thiopental 25-to50-mg increments until loss of consciousness

- Midazolam 1-mg increments or potent inhalational agent for hypertension
- Neuromuscular blockade with vecuronium (1 mg/kg) or pancuronium if pulse is less than 60 bpm
- Esmolol 10–20 mg for tachycardia

Maintenance before CPB

Anesthesia is maintained before CPB with incremental doses of benzodiazepines (midazolam), small amounts of additional narcotics, and varying concentrations of potent inhalational agents. Incision may not occur until 15–20 min after induction, and phenylephrine (50–100 μg) is frequently required to maintain an adequate perfusion pressure during skin preparation and draping. Because the concentrations of intravenous agents will have fallen from their induction peaks, additional narcotic (or increased volatile agent concentration) may be administered before incision to attenuate any hyperdynamic response. Ischemia must be treated aggressively with nitrates and β-blockers as indicated. Sternotomy and sternal retraction are the most stimulating portion of the cardiac operation. Nitrous oxide (N_2O) may be used in the prebypass period, though its use in the postbypass period is controversial. Until the depth of anesthesia can be appropriately adjusted, vasodilators or β-blockers may be used to reduce blood pressure after a particularly noxious surgical stimulus.

Preparation For CPB

After sternotomy, conduits for the aortocoronary artery bypass grafts are obtained, in the form of either saphenous veins from the legs and/or the internal mammary artery (IMA), usually from the left side of the chest. Before the start of CPB, the patient's blood must be anticoagulated with **intravenous heparin (300–400 units/kg).** Heparin enhances the intrinsic activity of antithrombin-III by a factor of 1000 and is rapidly reversible with protamine. Adequacy of anticoagulation is confirmed either by an activated clotting time (ACT) device or a heparin/protamine titration system. The ACT uses an activator of coagulation (diatomaceous earth or kaolin) within a standardized tube. Normal ACT values range from 100 to 150 sec, and CPB may be initiated when the ACT exceeds 400 sec. When anticoagulation is satisfactory, the surgeon places a large cannula in the ascending aorta to return blood from the CPB to the patient. A systolic blood pressure below 110 mm Hg is generally requested to prevent dissection of the aorta, a life-threatening complication. Additional anesthetic depth (or vasodilator) may be needed to lower the pressure, as manipulation of the aorta is quite stimulating. After insertion and deairing of the aortic cannula, it is connected to the arterial side of the CPB apparatus. When venous cannula(e) is (are) inserted via the right atrium, a substantial amount of blood is often lost and may be replaced from the CPB through the aortic line. Placement of a retrograde cardioplegia catheter into the coronary sinus is now standard practice at many institutions. The manipulations of the right heart commonly lead to supraventricular dysrhythmias. When the cannulae are in place and the ACT is acceptable, CPB may be initiated.

Mechanics and Physiology of CPB

CPB is a form of extracorporeal circulation used to maintain vital organ function during cardiac surgery. The CPB apparatus is run by a licensed perfusionist, who monitors the patient's vital signs as well as the function of the "pump" to ensure that homeostasis is maintained. The tubing and reservoirs of the bypass pump are primed with a crystalloid-based solution before initiation of CPB (Table 15.3). When patients go on bypass, their blood is diluted by the pump prime solution. Studies have shown that this hemodilution is not particularly harmful, since blood rheology and oxygen delivery may be improved, especially during hypothermia. The hematocrit should be maintained at 20% or greater during CPB and should be at least 20% before separation from CPB.

Table 15.3.
CPB "Priming" Solution for a 70-kg Adult

1500 ml Plasma-Lyte crystalloid solution
500 ml 6% hetastarch
25 gm (20%) mannitol
8,000–10,000 units heparin

Total volume: 2135 ml

Venous blood drains by gravity to the CPB reservoir. The volume of blood returned to the pump from the venous cannulae must approximate the amount pumped out via the aortic cannula, since a low venous return will drain the reservoir unless arterial flow is decreased. Poor venous return can usually be improved by adjusting the venous cannulae, or in some situations, merely raising the operating table.

Within the CPB, desaturated venous blood passes through an oxygenator, where CO_2 and oxygen are exchanged. Membrane oxygenator systems are most commonly used despite the greater cost, since trauma to the formed elements of the blood is significantly less than with a bubble-type oxygenator. The concentrations of O_2 and CO_2 are controlled by varying the oxygen flow and concentration to the oxygenator. After the blood is oxygenated, it is pumped through the arterial line to the aorta and then to the body (Fig. 15.3). The oxygenated blood may be warmed or cooled within the CPB before being returned to the patient. Most centers will employ moderate hypothermia (28–31°C) during CPB because the cerebral metabolic rate for oxygen ($CMRO_2$) is reduced by about 50%. On-line monitoring of mixed venous oxygen saturation, pH, and hematocrit is standard.

The flow generated by the arterial pump head is nonpulsatile; thus the only meaningful pressure value during CPB is the MAP. Ongoing cardiac activity may generate some pulsatile flow, but this is of secondary importance. An MAP between 50 and 90 mm Hg is generally acceptable during bypass. MAP is directly proportional to pump flow (usually > 2.0 liters/min/m^2) and may be modulated by vasoconstrictors, vasodilators, and altering the depth of anesthesia.

It is often necessary to arrest the contractile activity of the heart to permit an efficient operation. Cardioplegia solutions containing high concentrations of potassium have been developed to arrest the heart in diastole. Cardioplegia solutions may be injected into the aortic root after a cross clamp has been placed just proximal to the aortic cannula to prevent washout of the solution. Cardioplegia solutions may also be given in a "retrograde" fashion through a catheter placed in the coronary sinus.

Unfortunately, CPB is, in reality, a very "unphysiologic" event. Contact of the patient's blood with the components of

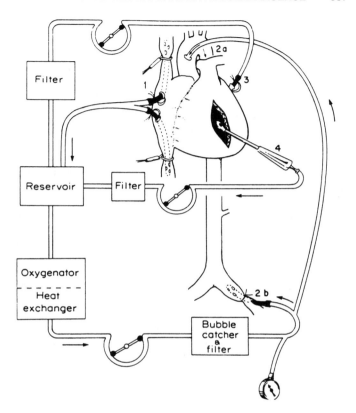

Figure 15.3. Cardiopulmonary bypass circuit. Blood flows from the right atrium or vena cava *(1)* to the cardiotomy reservoir of the bypass pump. The blood is oxygenated, warmed, or cooled, and then pumped into either the ascending aorta *(2a)* or the femoral artery *(2b)*. Blood also may be returned to the reservoir by way of a "vent" cannula in the left atrium or ventricle *(3)*, and "pump suckers" *(4)* used to clear the operative field. (Reproduced with permission from Hug CC. Anesthesia for adult cardiac surgery. In: Miller RD, ed. Anesthesia. 3rd ed. New York: Churchill Livingstone, 1990:1637 and from Nosé Y. Manual on artificial organs, vol 2. The oxygenator. St. Louis: CV Mosby, 1973.)

the bypass circuit sets off a chain of events including consumption of platelets, destruction of red blood cells, and activation of the inflammatory and kallikrein systems. For this reason, it is prudent to limit the "pump run" to as short a time as possible.

Maintenance of Anesthesia during CPB

When the perfusionist confirms that "full bypass" has been reached, the ventilator and pulse oximeter may be turned off. Although requirements certainly change during CPB, care must be taken to ensure an adequate level of anesthesia throughout the bypass run. The most common time for awareness to occur during surgery using cardiac bypass is during the rewarming phase. Though core temperature may be less than 30°C, warmed blood (>37°C) is being injected through the aortic cannula and distributed to the brain. Anesthetic requirements abruptly increase, and depth of anesthesia must be appropriate for the normothermic brain. Anesthetic depth may be maintained with intravenous agents, (benzodiazepines, narcotics), though if given in excessive amounts, these may prevent timely extubation. Most CPB pumps have a volatile anesthetic agent vaporizer in their circuit. An agent such as propofol may be considered, though it may be a better choice for the postbypass period. It is customary to maintain neuromuscular blockade during CPB, especially when hypothermia is used, to prevent shivering.

Preparation for Separation from CPB

Once the cardiac surgical procedure has been completed, the patient must be weaned from CPB. All transducers should be rezeroed, and reexpansion of the lungs may resume when the surgeon is satisfied that the surgical repair is adequate. Once operation on the heart itself is completed (distal anastomoses, valve placement), the aortic cross clamp is removed, and oxygenated blood washes out residual cardioplegia solution. A variety of cardiac rhythms may then ensue. If ventricular fibrillation occurs despite lidocaine treatment, internal DC cardioversion with 10–20 watts · sec of energy should be performed.

An appropriate heart rate and rhythm are essential to adequate postbypass cardiac function. Temporary pacing via epicardial wires is frequently required after cardiac surgery. Pacing the atria to a rate of 90–100 is desirable, though ventricular pacing may suffice if the atria are fibrillating or A-V conduction is abnormal. The patient should be normothermic, the hematocrit above 20%, and all electrolytes (Ca^{2+}, K^{+}, Mg^{2+}) at normal levels.

Separation from CPB

At the conclusion of CPB, the heart must be able to provide sufficient CO to maintain tissue homeostasis. All the components that determine CO (rate, rhythm, preload, and contractility) should be optimized so that the heart can take over the work load that was supplied by CPB during surgery. Inotropic support is occasionally necessary to assist the heart in making this transition. Factors that may predict a need for inotropic support include impaired ventricular function, unsatisfactory myocardial protection, and prolonged duration of operation.

Once ventilation of the lungs is resumed and an adequate cardiac rhythm is present, the perfusionist begins to occlude the venous drainage line, allowing the right heart to fill. If all is well, this volume will be pumped to the left heart, which will then begin to produce pulsatile flow throughout the systemic arterial tree. By observing the heart and invasive monitoring data, the surgeon and anesthesiologist can determine the optimal level of ventricular filling. The arterial line flow is gradually reduced, and if the heart appears to be functioning adequately, the pump is stopped, and the inflow and outflow lines are clamped. Decreased mixed venous oxygen saturation and elevated right heart pressures in the face of falling systemic pressures indicate impending cardiac failure. When this occurs, the perfusionist resumes full bypass flow, and inotropic support should be added as appropriate. A period of "rest" (10–15 min) is often beneficial to allow reestablishment of myocardial energy stores and satisfactory levels of inotropes.

Either natural (dopamine, epinephrine, norepinephrine) or synthetic (dobutamine, isoproterenol) catecholamines are the mainstays of inotropic therapy. Phosphodiesterase inhibitors (amrinone, milrinone) are powerful new additions to this armamentarium. Should pharmacologic inotropic support be inadequate to allow successful separation from CPB, an intraaortic balloon pump (IABP) may be considered. The IABP improves diastolic coronary perfusion, reduces afterload, and may allow a patient with a suboptimal revascularization or myocardial injury to overcome the temporary impairment and enjoy a successful recovery.

Hemostasis

After CPB is discontinued and the patient is stable, the bypass cannulae are removed. A calculated dose of **protamine** is given to reverse the effect of residual heparin. Though protamine neutralizes heparin on a 1:1 basis, the actual protamine dose given is somewhere between 50 and 90% of the total heparin dose, as heparin is metabolized to some extent during the operation. Adequacy of heparin reversal is measured by the ACT or in vitro heparin/protamine titration. Protamine must be given slowly to reduce the chances of adverse hemodynamic sequelae that include hypotension and pulmonary hypertension.

Many centers are now using antifibrinolytic agents in an attempt to reduce blood loss in cardiac surgical patients. **ε-Aminocaproic acid** is an older antifibrinolytic that may be given before bypass in anticipation of a prolonged bypass run or postoperative bleeding diathesis or after bypass if fibrinolysis is suspected or documented. **Aprotinin** was recently released for use in the United States. Along with its antifibrinolytic activity, aprotinin modulates the release of inflammatory mediators, including serine proteases and kallikreins. Aprotinin has been shown to dramatically reduce transfusion requirements in reoperative cardiac surgery patients, and further trials are investigating its use in other clinical situations. When aprotinin is used, ACT values (with diatomaceous earth systems) may be unreliable.

Once hemostasis is deemed adequate, the sternum is closed with wires, and the operation is completed. The CO may decrease with chest closure because of alterations in ventricular filling. This often responds to administration of additional volume or adjustments in levels of inotropic support. Once surgery is completed, the patient is transported directly to the ICU with full monitoring en route.

Timing of Extubation after Cardiac Surgery

As most cardiac anesthetics were historically based on a high-dose opioid technique, cardiac patients have routinely required mechanical ventilation following surgery. Routine overnight ventilation of postoperative cardiac surgery patients has largely fallen out of favor because of economic pressures. Cardiac patients at many institutions are now extubated within a few hours of surgery, without apparent adverse sequelae.

Optimal **candidates for early extubation** should have adequate ventricular function and be free from significant pulmonary disease. Patients with a reasonably short pump run (<2.0 hr) who separate from CPB with minimal inotropic support should at least be considered for early extubation. Sedation with a short-acting agent such as propofol after bypass may allow more rapid recovery and extubation once the conditions outlined in Table 15.4 are met. While no controlled trials have indicated whether outcome will be changed by this practice, early clinical experience is causing us to consider a greater number of patients for this type of management.

Anesthetic Management for Valvular Heart Surgery

The anesthetic management of the patient undergoing a valvular operation is in many ways similar to the anesthetic management for coronary artery bypass graft (CABG) operations, as described above. The "flows" of the pre- and postbypass periods are nearly identical, excepting the preparation of artery and vein for bypass grafting. The actual differences are a direct result of the consequences of the respective valvular defects, as outlined in the section on pathophysiology above. Monitoring considerations are generally the same as those used for CABG operations, although more patients may benefit from PA catheter placement, and TEE is used much more frequently. For example, TEE is routinely used in some centers to judge the adequacy of mitral valve repair.

Correction of the valvular lesion may involve repair (most frequently of the mitral valve) or replacement. Valve replacement may be with a tissue valve (porcine or pericardial) or a mechanical valve. Mechanical valves have the advantage of potentially lasting for the remainder of the patient's life, even those who are very young. Tissue valves tend to wear and degen-

Table 15.4.
Suggested Criteria for Early Extubation after Cardiac Surgery

Preoperative selection factors
Patient < 75 years of age undergoing a nonemergent revascularization procedure
Adequate ventricular function (ejection fraction ≥ 40% by cath or echo)
Concurrent valvular replacement or repair makes the patient a much less favorable candidate
No significant bronchospasm or obstructive pulmonary disease
Adequate renal function

Intraoperative selection factors
Short period on CPB (< 1.5 hr, cross-clamp time < 45 min)
Patient should separate from CPB with minimal inotropic support
Surgeon must be satisfied with adequacy of revascularization

Postoperative extubation parameters
Bladder temperature > 36°C
Awake, able to follow commands and protect the airway
Arterial blood gas: pH ≥ 7.30, pCO_2 ≤ 50 mm Hg, and pO_2 ≥ 80 mm Hg with FiO_2 not greater than 40%.
  PEEP not greater than 5 cm H_2O
  Spontaneous ventilation at a rate < 24/min
Hemodynamic stability characterized by
  Mean BP ≥ 70 mm Hg
  Urine output ≥1 ml/kg/hr
  Chest tube drainage ≤ 200 ml/hr for the two previous hours
  Cardiac index ≥ 2.0 liters/min on minimal inotropic support

---

erate over a 10- to 15-year period. One major disadvantage of mechanical valves is the requirement for long-term anticoagulation therapy (typically with warfarin) to prevent thrombosis on the valve surface.

Surgical correction of valvular cardiac pathology is truly "open heart" surgery; one or more cardiac chambers must be entered to perform the operation. The introduction of air into the heart is probably responsible for part of the increased morbidity and mortality of valvular surgery (postoperative neurologic dysfunction), compared with closed chamber procedures, such as CABG. Ejection of retained intracardiac air or debris into the cerebral or coronary circulations, particularly the right coronary artery (RCA), are associated with morbidity. Air in the RCA may lead to temporary but severe right heart dysfunction.

TEE is invaluable for documenting satisfactory "deairing" of the heart before separation from CPB.

Patients undergoing valvular surgery are also prone to hemorrhagic complications postoperatively, in part due to prolonged CPB times. Suture lines along the atrium (MVR) and aorta (AVR) are common sites for postoperative bleeding. Antifibrinolytics are often administered to these patients, and procoagulants should be available if needed after CPB.

Anesthetic Management of Specific Valvular Lesions

Aortic Stenosis. AS results from obstruction of the LV outflow tract, either at or below the level of the aortic valve. The cardiovascular management goals for patients with valvular AS are based on the pathophysiology discussed above and include

- Maintenance of a **sinus rhythm** with a **normal to decreased heart rate:** Patients with chronic AS and LVH may depend on their atrial "kick" for up to 40% of their cardiac output. Slower heart rates allow for a longer ejection time across the stenotic aortic valve as well as more time in diastole for coronary filling. Appearance of supraventricular dysrhythmias can be life-threatening and are usually treated with immediate cardioversion.
- **Maintenance of coronary perfusion** through **normal to increased diastolic blood pressure:** Afterload is fixed at a high level because of the stenotic valve, and higher perfusion pressures may be beneficial in supplying the subendocardial region of the hypertrophied ventricle. α-Adrenergic agents are often useful.
- **Maintenance of adequate CO** by **avoiding myocardial depressants and ensuring adequate preload:** Decreases in contractility are often poorly tolerated. A narcotic-based anesthetic technique should provide a slow HR with preservation of myocardial contractility and is often the technique of choice for these patients. Patients with valvular AS frequently have significant coronary disease, thus a combined valve replacement/CABG procedure is common. Fortunately, the management strategies for both conditions are similar.

AS may also arise from a dynamic, subvalvular obstruction, known as HCM, asymmetric septal hypertrophy (ASH), or

IHSS. This condition results from an asymmetric enlargement of the ventricular septum that encroaches on the LV outflow tract. This obstruction is worsened by decreasing LV volume or increasing the inotropic state of the heart. Myocardial depressants such as halothane or β-adrenergic blockers may increase forward flow. TEE can be an invaluable monitor in cases where myomectomy is performed to relieve the obstruction.

Aortic Regurgitation. AI leads to volume overload of the LV, and intraoperative management is geared toward preservation of the patient's own compensatory mechanisms.

- Maintain a **higher than normal heart rate (80–100 bpm):** Elevated heart rates allow less time for regurgitation of blood into the LV and thus yield a greater forward output. Atrial fibrillation is common yet is better tolerated than in AS.
- **Maintain or increase preload:** SV is augmented by increased LV preload. Nitroglycerin may be detrimental.
- **Reduce afterload:** Any reduction in impedance to forward flow should translate into higher CO. Caution must be exercised in the patient with coronary disease, since an adequate perfusion pressure must be maintained.
- **Avoid myocardial depression:** Patients with AI frequently have some impairment of LV function and often will not tolerate further reductions in inotropic state.

Induction and maintenance of anesthesia may rely more heavily on benzodiazepines (and other hypnotics) than on narcotics. Preservation of HR, contractility, and preload is more feasible with this technique. Volatile agents may be used if ventricular function is adequate.

Patients with a proximal aortic dissection may present with acute AI. If the dissection involves the cerebral vessels, circulatory arrest may be required to allow repair of the problem, and cannulation of the femoral vessels may be necessary. The patient is cooled on bypass to 15–18°C, barbiturate cerebral protection is given, and the pump is turned off while the repair is underway. Coagulopathy and cerebral dysfunction, however, are more common after this type of approach.

Mitral Stenosis. Left atrial dilation and pulmonary hypertension are common sequelae of chronic MS. A PA catheter is indicated in essentially all patients with significant MS. The TEE is invaluable if repair of the valve is considered. The management goals for MS include

- **Avoiding tachycardia** and **maintaining sinus rhythm** if possible: Slower heart rates allow more time for inflow from the left atrium to the LV. The atrial "kick" may be responsible for a large portion of ventricular filling and should be preserved.
- **Maintaining LV preload and contractility:** Adequate preload is necessary to maintain CO, though overaggressive expansion of the intravascular volume may quickly lead to pulmonary edema. Depression of contractility may aggravate this tendency.
- **Avoiding increases in PVR** and treating RV failure if it occurs.

Conditions such as hypoxia, hypercarbia, and acidosis will increase PVR and may lead to RV failure and inadequate filling of the left side of the heart.

Patients with coronary artery disease and MS may present for combined procedures. The tenets for valve replacement parallel the principles for CABG. Narcotic-based anesthetic techniques are good choices for patients with MS.

Mitral Regurgitation. Chronic **MR** results in an indolent progress of disease leading to LV dilation and symptoms of pulmonary edema. Acute, ischemic MR may lead to rapid deterioration, as compensatory mechanisms do not have adequate time to develop. The management goals for mitral regurgitation include

- Maintaining a **slightly elevated HR:** The regurgitant fraction may decrease if the time of each cardiac cycle is reduced. Sinus rhythm is desirable but not critical.
- **Reducing SVR:** More of the SV will be ejected in the antegrade direction if impedance to forward flow is reduced.
- **Maintaining adequate preload:** Chronic LV dilation is the rule, though caution against overload and pulmonary edema must be exercised. In some cases, overdistention may dilate the mitral annulus and increase the regurgitant fraction.
- **Avoiding myocardial depression:** Inotropic agents may increase forward flow in these patients, who frequently present with impaired LV function.

Tricuspid Regurgitation. The anesthetic management of the patient with tricuspid regurgitation is similar to the management of patients who present with MR. Generally, these patients are younger and may present with sequelae from endocarditis, occasionally from IV drug abuse, or congenital cardiac pathology. Monitoring of CVP is critical. Attempts should be made to **maintain a low PVR** to preserve RV output.

Tricuspid Stenosis. Tricuspid stenosis is quite rare in adult cardiac surgery, and management recommendations parallel those for MS, albeit applied to the right heart.

Anesthesia for Thoracic Transplantation Procedures

Cardiac Transplantation

Orthotopic heart transplantation has become an accepted procedure for treatment of end-stage cardiac pathology. Advances in surgical, anesthetic, and immunosuppressive techniques have pushed 1-year survival rates above 90%, with similar improvements in long-term outcome. Regardless of etiology, perioperative care revolves around preservation of cardiovascular homeostasis until the patient is placed on CPB.

While all heart transplant recipients are extremely ill, some patients will arrive from home for the procedure, while other recipients may be in extremis, on full ventilatory, inotropic, and mechanical cardiac support. **Preoperative preparation** must be individualized, and ample information should be available in the medical record. **Judicious intravenous premedication** in a monitored setting is most appropriate. Full invasive monitoring is the rule, and a PA catheter with continuous display of mixed venous oxygen saturation may be helpful. Sterile technique is critical because the patients will be immunocompromised.

A "high-dose" narcotic **induction technique** is often appropriate, with incremental doses of benzodiazepine to ensure amnesia. Pharmacologic support of blood pressure is frequently required. Inotropic support should be continued until the patient is placed on CPB as the donor heart enters the operating room (Fig. 15.4).

After the new heart is reperfused and "deaired," the patient is weaned from CPB. The usual cause of failure to wean from bypass is right heart failure, and isoproterenol and dopamine are useful for their inotropic and chronotropic effects. Discussions of the postoperative care and immunosuppressive therapy

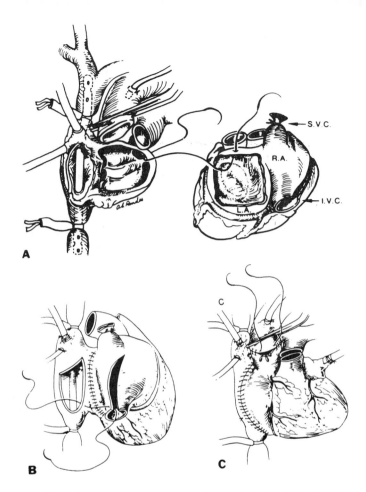

Figure 15.4. Operation for orthotopic heart transplantation. **A,** Aortic and (superior and inferior) vena caval cannulae are placed, and the patient is placed on CPB. The recipient heart is excised as shown, and the left atrial anastomosis is begun aligning the recipient left superior pulmonary vein with the donor left atrial appendage. **B,** Right atrial anastomosis follows completion of the left atrial suture line. **C,** After completion of the atrial and aortic anastomoses, the pulmonary arterial anastomosis must be completed. This is performed last to facilitate "deairing" after removal of the aortic cross-clamp. (Reproduced with permission from Baldwim JC, Stinson EB, Oyer PE, Starnes V, Shumway NE. Cardiac transplantation and follow-up care. In: Hurst JW, ed. The heart, arteries, and veins. 7th ed. New York: McGraw-Hill, 1990:2250.)

of these patients may be found in the selected readings at the end of this chapter.

Pulmonary Transplantation

A growing number of patients with end-stage lung disease are undergoing pulmonary transplantation. Though early pulmonary transplants were actually heart-lung procedures, novel surgical techniques have led to the growth of single lung and bilateral single lung transplants.

Pulmonary transplants are performed through a thoracotomy incision and can usually be performed without bypass, although CPB "standby" is mandatory should oxygenation fail on "one-lung" anesthesia. Full invasive monitoring is standard, and tracheal extubation is rarely considered until 24 hours after surgery.

Anesthesia for Electrophysiologic Procedures

Placement of a **permanent electronic pacemaker** may be required for patients with damage to the intracardiac conduction system or those who develop complete heart block or sick sinus syndrome after cardiac surgery (particularly mitral valve procedures). This is usually accomplished under local anesthesia in the cardiac catheterization laboratory. Rarely, a patient will be brought to the operating room for pacemaker placement, but general anesthesia is rarely needed.

Since their introduction into clinical practice in the 1980s, **automatic implantable cardioverter-defibrillators (AICD)** have been implanted into a number of patients with inducible ventricular tachydysrhythmias. The most recent generation of AICD is a device about the size of a pacemaker that is inserted in the electrophysiology laboratory. A defibrillator "patch" is placed in the subcutaneous tissue, and sensing and firing leads are placed transvenously under fluoroscopic guidance. Most of these procedures are still performed under **general anesthesia,** as ventricular fibrillation must be induced to test the device (Fig. 15.5). Selected patients may tolerate monitored anesthesia care (**MAC**) with deep sedation before testing the appliance. An **arterial line** is often placed to monitor blood pressure, and many clinicians place a **central line** as a portal for rapid administration of cardioactive drugs. Since many patients requiring

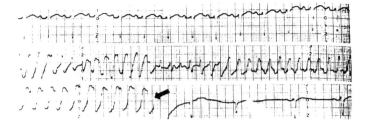

Figure 15.5. Testing of the automatic implantable cardioverter-defibrillator (AICD), showing "automatic" conversion of ventricular fibrillation to sinus rhythm. *Upper strip,* baseline (sinus) rhythm; *Middle strip,* ventricular fibrillation; *Lower strip,* 25-joule discharge *(arrow)* from the AICD successfully converts ventricular fibrillation to sinus rhythm. (Reproduced with permission from Mirowski M. The implantable cardioverter-defibrillator. In: Hurst JW, ed. The heart, arteries, and veins. 7th ed. New York: McGraw-Hill, 1990:2112.)

AICD have ischemic cardiomyopathy, etomidate is a reasonable choice as an induction agent, and a balanced technique using low-dose isoflurane is acceptable. Neuromuscular blockade will prevent excessive movement if external defibrillation is required. The patient should be extubated at the conclusion of the procedure and may be monitored by ECG telemetry postoperatively.

Diabetes, hypertension, COPD, and chronic renal insufficiency are common in patients with vascular disease. These disease processes must be controlled or optimized before elective surgery and require careful management throughout the perioperative period.

The physical examination should help reveal significant cardiopulmonary pathology and identify perioperative risk factors. Documentation of an adequate hemoglobin concentration and baseline renal function is essential. A 12-lead ECG and a CXR are obtained in essentially all patients scheduled for major vascular surgery.

Cardiac Screening Tests

Several "noninvasive" screening tests have been developed to detect those patients at risk for adverse cardiac outcome who might benefit from further diagnostic or therapeutic intervention before their surgical procedure. Many vascular patients cannot exercise enough to provide a meaningful result from exercise or "stress" ECG testing. Several newer tests may be of value when applied to high-risk patient groups such as those undergoing vascular surgery, though false positives and false negatives remain a problem.

Dipyridamole-Thallium Scanning. The dipyridamole-thallium test uses the property of thallium-201 to localize in the myocardium along the routes of coronary perfusion. Dipyridamole is an indirect vasodilator that may cause a "steal" of blood flow from areas distal to a coronary stenosis. Areas supplied by a stenotic coronary artery will appear cold on initial scanning, suggesting ischemia. A repeat scan is performed 3–4 hours later, and an area that "reperfuses" at that time is considered to be myocardium at risk for perioperative ischemia. Areas that remain "cold" are thought to represent zones of prior infarction. If a significant amount of myocardium is at risk, the patient will be referred for cardiac catheterization. False positives have been more of a problem than false negatives in early studies, though in properly selected populations, sensitivity and specificity should exceed 80%.

ANESTHESIA FOR VASCULAR SURGERY

Preoperative Evaluation

Preanesthetic evaluation of a "noncardiac" surgery patient should identify factors that will increase the risk of adverse outcome in the perioperative period and determine whether the patient is in optimal condition. The prevalence of significant cardiac disease in vascular surgery patients may exceed 50%, and most of the major complications and mortality associated with vascular surgery are directly related to the cardiovascular system. Mortality for major vascular surgery is 2–3 times higher than that for cardiac surgery because the patient's cardiac disease will not be repaired at the end of the case. Between 5 and 7% of patients with significant CASHD undergoing major "noncardiac" surgical procedures will sustain a perioperative MI, associated with a mortality of 38–70%. Patients who have sustained a prior MI are also at increased risk for perioperative reinfarction. That risk may be as high as 37% in those patients with an MI in the past 3 months, decreasing to the "baseline" level of about 6% in patients whose MIs are more than 6 months remote.

History and Physical Examination

The preoperative evaluation of the vascular surgery patient is in many ways similar to that described for cardiac surgical patients. The preanesthetic history should elicit symptomatology of CASHD, including angina and anginal equivalents such as dyspnea on exertion. Signs and symptoms of CHF are particularly ominous predictors of perioperative morbidity and mortality. Most patients with significant cardiac pathology will describe some symptomatology related to their disease process. Patients with normal exercise tolerance who give no history suggesting myocardial disease are unlikely to require or benefit from more sophisticated cardiac testing before their surgery. A significant number of vascular patients, however, are **unable to exert themselves sufficiently** to produce cardiac symptomatology, even though they may have critical cardiac pathology. Recent evidence also suggests that a large portion of myocardial ischemia, especially in the postoperative period, may occur without symptomatology. This **"silent ischemia"** is detectable by ambulatory Holter ECG monitoring.

Ambulatory ECG Monitoring. Several centers are using ambulatory Holter ECG monitoring as a screening test in patients at risk for myocardial ischemia. Patients wear the monitor for 24 hours while pursuing their usual activities, keeping a diary of symptomatology. The tracings are then analyzed for ST abnormalities, a positive test read as ST changes of greater than 1 mm from baseline for some predetermined amount of time during the testing period. Once the Holter monitors are purchased, this may be one of the more cost-effective tests available.

Stress Echocardiography. The 2-dimensional echocardiogram provides a wealth of information about myocardial anatomy and function. Recently, patients have been given pharmacologic stressors while undergoing echocardiographic imaging in an attempt to identify those at risk for perioperative cardiac complications. Areas of the heart supplied by significantly diseased vessels will exhibit regional wall motion abnormalities (RWMA) when the heart is stressed with increases in HR and BP using dobutamine. The sensitivity and specificity of this test approaches (and may exceed) that of thallium screening, and dobutamine stress echocardiography may provide the most accurate prediction of cardiac risk.

Patients who are found to have "positive" noninvasive tests, or those with significant cardiac symptomatology, may be referred for cardiac catheterization. Although expensive and not without risk, catheterization allows precise definition of coronary anatomy and identifies patients who may benefit from revascularization before their noncardiac surgical procedure. Survival may be improved in "high-risk" patients who undergo CABG before their noncardiac surgical procedure, though the decision to proceed with revascularization is frequently controversial. The risks associated with revascularization, when added to those inherent to the noncardiac procedure, may not be much lower than if the patient proceeded directly to surgery without CABG. There are few data in the literature to support improved outcome in patients who have undergone percutaneous transluminal coronary angioplasty (PTCA) before their surgical procedure, although many cardiologists and surgeons feel PTCA does confer some protection.

Special Considerations for Vascular Surgery Patients Admitted the Morning of Surgery

A growing number of vascular patients are being admitted to the hospital on the morning of the scheduled surgery. For now, these patients tend to be reasonably "fit" ones, as more critically ill patients will have been hospitalized for a time before their surgery. Morning-admit patients must be relied upon to take appropriate medication before arrival at the hospital. It may be more difficult to track down preoperative test data and consultations in this situation, but the information must be obtained before anesthesia.

Premedication

Sedative premedication for patients undergoing vascular surgery tends to be lighter than that prescribed for cardiac surgery patients. Small incremental doses of intravenous benzodiaze-

pine and narcotic usually suffice for insertion of invasive monitoring lines preoperatively. As it is ordinarily the goal to extubate most vascular patients at the conclusion of surgery,
long-acting agents traditionally used for cardiac patients may
not be wise choices. Most of the patient's chronic medications,
including insulin, should be continued through the perioperative period, as described in the previous section.

Monitoring the Vascular Surgery Patient

ECG

Monitoring for myocardial ischemia is of particular importance
in the vascular surgery population. Most institutions will monitor at least two ECG leads in the operating room. Traditionally,
lead II is monitored for dysrhythmias and inferior myocardial
ischemia, while **lead V5** tracings are scanned for anterolateral
ischemia. While 80% of ischemic episodes can be detected in
these two leads, 96% of ischemic episodes may be detected with
leads II, V4, and V5. Computerized ST-segment monitoring
should increase awareness of intraoperative ischemia on a monitor screen where as many as 8 waves may be packed together.
It has been difficult to document that improved postoperative
outcome can be attributed to earlier recognition and treatment
of these ischemic episodes.

Direct Arterial Pressure Monitoring

The magnitude of surgical trespass and severity of concomitant
disease processes frequently mandate the use of invasive cardiovascular monitoring in vascular surgery patients. Indications for
placement of an **arterial line** include situations in which cardiovascular instability is anticipated (e.g., aortic surgery). Many anesthesiologists will also place an arterial line for less invasive
procedures in a patient with significant cardiopulmonary disease, hypertension, or obesity, where noninvasive BP monitoring might be less than adequate. Long cases requiring frequent
blood sampling also argue for placement of an arterial catheter.
Complications from arterial line placement by experienced personnel are extremely rare, but the risk of thrombosis is increased by the duration of vascular cannulation and the size of
the catheter. The Allen test to assess collateral arterial flow has

not been found to predict ischemic complications in recent studies. If the radial artery cannot be cannulated, the ulnar or axillary artery may be a second choice, as femoral line placement is unsatisfactory for most vascular surgical procedures.

Monitoring of Central Venous and Pulmonary Artery Pressures

The published indications for **accessing the central circulation** include operations in which major fluid shifts are anticipated, the use of vasoactive drugs is likely, and peripheral access is inadequate for the proposed procedure. The choice of a PA catheter instead of a CVP line is considerably more controversial. Placement of a **PA catheter** may be considered if the patient has significant LV dysfunction, severe ischemic heart disease, or severe pulmonary disease, especially when associated with pulmonary hypertension. In those circumstances, variations in right heart filling pressures may inaccurately reflect actual left side filling pressures. The ability to quantify cardiac function by means of thermal dilution cardiac outputs is perhaps the major advantage of PA catheterization. The appearance of a "V-wave" on the PA pressure tracing has not been found to correlate with other determinants of myocardial ischemia. The improved outcomes cited in older studies that argued for use of a PA catheter probably resulted from more rigid hemodynamic control rather than from use of any particular monitor. A CVP catheter should predict left-sided filling pressures with reasonable accuracy in patients with an LV ejection fraction of more than 50% and without significant pulmonary disease. There are no outcome data to support the routine use of PA catheters for either aortic or cardiac surgery.

The most common complication of CVP and PA catheterization is inadvertent arterial puncture, especially with an IJ approach. Subclavian vein catheterization is more often associated with pneumothorax or hemothorax than is the IJ technique. Embolism of wire or catheter fragments is easily preventable by following accepted principles of practice. PA rupture is a rare but potentially fatal (45%) complication unique to PA catheterization. The dysrhythmias seen with passage of the PA catheter have not been shown to contribute to morbidity.

Transesophageal Echocardiography

TEE is being used more frequently during noncardiac surgery because it has proven to be an accurate, real-time monitor of cardiac function and a sensitive indicator of myocardial ischemia. Venticular RWMAs result from ischemia and may be visualized using a transgastric short-axis view that shows a portion of the distribution of all three major coronary arteries. This is also an excellent view of the heart for evaluation of ventricular volume status.

Limitations to TEE monitoring include the expenses for acquisition of the TEE console and probe and having personnel with the expertise necessary for interpretation of intraoperative images. While TEE is an extremely sensitive detector of perioperative ischemia, its specificity may be much lower, and its predictive value for adverse cardiac outcome has yet to be definitely established. Segments of myocardium that are reperfused after ischemia may take days to recover their systolic function. RWMAs may also be associated with the changes in afterload characteristic of aortic surgery, rather than actual ischemia. Despite this, intraoperative detection of new and persistent RWMAs during peripheral vascular surgery has been associated with increased cardiac morbidity.

Anesthesia for Aortic Reconstructive Surgery

Careful preoperative preparation is essential in elderly and debilitated patients who may undergo aortic reconstructive surgery.

Choice of Anesthetic Technique

There are currently no conclusive, large-scale, randomized outcome studies in the literature documenting the superiority of either regional or general anesthetic techniques for aortic surgery. For abdominal aortic surgery patients, most regional techniques are combined with a "light" general anesthetic, as a block alone is often poorly tolerated. Regional techniques have long been felt to offer protection against the cardiovascular insults inherent with major vascular surgery.

Epidural blockade with local anesthetic produces decreases in myocardial workload, oxygen consumption, preload, and afterload. Conflicting data have been reported as to whether neuraxis blockade may decrease the incidence of myocardial ischemia and adverse outcome in patients undergoing major vascular surgery. Patients receiving epidural narcotic or local anesthetics in the perioperative period tend to have better pulmonary function than similar patients not receiving epidural analgesia. While regional techniques appear to provide some control of the neuroendocrine "stress" response to surgery, this has not been definitely linked to improved cardiac outcome. Blockade of sympathetic fibers may impair myocardial contractility and produce hypotension in some patients. If spinal opioids are administered, the potential for respiratory depression from the cephalad spread of narcotic must be considered. The potential for epidural hematoma always exists in patients who will receive heparin intraoperatively, though the likelihood of this complication is actually quite low. Some practitioners will postpone elective surgery for 24 hours if a "bloody tap" occurs during epidural placement. Intrathecal preservative-free morphine (0.25–1.0 mg) is one alternative to epidural analgesia in aortic surgery patients.

Induction and Maintenance

Patients for most major vascular procedures, including aortic surgery, may be anesthetized with a "balanced" general technique. Sodium thiopental (3–5 mg/kg) may be used for induction, or etomidate (0.15–0.3 mg/kg) may be considered in patients with limited cardiovascular reserve. Narcotic (fentanyl, 3–5 μg/kg) should be given before laryngoscopy to prevent hypertension. A nondepolarizing muscle relaxant such as pancuronium, vecuronium, or rocuronium will facilitate tracheal intubation. Anesthesia may be maintained with incremental injection or infusion of fentanyl (1–3 μg/kg/hr) in combination with isoflurane, air, and oxygen. N_2O may be used in selected patients at concentrations of 50% or less, though many clinicians avoid N_2O because of its potential for bowel distention. Most patients may be extubated in the operating room or PACU, but those with limited reserve might benefit from overnight sedation and mechanical ventilation.

Intraoperative Management

Application of the aortic cross-clamp, especially to the suprarenal aorta, frequently results in dramatic hemodynamic consequences. Afterload is increased, and preload is often decreased because of reductions in venous return from the lower extremities. Systemic blood pressure may rise dramatically, and increased myocardial oxygen consumption results from elevations in LV wall tension. Patients with suprarenal or thoracoabdominal aneurysms often exhibit much greater swings in blood pressure with aortic clamping and unclamping than those with pathology limited to the infrarenal aorta. Patients with aortoiliac occlusive disease will tend to have well-developed collateral vessels around their abdominal aortas, and application of the clamp will have minimal hemodynamic effects. Unfortunately, the response to aortic clamping is difficult to predict. Minimizing these hemodynamic swings should help to preserve myocardial O_2 supply and demand ratios and may reduce the risk of perioperative cardiac complications.

The surgeon will request intravenous heparinization, usually 100 U/kg, approximately 3 min before aortic cross-clamping. It is often beneficial to administer a vasodilator (e.g., sodium nitroprusside) or increase the concentration of inhaled anesthetic at this juncture to attenuate any adverse hemodynamic responses from cross-clamp application. Augmentation of intravascular volume during placement of the aortic graft should at least replace blood loss from the surgical field. After the aortic repair, removal of the cross-clamp may lead to profound hypotension and decreased coronary blood flow. Adequate expansion of the intravascular volume may mitigate any decreases in blood pressure. There are no data to support the use of colloid solutions over crystalloid for this purpose. With release of the clamp, small boluses of phenylephrine (50–100 μg) may be given to maintain perfusion pressure until adequate preload can be established. Sodium bicarbonate should be administered based on the arterial pH, since acidosis may ensue with reperfusion of the ischemic lower extremities. Blood-scavenging devices may reduce or eliminate the need for allogeneic blood transfusion.

Renal Protection. Infrarenal aortic clamping produces a significant decrease in renal blood flow and glomerular filtration rate in spite of normal perfusion pressure. Some degree of acute renal failure (ARF) occurs in up to 50% of patients undergoing major cardiovascular surgery. While preexisting renal dysfunction is a risk factor for the development of ARF, diabetes, CHF, dehydration, and the presence of large contrast dye loads may also be important. All efforts should be directed to avoid or minimize systemic hypoperfusion and its renal consequence, acute oliguria. **Mannitol** has been shown to maintain renal tubular flow in animal models. Renal-dose **dopamine** improves urine flow and glomerular filtration but is not effective in reversing cross-clamp-induced renal failure. Although furosemide is considered a nephrotoxin, it is used by some clinicians to increase urine flow or in an attempt to convert oliguric ARF to nonoliguric ARF after aortic surgery. A promising dopamine-1-receptor agonist, fenoldopam, is currently under investigation. Though there are few human outcome data on this subject, most cardiovascular anesthesiologists will prophylactically institute mannitol and/or dopamine infusions during aortic surgery. If pharmacologic renal protection is chosen, it should be started well before the application of the aortic cross-clamp.

Special Considerations for Patients with Thoracic and Thoracoabdominal Aortic Aneurysms

Patients with thoracoabdominal aortic aneurysms are more prone to hemodynamic lability and cardiac and renal complications than those with aortic disease limited to the abdomen. The thoracic portion of the aneurysm is typically approached through a left thoracotomy incision, which is extended to the abdomen as necessary. Exposure of the thoracic aorta may be facilitated by collapse of the left lung using a double-lumen endotracheal tube or bronchial blocking device. The incidence of spinal cord ischemia and neurologic deficit is also much higher in patients after operation on the thoracic aorta. Identification and preservation of the spinal artery of Adamkiewicz is theoretically attractive but technically difficult. **Spinal drainage catheters** are used at some centers to keep cerebrospinal fluid pressure below 10 cm H_2O during aortic occlusion to ensure the spinal cord perfusion pressure, though outcome data for this practice in humans are scant. Stable hemodynamics and a short cross-clamp time are probably the best insurance against these complications.

Aortic aneurysms involving the proximal aorta are approached through a median sternotomy. If disease involves the ascending aorta, use of CPB is necessary because the aortic root is typically replaced along with reimplantation of the coronary arteries. If the cerebral vessels are involved, replacement of the aorta under deep hypothermia and circulatory arrest (DHCA) may be necessary. Hypothermia lowers the $CMRO_2$ of neuronal tissue by decreasing body temperature and will confer some protection against cerebral ischemia. The allowable period of ischemia may be extended by deep hypothermia, and repair of the arch may be more safely undertaken. Neurologic and hematologic complications related to this technique, however, limit its application. If disease is confined to the descending aorta, replacement surgery is similar to that described for thoracoabdominal aneurysms.

Special Considerations for Patients with Ruptured Aortic Aneurysms

Patients presenting with aortic rupture or dissection are also at much higher risk for cardiac, renal, and neurologic complications. These patients are frequently hypotensive or even moribund on their arrival in the operating room, and preoperative evaluation must not delay resuscitation. There is rarely sufficient time for preoperative consultation. Control of the blood pressure is of paramount importance. If systemic pressures are elevated, vasodilators may reduce the extent of dissection. Low systemic pressures should suggest profound hypovolemic shock. With aortic rupture, return of adequate hemodynamics will not occur until the aorta has been clamped, and therefore, under these circumstances, anesthesia should be induced with minimal drugs while the patient is being resuscitated. Vasoconstrictors and inotropic agents should be readily available. Mortality rates for emergent aortic surgery exceed 50% in some series.

Anesthesia for Peripeheral Arterial Revascularization

Preoperative Considerations

Patients undergoing peripheral revascularization procedures are unquestionably at risk for the same concurrent disease processes as aortic surgery patients. Fortunately, the hemodynamic insults of peripheral revascularization (including femoral-popliteal and distal bypass grafting) are usually much less significant than those brought on by aortic cross-clamping. The duration of distal bypass procedures may surpass 5 or 6 hours. Preoperative preparation is essentially identical to that described for aortic surgery patients, although it is extremely uncommon to electively ventilate these patients in the postoperative period.

Monitoring

Along with ASA standard monitors, an arterial line is helpful in some patients for monitoring of systemic blood pressures and blood sampling during these frequently prolonged procedures. A Foley catheter is routinely inserted. While central pressure monitoring is essentially mandatory for aortic surgery, the decision to place a CVP line for peripheral procedures depends on the adequacy of peripheral access, the likely duration of surgery, and the acuity of the patient's illness. PA catheterization is rarely, if ever, necessary, and TEE monitoring is rarely indicated.

Choice of Anesthetic Technique

The choice of anesthetic in peripheral vascular procedures is dictated by the length of the planned surgery, the speed of the vascular surgeon, and the patient's stated preference. Unlike aortic surgery, regional anesthesia alone may be appropriate for many patients. Vascular surgery patients have been shown to be hypercoagulable compared with age-matched controls, and recent studies have found that modulation of the "stress" response to surgery with a regional anesthetic technique may favorably affect the coagulation and fibrinolytic cascade. Fewer reoperations for limb ischemia in peripheral revascularization patients may result from reductions in this "stress" response with central neuraxis blockade. Plasma catecholamine levels are lower in patients receiving epidural anesthesia, and decreased levels of plasminogen activator inhibitor (PAI) have been reported in patients who received an epidural for peripheral revascularization. Patients with elevated PAI levels have a higher incidence of postoperative thrombotic complications. No difference in cardiac outcomes has been reported when regional anesthesia is compared with a general anesthetic in peripheral vascular surgery patients.

Perioperative Management

Induction of general anesthesia may be accomplished with any number of drugs, and a balanced technique using O_2, N_2O, narcotic, and low-dose isoflurane is satisfactory for maintenance of anesthesia. Neuromuscular blockade is not usually necessary for peripheral revascularization. Surgical stimulation is fairly light for most of the procedure, and extubation in the operating room is a very reasonable goal. Hemodynamic perturbations are minimal with clamping of peripheral arteries, which are at least partially occluded in most patients.

The choice of local anesthetic for spinal anesthesia depends on the anticipated duration of the surgical procedure. Lidocaine with epinephrine may be acceptable for a fast surgeon performing a femoral-popliteal bypass, though bupivicaine and tetracaine may be more reasonable choices. Narcotic (fentanyl or morphine) may also be injected with the local anesthetic for postoperative analgesia. Hypotension should be aggressively treated with vasoconstrictor agents. The advisability of "preloading" with IV fluid before neuraxis blockade has been questioned in recent studies and may be poorly tolerated by a patient with impaired cardiac function.

Epidural blockade has the advantage of more gradual onset of sympathectomy than with a subarachnoid block, and the catheter may be redosed in a lengthy case. Less profound block of sacral segments may be problematic, however. Lidocaine and bupivicaine are the most frequently chosen agents. Most patients undergoing peripheral vascular surgery should not require ICU admission, unless perioperative events warrant such close observation.

Anesthesia for Carotid Endarterectomy

Preoperative Considerations

Patients scheduled for carotid endarterectomy (CEA) have an extremely high incidence of concomitant coronary artery disease. Some patients who are scheduled for endarterectomy actually present to the hospital for evaluation of CASHD and during their workup are found to have critical carotid stenosis. Preoperative evaluation is similar to that described above for other cardiovascular patients. Special attention must be paid to the preoperative neurologic status, and any deficits should be carefully documented in the preanesthetic evaluation.

Monitoring

In addition to ASA standard monitors, it was routine for every patient who underwent carotid endarterectomy to be monitored with an arterial line and to spend at least the first postoperative night in the ICU. Under economic pressures, this practice has evolved to a point where most CEA patients are not admitted to the ICU. Arterial catheters are placed only in selected patients with significant hypertension, coronary artery disease, or valvular heart disease. Central venous access is rarely necessary, though secure IV access for administration of vasoactive medications is mandatory. CVP lines must not impinge on the surgical field.

CNS Monitoring. Many modalities are available to monitor the brain during anesthesia and surgery in an attempt to protect against adverse neurologic outcomes. The electroencephalogram (EEG) can be used to detect slowing or asymmetry in cortical signals, which may reflect regional reductions in cerebral blood flow (CBF). In its unprocessed form, the EEG is difficult to interpret, and "anesthesiologist-friendly" models that process raw EEG data and transform it into understandable displays may be less sensitive. A wide variety of anesthetic agents and environmental factors also interfere with the EEG signal. Outcome studies have not supported the use of any cerebral monitor in vascular surgery patients, although some surgeons use the EEG to assess the need for intraluminal shunting during carotid clamping. Measurement of CBF is cumbersome and has not been shown to correlate with clinical outcome. Indeed, the optimal monitor of cerebral function may be the awake patient's brain. The adequacy of CBF is all but assured if the patient is mentating, though outcome studies validating improved neurologic outcome in patients undergoing carotid surgery do not exist at this time.

Protection against cerebral ischemia during carotid surgery may be afforded by placement of an intraluminal shunt during endarterectomy, though the decision to place a shunt is largely a matter of the surgeon's preference. No particular pharmacologic intervention provides definitive cerebral protection against the kind of global cerebral ischemia that may occur during CEA, and this type of therapy cannot be used in the awake patient.

Choice of Anesthetic Technique

There have been no definitive outcome studies showing that either regional or general anesthesia results in improved cardiac or neurologic outcome in carotid surgery. Patients undergoing CEA may be managed under regional (cervical plexus block) or local (field block) anesthesia, though careful patient selection is essential. Patients who are claustrophobic or who cannot lie flat will not tolerate an "awake" CEA. Patients who receive a regional anesthetic may require fewer vasoactive drugs postoperatively, though this, like almost everything else in vascular anesthesia, is controversial. The advantages of local or regional anesthesia in carotid patients include the ability to use the awake patient's neurologic status as a guide to whether intraluminal shunting is necessary. Using these techniques, as many as 96% of patients may avoid shunting and its attendant risks. Patients who have mental status changes with carotid clamping may be at risk for postoperative neurologic events and may benefit from closer observation and early therapeutic intervention postoperatively.

Perioperative Management

Induction and maintenance of **general anesthesia** should emphasize control of the systemic blood pressure. Patients with carotid disease are frequently hypertensive, and lability of blood pressure may be problematic. Most clinicians will attempt to maintain blood pressure on the high side to ensure cerebral perfusion prior to carotid clamping. Carotid occlusion below the carotid sinus may result in a compensatory rise in blood pressure, occasionally accompanied by a reflex bradycardia. Vasoactive agents (phenylephrine, nitroprusside, or nitroglycerin) are frequently required for blood pressure control. Rapid awakening at the conclusion of the procedure is essential to allow evaluation of neurologic status if a general anesthetic is provided.

If a **regional technique** is chosen, supplemental oxygen is mandatory. Sedation should be kept to a minimum, and small increments of narcotic and benzodiazepine should be adequate. During clamping of the carotid artery, patients may lose consciousness, become confused, or seize until flow is restored by an intraluminal shunt. Airway support may also be necessary; it is thus essential to have extra personnel available at this critical juncture.

Blood pressure will frequently normalize after removal of the stenotic plaque and restoration of carotid flow. After cerebral reperfusion, systemic blood pressure should be maintained in the normal-to-low range because cerebral autoregulation distal to the carotid stenosis may be altered from prior hypoperfusion. Vasoactive drips may be necessary early in the postoperative period, though if weaned aggressively in the recovery room, the patient should not require ICU admission. The patient should be observed long enough to detect any postoperative complications such as hematoma or neurologic deficit. If a neck hematoma occurs, it must be frequently evaluated, since airway compromise can ensue.

Suggested Readings

Hug CC. Anesthesia for adult cardiac surgery. *In:* Miller RD, ed. Anesthesia, vol. 2. 3rd ed. New York: Churchill Livingstone, 1990.

Hurst JW, ed. The heart. 7th ed. New York: McGraw Hill, 1990.

Kaplan JA, ed. Cardiac anesthesia. 3rd ed. Philadelphia: WB Saunders, 1993.

Aho M, Erkola O, Kallio A, et al. Dexmedetomidine infusion for maintenance of anesthesia in patients undergoing abdominal hysterectomy. Anesth Analg 1992;75:940–946.

Eagle KA, Coley CM, Newell JB, et al. Combining clinical and thallium data optimizes preoperative assessment of cardiac risk before major vascular surgery. Ann Intern Med 1989;110:859–866.

Foster ED, Davis KB, Carpenter JA, et al. Risk of non-cardiac operation in patients with defined coronary disease: the coronary artery surgery study (CASS) registry experience. Ann Thorac Surg 1986;41:42–50.

Hertzer NR, Beven EG, Young JR, et. al. Coronary artery disease in peripheral vascular patients. A classification of 1000 coronary angiograms and results of surgical management. Ann Surg 1984;199:223–233.

Leung JM, Stanley T, Mathew J, et al. An initial multicenter, randomized controlled trial on the safety and efficacy of acadesine in patients undergoing coronary artery bypass grafting. Anesth Analg 1994;78:420–434.

Mangano DT. Perioperative cardiac morbidity. Anesthesiology 1990;72:153–184.

Mantha S, Roizen MF, Barnard J, et al. Relative effectiveness of four preoperative tests for predicting adverse cardiac outcomes after vascular surgery: a meta-analysis. Anesth Analg 1994;79:422–433.

Rao TLK, Jacobs KH, El-Etr AA. Reinfarction following anesthesia in patients with myocardial infarction. Anesthesiology 1983;59:499–505.

Rosenfeld BA, Beattie C, Christopherson R, et al. The effects of different anesthetic regimens on fibrinolysis and the development of postoperative arterial thrombosis. Anesthesiology 1993;79:435–443.

Tuman KJ, McCarthy RJ, March RJ, et al. Effects of epidural anesthesia and analgesia on coagulation and outcome after major vascular surgery. Anesth Analg 1991;73:696–704.

Yeager MP, Glass DD, Neff RK, et al. Epidural anesthesia and analgesia in high-risk surgical patients. Anesthesiology 1987;66:729–736.

Chapter 16

Trauma and Burns

Overview (1)

1. Leading cause of death in first three decades of life
2. Fourth leading cause of death in the U.S.
3. Traumatic death in the U.S. claims more than 140,000 lives per year
4. Annual cost in the U.S. more than $130 billion
5. Trauma patients now occupy one of every eight hospital beds
6. Results in more work-years of life lost than all forms of heart disease and cancer combined

Unique Anesthetic Considerations

Lack of Comprehensive Preoperative Anesthetic Evaluation

1. Quick review of emergency room data
2. When possible, perform an "AMPLE" history (2)—allergies, medications, past illnesses, last meal, events/environment related to injury
3. Airway assessment, cardiopulmonary examination

Airway Considerations

I. Indications for intubation
   A. Airway protection (altered mental status, full stomach, bleeding)
   B. Airway obstruction
   C. Mechanical ventilation (acute or impending ventilatory failure, need to hyperventilate for elevated intracranial pressure, etc.)

    D. Tracheobronchial toilet (inability to clear secretions)

    E. Oxygenation improvement (reliable delivery of high inspired oxygen concentrations or distending airway pressure)

II. Factors complicating intubation

    A. Cervical spine trauma

Immobilization: Soft and hard collars allow significant neck flexion, extension, and rotation. Manual inline traction applied by an assistant during intubation reduces neck movement but may increase the risk of distraction or lengthening of the spinal cord at the fracture site. The combination of a hard collar, bilateral head sand bags, and secure taping of the head to a rigid board affords the best protection from damage to an unstable spine.

Radiographic evaluation: Cross-table lateral view (CTLV) should be obtained, which shows all seven cervical vertebrae clearly (74–82% sensitivity in ruling out cervical spine fracture). Sensitivity can be increased to 93% by adding an anteroposterior view (to assess vertical alignment of the spinous and articular processes and abnormalities in joint and disc spaces) and an odontoid view (to assess integrity of atlantooccipital and atlantoaxial joints and the odontoid process (3)). In general, a CTLV alone is inadequate to safely clear the cervical spine of instability, and precautions should continue if anteroposterior and odontoid views cannot be obtained prior to intubation.

Intubation plan: Awake intubation with avoidance of neck manipulation permits checking gross neurologic function directly after intubation and before administration of anesthetic or sedative agents. Options include awake oral or nasal fiberoptic intubation and awake blind nasal intubation. Fiberoptic intubation may be difficult if blood is present in the pharynx and in uncooperative patients.

    B. Full stomach

All trauma patients are considered to have "full stomachs" because of recent oral intake, presence of blood in the stomach (from trauma, swallowed blood), and delayed gastric emptying (from trauma, pain, anxiety, or alcohol). This results in an increased risk of aspiration of gastric contents during intubation. Studies suggest that severity of pulmonary injury from aspiration is related to acidity and volume of stomach contents (greatest risk pH < 2.5, volume > 25 ml).

Preoperative preparation: If time is available, treatment with H_2-blockers (to decrease gastric acidity), metaclopromide (to speed gastric emptying), or a nonparticulate antacid like sodium citrate (to neutralize acid present in the stomach) reduces the risk of pulmonary damage if aspiration occurs during intubation.

Intubation plan: Awake techniques under local anesthesia (blind nasal versus topicalized oral intubation) or a rapid sequence intubation with cricoid pressure; (tracheal topicalization may eliminate protective airway reflexes and increase risk of aspiration, especially in patients with altered mental status).

C. Facial fractures

Preoperative assessment: All patients with facial fractures secondary to blunt trauma are at risk for concomitant cervical spine fracture. Check for signs of basilar skull fracture (CSF rhinorrhea, raccoon eyes, Battle's sign) and for broken teeth, dentures, caps, crowns, and bone fragments, which can be aspirated during intubation. Missing teeth or dental work should be accounted for via facial and chest radiographs, when possible.

Intubation plan: Nasal intubation is relatively contraindicated in patients with Lefort II or III fractures, because of the risk of disruption of the cribriform plate by the endotracheal tube and the potential for passage of the tube into the brain substance. Cerebrospinal fluid leakage is possible, increasing the likelihood of CNS infection when a nasal endotracheal tube is in place. Attempt oral intubation, though this may be complicated by loss of normal anatomical landmarks. With acute airway obstruction from extensive bony or soft tissue injury, intubation may be facilitated by grasping the tongue firmly with a towel clip or clamp and forcibly withdrawing it from the mouth. Traction on the tongue helps relieve the airway obstruction, and the tongue can be followed to its base as a landmark in identifying the epiglottis and vocal cords. Tracheostomy or cricothyroidotomy should always be considered when extreme traumatic airway distortion makes successful intubation unlikely.

D. Head injury (HI)

Preoperative assessment: In the presence of HI, always consider concomitant cervical spine fracture. Obtundation and elevated intracranial pressure (ICP) are indications for intubation for airway protection and hyperventilation. Patients may have received mannitol to lower ICP and are at risk for hypovolemia, which may become evident when sedatives are administered. Sedatives and narcotics should be avoided in patients with altered mental status unless intubation and mechanical ventilation are planned. Respiratory depression in a spontaneously breathing patient results in hypercarbia, increased cerebral blood flow, and increased ICP.

Intubation plan: Airway management goals include smooth, rapid oral intubation after intravenous administration of cerebral protective agents (sodium thiopental, lidocaine, benzodiazepines, and/or narcotics) and a rapid-acting muscle relaxant (succinylcholine). Although succinylcholine may increase ICP, this is offset by the ICP-lowering effects of induction agents. Since these patients are at risk for aspiration of gastric contents, succinylcholine remains the most reliable short-acting muscle relaxant, minimizing the time that the airway remains unprotected. Coughing, bucking, gagging, and straining can elevate ICP markedly and should be avoided. After intubation, the anesthesiologist and neurosurgeon should discuss further sedation and/or muscle relaxation plans. Short-acting agents can be used if the neurosurgeon requires continued evaluation of the patient's mental status. Otherwise, patients should be well-sedated to avoid elevated ICP from reaction to the endotracheal tube.

E. *Open globe eye injury*

Succinylcholine has the quickest onset and shortest duration of action of currently used muscle relaxants. An unfortunate side effect is increased intraocular pressure, which may lead to extrusion of vitreous contents.

In patients with open globe eye injury, its use remains controversial, although it has been used successfully in several published series of cases.

Hemorrhagic Shock

Hemorrhagic shock is the most common form of shock in trauma patients; final common pathway is inadequate blood flow and tissue oxygenation.

I. Classification of hemorrhage (4)

Class I: loss of up to 15% blood volume: clinical signs—minimal physiologic changes

Class II: loss of 15–30% blood volume: clinical signs—moderate increase in heart rate, decrease in pulse pressure, slightly delayed capillary refill, mildly depressed urine output, postural hypotension, mild CNS changes (anxiety, hostility)

Class III: loss of 30–40% blood volume: clinical signs—tachycardia; systolic and diastolic hypotension; delayed capillary refill (> 2 seconds); decreased urine output; and agitated, somewhat clouded consciousness

Class IV: loss of 40% or more of blood volume: clinical signs—frank shock; tachycardia; hypotension or full cardiac arrest; obtundation; anuria; cool, clammy ashen skin

II. Pathophysiology

A. Cardiovascular response

1. Acute decrease in venous return (decreased preload secondary to hypovolemia); compensatory venoconstriction

2. Cardiac output (CO) decreases transiently with acute loss of preload; followed by reflex cardiovascular compensation for hemorrhage (tachycardia), increased ejection fraction via sympathetic stimulation

3. Reflex constriction of peripheral vessels, increased systemic resistance (SVR)

4. Microcirculation: Central aortic blood pressure is maintained at the expense of reduced flow through splanchnic, renal and cutaneous capillary beds. Arteriolar vasoconstriction is eventually released during prolonged shock (diminished SVR), while venoconstriction is maintained much longer. This venocon-

striction results in a rise in intracapillary pressure and a predisposition to edema formation. Continued blood loss, intravascular fluid loss to the interstitium, and an decreased SVR result in profound hypotension.

B. Respiratory response
1. Reduced pulmonary blood flow produces increased dead-space ventilation, with subsequent increases in minute ventilatory requirements.
2. Reduced respiratory muscle blood flow results in respiratory muscle failure.
3. Arterial blood gases
   a. Metabolic acidemia from hypoperfusion and lacticacidemia
   b. Hypocarbia secondary to hyperventilation from pain, agitation, head injury, and respiratory compensation of metabolic acidemia
   c. Hypoxemia from lung injury and splinting from pain
   d. Respiratory acidemia with impaired CO_2 excretion due to prolonged, severe hypovolemia and reduced cardiac output

C. Renal response
1. Renal blood flow (RBF) is reduced to preserve central perfusion
2. Glomerular afferents vasodilate, while efferents constrict in an effort to maintain glomerular filtration rate (GFR)
3. Release of stress hormones mediates decreased GFR, RBF, and urine output (UOP)
4. Decreased GFR, tubular damage, and precipitation of toxins (myoglobin, free hemoglobin) results in acute tubular necrosis and acute renal failure (oliguric or nonoliguric)

D. Metabolic response
1. Sympathetic stimulation: Release of epinephrine results in decreased renal, splanchnic, and cutaneous perfusion.
2. ACTH release from the pituitary stimulates cortisol release.
3. Increased glucagon and decreased insulin release

from the pancreas results in hyperglycemia ("diabetes of trauma").

4. β-Adrenergic stimulation causes hypokalemia and lipolysis.

5. Profound lactic acidemia results from uncorrected hypovolemia.

III. Treatment (rapid, aggressive fluid resuscitation)

A. *IV access:* Establish venous access with at least two upper extremity large-bore (14–16 gauge) IVs. If necessary, proceed to central access if peripheral IVs are unobtainable. The subclavian vein is the most accessible in the hypovolemic patient because it remains stented open by its adherence to the clavicle despite low central pressures. Avoid lower extremity access in patients with abdominal trauma, because of the possibility of traumatic or surgical disruption of the inferior vena cava.

B. Fluid replacement calculations:

1. Estimate approximate percentage of blood volume lost, using clinical signs (See Classification of hemorrhage)

2. Calculate estimated blood lost (EBL) with the following formula:

$$EBL = \text{estimated blood volume (EBV)} \times$$
$$\text{(percentage blood volume lost)};$$

EBV is approximately 70 ml/kg in adults
(e.g., EBL for an 80-kg patient with a 25% blood volume loss = $80 \times 70 \times 0.25 = 850$ ml)

3. Calculate replacement required, depending on solution chosen (see below)

C. Types of fluid replacement

1. *Isotonic crystalloid solution* requires 3 ml replacement per ml of blood loss, since only a portion remains intravascular. (Replacing 850 ml blood loss requires approximately 2500 ml crystalloid.)

2. *Colloid*
   • 5% albumin—replace 1 ml per ml EBL; 50% remains intravascularly after 16 hours (5)
   • 6% hetastarch—replace 1 ml per ml EBL; 50% remains intravascularly after 24 hours (6)

3. *Blood products*

a. *Whole blood* (WB) versus *packed red blood cells* (PRBC)

Fresh WB contains RBCs, plasma, and platelets in a preservative solution, while a PRBC unit contains only RBCs in concentrated form. Advantages to using fresh WB include fewer donor exposures for the recipient when plasma or platelets are also required and a reduced risk of developing a massive transfusion-related coagulopathy. *Stored WB* is deficient in the labile clotting factors (V, VIII), and platelets are not functional. The main advantage of PRBC is a more efficient use of blood components (plasma and platelets can be directed to patients who specifically need them). The only indication for blood transfusion is to increase the Hct and oxygen-carrying capacity. Blood products should never be given for volume replacement alone.

b. *Fresh frozen plasma (FFP)*

FFP contains plasma, including all coagulation factors, but no platelets. Besides treating specific factor deficiencies and disorders, FFP is indicated for treating a clinically evident, dilutional coagulopathy following massive blood transfusion. Every attempt should be made to document abnormal clotting studies (PT, APTT, thromboelastogram) before FFP administration.

c. *Platelet concentrates* (random donor)

Each unit is prepared from a single unit of WB. Transfusion of one unit is expected to raise the platelet count of an adult by $5000–10,000/\mu l$. Platelets should not be administered through a filter with a pore size smaller than 170 μm, because a significant number of platelets will be lost. During massive transfusion of blood, a dilutional thrombocytopenia commonly ensues, making platelet transfusion necessary. Hypothermia will also decrease the effectiveness of circulating platelets, making correction of the coagulopathy extremely difficult.

d. *Cryoprecipitate*

Cryoprecipitate contains factor VIII:C, factor VIII:VWF, fibrinogen, factor XIII, and fibronectin. Cryoprecipitate is used to replace fibrinogen during massive transfusion or with fibrinogen consumption during DIC. Plasma fibrinogen levels should be measured during massive transfusion, and decreased fibrinogen may produce increases in both PT and APTT.

Specific Injuries

I. Head, facial injuries (see above)
II. Neck injuries
   A. *Cervical spine injury* (See airway management section)

Spinal shock immediately follows cervical spinal cord injury and lasts from a few days to several weeks after onset of quadriplegia. Fluid requirements may be massive, due to a functional sympathectomy from the injury. Ventilatory function should be assessed acutely by history, physical examination, arterial blood gas measurement, and maneuvers that determine ventilatory strength. A vital capacity (VC) of 15 ml/kg or a negative inspiratory force (NIF) of $-$ 20 cm H_2O indicates sufficient strength to support spontaneous ventilation and generate a cough forceful enough to clear secretions. Ventilatory function can be affected by diaphragmatic paralysis (high cervical lesion involving the phrenic nerve $C_{3,4,5}$), chest wall paralysis (thoracic segment involvement), and deceased functional residual capacity (mechanical effects of abdominal distention, gastric atony, or paralytic ileus).

   B. *Tracheobronchial tree disruption*

Hoarseness, dyspnea, dysphasia, subcutaneous emphysema, and mediastinal air on chest radiograph suggest laryngotracheal injury. This may be manifested clinically when positive pressure ventilation is initiated and a simple pneumothorax (PTX) is converted to a tension PTX with subsequent hypoxemia, hypercarbia, and hypotension. The presence of these clinical signs should result in a high level of suspicion. A chest tube should be placed promptly once the diagnosis of tension PTX has been made.

C. *Expanding neck hematoma*

Early intubation should be performed to prevent airway obstruction. Intubation may be difficult because of the distortion of pharyngeal anatomy. Awake intubation may be preferable. Beware of relative hypovolemia secondary to significant hemorrhage. Gross evaluation of neurologic function and mental status should take place before intubation whenever possible.

III. Chest injury

A. Pleural space injury

1. *Pulmonary contusion* occurs with blast injury and blunt trauma, commonly results in tachypnea, dyspnea, and hypoxemia. Treatment is supportive (supplemental oxygen, continuous positive airway pressure, CPAP, intubation, and mechanical ventilation in severe cases).

2. *Pneumothorax* (PTX) classically presents as absent or decreased breath sounds, tympanic percussion, distant or shifted cardiac sounds, engorged neck veins and elevated CVP, tracheal deviation, hypoxemia, hypotension, or increased airway pressure during mechanical ventilation. Definitive treatment is chest tube placement, but it can be treated emergently by placing a 14-gauge angiocatheter through the anterior chest wall in the second intercostal space at the midclavicular line, directly above the third rib. Connecting the catheter hub with extension tubing to a syringe barrel partially filled with fluid will allow visualization of bubbles as intrapleural air escapes and the tension PTX is relieved. This confirms the diagnosis and correct placement of the catheter. During anesthesia, be aware that nitrous oxide can enlarge an undecompressed PTX by diffusing into the enclosed space.

3. *Hemothorax* signs are similar to those of PTX, except neck veins are flat and the involved hemothorax is dull to percussion. Treatment differs from that for

PTX in that early decompression of the hemothorax will negate the tamponading effect on the bleeding source, resulting in additional hemorrhage. Thus, the first line of treatment is fluid resuscitation followed by chest tube placement with a collecting system that allows for collection and autotransfusion of drained blood.

B. Mediastinal injury

1. *Pericardial tamponade* (PCT) occurs when blood or fluid collects within an intact pericardial sac. It results in raised intrapericardial pressure, which restricts filling of the cardiac chambers and produces reduced cardiac output. Treatment consists of keeping the patient's heart "fast and full." Administer fluid to raise central venous pressure (CVP) above pericardial pressure. Inotropes are rarely needed in the absence of cardiac failure, because of the existing maximal level of endogenous sympathetic stimulation. Percutaneous pericardiocentesis and removal of some fluid can be performed in the awake patient prior to induction of anesthesia, to improve myocardial function. The definitive surgical procedure is the pericardial window. (An experienced surgeon can perform this procedure using local anesthesia and sedation.)

2. *Myocardial contusion* should be strongly considered when any blunt chest trauma is present. Signs include cardiac dysrhythmias or angina that does not respond to nitroglycerin. Diagnosis is difficult and usually based on electrocardiogram findings and positive CPK isoenzyme. Echocardiography is extremely useful in identifying regional ventricular wall abnormalities and effusions associated with myocardial contusion.

3. *Great vessel injury*

Aortic transection usually results in rapid exsanguination. Lesser aortic injury may lead to an intimal tear with formation of a dissecting aneurysm. Traumatic aortic rupture should be considered in any patient with a history of blunt or penetrating chest injury and symptoms of retrosternal or interscapular pain, dyspnea or hoarseness (secondary to traction on recurrent laryngeal nerves from an expanding aneurysm), or ischemia-type extremity pain. Signs include a harsh, systolic murmur heard over the precordium or interscapular region; wide variance of blood pressure measurements between two extremities; carotid bruit or decreased carotid pulses; or a pulsatile mass at the base of the neck. Any trauma patient with a widened mediastinum on chest radiograph should receive an aortogram to rule out great vessel injury. Treatment goals include fluid resuscitation and avoidance of tachycardia and hypertension, which can worsen aortic wall stress.

C. Chest wall injuries

   1. *First, second, or third rib fractures* of these well-protected ribs requires extreme force. Blunt trauma of this magnitude is often associated with other serious chest trauma such as disruption of the aortic arch.

   2. *Flail chest* is defined as multiple fractures of three or more adjacent ribs resulting in a free segment of chest wall. No longer under chest muscle control, the flail segment moves with changes in pleural pressure. The segment will move in during inspiration and out during expiration (termed "paradoxic" movement). Shunting due to underlying lung contusion and atelectasis results in hypoxemia. Treatment is supportive with supplemental oxygen, continuous positive airway pressure, adequate analgesia, aggressive tracheobronchial toilet, and in severe cases, mechanical ventilation to reduce the work of breathing.

IV. *Abdominal injuries* can occur in the peritoneal cavity, retroperitoneal space, or pelvis. Large amounts of blood can be sequestered in the abdominal cavity, and the tamponading effect of the abdominal wall may be lost even before surgical incision. Muscle relaxants used on induction of anesthesia decrease abdominal wall tension. In extreme cases, the abdomen should be prepared and draped and a surgeon be present, gowned, and gloved before induction. Be prepared for sudden, massive blood loss at induction and again at incision.

V. *Extremity injuries*

Significant occult hemorrhage can occur with major fractures, from lacerated blood vessels and rupture of interosseous blood vessels. In addition to hypovolemia, other complications of long bone fractures include neurovascular injury, fat emboli, and compartment syndrome. Decreased pulses distal to the fracture site may indicate compartment syndrome or neurovascular injury. Extensive crush injuries to muscle may result in myoglobinuria and acute renal failure.

BURN INJURY

Overview

Outcome

CA_{50} (percentage body surface burned that results in death in 50% of patients) is approximately 80%

Assessment of Burn Injury

I. Depth
  A. *Superficial partial thickness* involves mainly epidermis.
  B. *Deep partial thickness* involves variable depth of dermis but spares hair follicles and sebaceous glands.
  C. *Full thickness* involves deep dermis, with destruction of hair follicles and sebaceous glands.
II. *Extent*

Estimate percentage of body surface area burned by the "*rule of nines*" (9% for surface area of head and neck, each upper extremity, each anterior portion of lower extremity, each posterior portion of lower extremity, 18% for both anterior torso and posterior torso, 1% for genital region).

Classification of Burn Injury

I. *Major burn injury*
  A. Burn > 25% total body surface area (TBSA)

B. Children < 10 years old with burns > 20% TBSA
C. Full-thickness burns > 10% TBSA
D. Burns involving face, eyes, hands, feet, or perineum likely to result in functional or cosmetic impairment
E. All significant high voltage electrical burns
F. *Complicated burns*
1. Inhalation injury
2. Major trauma
3. Associated illness

II. *Minor burn injury*
A. Burns < 15% TBSA
B. Children < 10 years old with burns < 10% TBSA
C. Full-thickness burns < 2% TBSA

Pathophysiology of Burn Injury

Dermatologic

Breakdown of protective barrier normally provided by intact skin

1. *Thermoregulatory dysfunction*—potential for hypothermia
2. *Fluid/electrolyte disturbances*—potential for hypovolemia
3. *Disrupted barrier* to infection
4. *Loss of protective surface* covering—potential for trauma to underlying structures

Cardiac

A. Early phase (0–48 hours postinjury)
1. Decreased cardiac output (reduced circulating blood volume, possible release of myocardial depressant factor with large burns)
2. Decreased preload (increased vascular permeability and third-spacing, release of endogenous vasodilating mediators, loss of fluid across burned areas)
B. Late phase (> 48 hours postinjury)
1. Increased cardiac output from increased SV and heart rate (hypermetabolic state, 2- to 3-fold increase)
2. Unpredictable changes in SVR (increased levels of circulating catecholamines versus increased incidence of sepsis)

Pulmonary

A. Early phase (0–48 hours postinjury)
 1. Smoke toxicity (direct injury)
  a. *Upper airway obstruction* secondary to edema
  b. *Lower airway obstruction* secondary to bronchospasm, edema, inhalation of particulate matter, and cell necrosis producing hypoxemia
  c. *Decreased lung-thorax compliance* from increased lung water, alveolar collapse and reduced chest wall excursion from burn eschar results in decreased FRC and increased work of breathing
 2. Carbon monoxide (CO) toxicity
  a. Markedly reduced arterial oxygen content (CO-hemoglobin affinity 210 times that of O_2-hemoglobin)
  b. Leftward shift of oxyhemoglobin dissociation curve (reduced oxygen delivery to tissues)
  c. CO binds to cytochrome system, interfering with O_2 utilization for oxidative phosphorylation
B. Late phase
 1. Increased incidence of ARDS
 2. High incidence of sepsis after tracheostomy
 3. Chronic pulmonary fibrosis

Gastrointestinal

1. Paralytic ileus (usually resolving within 24 hours)
2. Increased incidence of gastric stress ulcer (especially with sepsis)

Hepatic

A. Early phase
 1. Decreased hepatic function (hypoxemia, hypotension, and hepatocellular damage from inhaled or absorbed chemical toxins)
 2. Elevated hepatic enzymes and bilirubin level
B. Late phase
 1. Increased hepatic function (hypermetabolism, enzyme induction, increased cardiac output)
 2. Elevated hepatic enzymes and bilirubin level(especially with sepsis)

Renal

A. Early phase
  1. Decreased GFR, RBF, urine output
  2. Myoglobinuria, hemoglobinuria (especially with electrical injury)
B. Late phase
  1. GFR, RBF, and urine output increase (primarily as a result of increased cardiac output)
  2. Tubular dysfunction (decreased ability to concentrate urine; seen most commonly in burns $>$ 40% TBSA)

Neurologic

1. Encephalopathy (hypoxic, neurotoxic)
2. Seizure (increased CNS irritability)
3. Increased ICP
4. ICU psychosis

Metabolic

1. Catecholamine-mediated hypermetabolism, hyperdynamic circulation
2. Negative nitrogen balance (catabolism, loss of protein through burn wound)
3. Increased oxygen consumption, carbon dioxide production
4. Abolished/diminished thermoregulatory mechanisms

Endocrine

1. Massive release of stress hormones (ACTH, renin, angiotensin, cortisol, ADH)
2. Increased calcitonin levels, normal parathyroid hormone levels; decreased ionized calcium
3. Paradoxic reduction of T_3 and T_4, normal TSH levels
4. Hyperglycemia (stress response, unpredictable insulin level and function)

Hematopoietic

A. Early phase
  1. Thrombocytopenia (dilutional, platelet aggregation)
  2. Decreased factors V and VIII and fibrinogen levels

  3. Increased levels of fibrin split products
  4. Hemoconcentration (third-spacing of fluids)
B. Late phase
  1. Thrombocytosis (reactive)
  2. Increase in factors V and VIII and fibrinogen levels
  3. Anemia (increased RBC destruction, decreased hematopoiesis)
  4. Increased incidence of sepsis and disseminated intravascular coagulation (DIC)

Immunologic

1. T cell function and number depressed
2. Depressed chemotactic and bacteriocidal activity of neutrophils

Unique Anesthetic Concerns with Burn Injury

Airway Management

Potential for airway obstruction, carbon monoxide (CO) poisoning, inhalation injury

1. *History*—routine, plus specific questions about loss of consciousness, thermal injury in an enclosed space (increased risk of inhalation injury), inhalation of noxious chemicals
2. *Physical examination*—cardiopulmonary examination, plus careful airway examination including check for facial burns, singed facial or nasal hairs, erythema or swelling of oro- or nasopharynx, hoarseness, grunting, stridor, tachypnea, expectoration of carbonaceous sputum
3. *Laboratory tests*—routine plus ABG with measured carboxyhemoglobin and methemoglobin levels, chest x-ray
4. Immediate placement of humidified 100% oxygen delivery system on any patient suspected of CO poisoning and/or inhalation injury
5. Fiberoptic examination of glottis and tracheobronchial tree if inhalation injury is in question
6. Early prophylactic intubation when airway involvement is suspected or when massive fluid resuscitation is expected (potential for airway edema)
7. Mechanical ventilation and supportive therapy when appropriate

Fluid Resuscitation

Potential for hypovolemia

1. Loss of fluid across burn wound and increase in systemic capillary permeability (with burns larger than 30% TBSA)
2. Intravenous therapies (7)—first 24 hours, based on weight and percentage TBSA injured (all formulas give half calculated volume in first 8 hours, the remainder of volume in the following 16 hours; recommendations for fluid resuscitation vary widely)
   a. *Parkland formula*—Ringer's lactate, 4 ml/kg/percentage burn; for example, a 70-kg patient with a 25% TBSA burn requires 7000 ml of Ringer's lactate in the first 24 hours
   b. *Brooke formula*—Ringer's lactate 1.5 ml/kg/percentage burn, colloid solution 0.5 ml/kg/percentage burn, D_5W 2000 ml; for example, a 70-kg patient with a 25% TBSA burn requires 2625 ml of Ringer's lactate, 875 ml of colloid, and 2000 ml of D_5W in the first 24 hours
3. Patients with fluid requirements greater than calculated needs
   a. Electrical injury (deep tissue damage is more important in determining fluid requirements than are superficial burns)
   b. Inhalation injury (additional loss of vascular membrane integrity with increased third-spacing)
   c. Patients in whom resuscitation is delayed
4. Indicators of adequate resuscitation
   a. Normal acid-base balance—most important indicator of adequate perfusion
   b. Relative hemodynamic stability—no need for excessive pressor therapy
   c. State of sensorium—unreliable with sedation, sepsis, and encephalopathy
   d. Hourly urine output (minimum 0.5–1 ml/kg/hr)

Potential for Hypothermia

1. Loss of heat through all forms of heat transfer (conduction, radiation, convection, evaporation)
   a. Loss of protective skin covering and subcutaneous tissue (decreased insulation)

    b. Massive fluid resuscitation, often with nonwarmed solutions
2. Prophylaxis—warm ambient temperature, warmed solutions, warmed humidified ventilatory gases, covering of exposed surfaces

Potential for Infection

1. Strict aseptic technique
2. Early removal of nonessential transcutaneous catheters
3. Topical antibiotics
    a. Mafenide acetate (painful on application; acts as carbonic anhydrase inhibitor and promotes diuresis)
    b. Silver sulfadiazine (causes transient leukopenia, silver tissue deposits)
    c. 0.5% $AgNO_3$ (causes hyponatremia, black staining on contact)
    d. Betaine (results in metabolic acidosis, elevated serum iodine levels)
4. Systemic antibiotics, when appropriate
5. Aggressive surgical debridement and coverage with allograft

Potential for Excessive Intraoperative Bleeding with Skin Grafting

1. Estimate 1–4 ml blood loss per cm^2 skin excision
2. Use urine output, blood pressure, pulse, CVP, hematocrit, and intraoperative blood loss estimates to guide therapy
3. Epinephrine soaks applied to tissue beds (10 μg/ml solution of epinephrine in 0.9% NaCI solution) for hemostasis

Potential for Carbon Monoxide (CO) Poisoning

1. Despite well-oxygenated, well-perfused "cherry red" appearance, patient may be hypoxemic.
2. Pulse oximeter is insensitive to detection of carboxyhemoglobin (COHb) and will continue to give normal oxygen saturation readings in the face of profound desaturation.
3. Arterial blood gas analysis will often show a normal PaO_2, which will not correlate with a grossly decreased measured arterial oxygen saturation, SaO_2 (e.g., a PaO_2 of 70 with an SaO_2 of 70%). A COHb saturation level will usually be ele-

vated a corresponding amount (i.e., COHb ≈ 25% with this example).

4. All patients with suspected or diagnosed CO should be treated with 100% oxygen, which will decrease the half-life of COHb to 40 minutes from 250 minutes, when breathing room air. Hyperbaric oxygen therapy should be considered, if available, for severe cases of CO poisoning.

Monitoring and Vascular Access

1. Difficulty identifying intravenous access sites in burned tissue
2. Potential for infection with indwelling catheters
3. Need for large bore IVs for fluid resuscitation
4. Difficulty securing intravascular catheters to burned tissue (may require suturing in place); avoid traversing burned tissue with catheters whenever possible
5. With burns of chest and extremities, reliable application of blood pressure cuff and ECG electrodes becomes difficult (may require intraarterial blood pressure monitoring and sterile needle electrodes or stapling of electrodes to eschar for ECG monitoring)

Altered Pharmacokinetics/Pharmacodynamics

1. Cardiovascular factors—In general, changes in hepatic and renal blood flow parallel the changes in drug metabolism and elimination.
2. Protein-binding factors (8)
   a. Increased levels of α_1 acid glycoprotein ($\alpha_1$ag) result in increased binding of $\alpha_1$ag-bound drugs such as nondepolarizing agents and antiepileptics.
   b. Decreased levels of albumin result in decreased binding of albumin-bound drugs such as benzodiazepines and antiepileptics.
3. Other factors affecting drug metabolism: sepsis, concomitant drugs that induce or inhibit drug metabolism, hepatotoxic/nephrotoxic drugs, preexisting systemic disease
4. Examples
   a. *Succinylcholine*—induces massive potassium release from the muscle cell, which may result in lethal hyperkalemia; mechanism postulated to be denervation-type supersensi-

tivity; use is contraindicated after the first 24 hours post-injury

b. *Nondepolarizing muscle relaxants (NDMR)*—increased requirements, especially if burn exceeds 40% TBSA; not explained by increased volume of distribution, increased plasma binding, or increased loss through burn wound; proliferation of receptors or decreased sensitivity of receptors to nondepolarizing muscle relaxants may explain the increased NDMR requirement

c. *Anxiolytics:* diazepam and chlordiazepoxide have a prolonged effect after repeated doses; lorazepam maintains a normal duration of action; midazolam, with a shorter duration of action, may hasten postoperative neurologic assessment

d. *Induction agents: thiopental*—increased requirements during chronic phase; *ketamine*—popular because of its sympathetic stimulating and analgesic properties; beware of its cardiac depressant effects in the presence of hypovolemia or in patients who already have maximal sympathetic stimulation; *narcotics*—increased requirement during chronic phase; useful in the hemodynamically unstable burn patient

e. *Inhalation agents* can be used safely in hemodynamically stable burn-injured patients. They have the advantage of being rapidly eliminated if cardiovascular instability ensues (unlike intravenous agents). N_2O is often used in burn centers for dressing changes because it provides good analgesia with minimal hemodynamic changes.

PATIENT PREPARATION AND ROOM SETUP FOR TRAUMA

Premedication

1. *Anticholinergics* are useful when administered IM as antisialagogues, especially when use of ketamine is anticipated; vagolytic effects make tachycardia an unreliable indicator of volume status

2. *H_2-blockers* (PO) require up to 90 minutes to take effect and have no effect on acidity and stomach contents previously present.

3. *Metoclopramide* (PO) requires 30–60 minutes to take effect,

(IV) 1–3 minutes; may facilitate gastric emptying; should not be used with bowel obstruction or perforation.

4. *Antacids*—Nonparticulate antacids such as bicitrate and sodium bicarbonate given within 30 minutes of induction will increase gastric pH.

Rapid Sequence Induction/Emergence

1. Evaluate airway and estimate predicted ease of intubation by physical examination.

2. Preoxygenate (denitrogenate) with 100% oxygen. Complete denitrogenation can be assessed by gas-analyzer measurement of expired N_2.

3. Avoid positive pressure ventilation until patient is intubated.

4. Classically, use barbiturate (thiopental 3–5 mg/kg) and succinylcholine (1.5 mg/kg); prior precurarization is controversial; avoid succinylcholine in burn patients after the first 24 hours following injury. Use ketamine (1–2 mg/kg) or etomidate 0.1–0.3 mg/kg) if hypovolemia is suspected.

5. Backward pressure on the cricoid cartilage (Sellick maneuver) should be maintained by an assistant from the moment of induction until correct placement of the ETT has been confirmed and the cuff inflated. The cricoid is the only complete cartilaginous ring in the trachea, and firm pressure here causes occlusion of the esophagus and helps prevent passive regurgitation. There is a risk of esophageal rupture if the esophagus is occluded by cricoid pressure during active vomiting.

6. After intubation, an oral or nasal gastric tube (NGT) can be placed (if not contraindicated by facial or skull fractures) in an attempt to partially empty the stomach prior to emergence. An NGT placed before induction can not be considered a reliable means of completely emptying the stomach, and full-stomach precautions should be maintained. Whether or not an NGT in place before induction should be removed before performing a rapid sequence induction remains controversial.

7. If rapid sequence intubation is indicated, it is mandatory that patients remain intubated until they show full recovery of airway reflexes and are awake and responding to command.

Esophageal Obturators

Esophageal obturators may be placed by emergency medical personnel in the field, to assist ventilation. An esophageal obturator must never be removed until endotracheal intubation is accomplished, because of the nearly 100% incidence of vomiting on removal of the device. During induction, an endotracheal tube placed inadvertently in the esophagus should similarly be left in place with cuff inflated while a second tube is used to secure the airway.

Trendelenburg

Head-down positioning can be used to increase venous return from the lower extremities while fluid resuscitation continues. Although this will increase ICP in patients with head injuries, it may be necessary for limited periods to permit cardiovascular resuscitation.

Military Antishock Trousers (MAST)

MAST probably function by increasing lower extremity venous return and increasing SVR. When inflated, MAST can increase bleeding in thoracic or abdominal injuries. Elevated intragastric pressure increases the risk for aspiration. Increased intraabdominal pressure and restricted diaphragmatic excursion decrease FRC, predisposing to hypoxemia and increased work of breathing, and can cause increased resistance to positive pressure ventilation.

Operating Room Preparation

Trauma centers should always have an OR set up to receive patients.
Acronym: (S.O.A.P.—M.I.—filthy hair)
Suction/**O**xygen/**A**irway/**P**harmacy/**M**onitors/**I**V/**F**luid/**H**eat

   I. Suction—easy one-handed access to a wide-bore suction apparatus
  II. Oxygen—oxygen delivery system
      A. Anesthesia machine checked and functioning properly
      B. Backup means of delivering positive pressure ventilation

      1. Ambu-bag, Laerdal bag, or a Jackson-Reese circuit
      2. Full oxygen tank with tank key
      3. Adequate length of tubing to connect tank to bag or circuit

III. Airway—equipment for maintaining an artificial airway
  A. Variety of laryngoscope blades, including curved and straight no. 3 blades
  B. Two or more laryngoscope handles
  C. Endotracheal tubes (ETT)
    1. Styletted 7.5 (adult female) or 8.0 (adult male) ETT with cuff checked and syringe for cuff inflation attached
    2. Full set of backup ETTS, including pediatric sizes for cases of unanticipated airway swelling, compression, or other compromise
  D. Oral and soft nasal airways
  E. Masks
  F. Emergency access to cricothyrotomy kit (including jet ventilator setup)
  G. Emergency access to a flexible fiberoptic bronchoscope
  H. Long guidewire for retrograde identification of the larynx and intubation

IV. Pharmacy
  A. Induction agents
    1. Ketamine is sympathomimetic but may exhibit cardiovascular depression.
    2. Etomidate causes less hemodynamic instability than barbiturates.
    3. Barbiturates are used in reduced dosage because of their cardiac depressant effects.
  B. Narcotics have unique hemodynamic stability but can cause bradycardia. They can potentiate hypotension when combined with sedative-hypnotics.
  C. Muscle relaxants
    1. Succinylcholine (see "Rapid Sequence Induction")
    2. Nondepolarizer—component of "balanced" anesthetic in patients whose hemodynamic instability often prevents deep anesthesia
  D. Amnestics
    1. Scopolamine

  2. Benzodiazepines—may produce hypotension when combined with narcotics
E. Resuscitative drugs
  1. Atropine
  2. Epinephrine—bolus and infusion
  3. Vasoconstrictors

    Indirect-acting agents (e.g., ephedrine) that depend on liberating stored catecholamines may be less effective than direct-acting agents like phenylephrine. Hypotension secondary to hypovolemia should be treated with volume replacement. Vasopressors should be used sparingly and only as a bridge until fluid resuscitation can be completed.

  4. Sodium bicarbonate (NaHCO$_3$)

    Hypoperfusion leads to lactic acidosis, but it has not been shown that treatment with sodium bicarbonate affects outcome. ATLS suggests that shock patients with persistent acidosis be treated with additional fluids and not sodium bicarbonate unless the pH is less than 7.20. To calculate total base deficit, first calculate the total extracellular fluid content, then multiply by the measured base deficit. NaHCO$_3$ proponents recommend administering half the calculated deficit initially and then drawing new blood samples. Metabolism of citrate used as an anticoagulant in blood products may result in metabolic alkalosis after massive transfusion. Unnecessary administration of NaHCO$_3$ may worsen the alkalosis in the postoperative period.

  5. Calcium levels can be transiently lowered by massive transfusion of citrated blood. The acute decline in ionized calcium is directly related to the rate of citrated blood infusion and not the total amount of blood infused. Citrate is metabolized rapidly by the liver after transfusion, liberating its calcium. Significant decreases in ionized calcium can produce hypotension from diminished myocardial contractility and can interfere with coagulation. Rapid replacement of calcium and hypercalcemia can lead to cardiac complications. In the absence of prolonged QT waves on ECG or mea-

sured inadequate calcium values along with hypotension, the replacement of calcium is probably not indicated. Citrate metabolism is slowed by hypothermia, acidosis, and liver disease (hypomagnesemia and resultant ventricular dysrhythmias can also result from citrate infusions).

V. Monitors
  A. Routine: ECG, blood pressure cuff, pulse oximeter, exhaled CO_2 analyzer, precordial stethoscope, temperature probe, and oxygen analyzer
  B. Transducers for arterial and central venous pressures
  C. Defibrillator

VI. IV—a variety of catheters for peripheral IV, central venous, and arterial cannulation

VII. Fluids including isotonic crystalloid (normal saline or Ringer's lactate) and colloids (hetastarch and 5% albumin), should be readily available.

VIII. Heat
  A. Blood/fluid warmers
  B. Airway circuit-heated humidifier or "artificial nose" (heat and moisture exchanger-filter)
  C. Extremity wraps/head wrap
  D. Forced-air warming blanket
  E. Heating lights
  F. Increase OR temperature
  G. Irrigation at surgical site with warmed solutions

References

1. Lucas CE, Ledgerwood AM. Hemodynamic management of the injured. In: Capan LM, Miller SM, Turndorf H, et al. Trauma: Anesthesia and Intensive Care. Philadelphia: JB Lippincott, 1991:4–18.
2. American College of Surgeons. Advanced Trauma Life Support Student Manual. Chicago, 1989:20.
3. Crosby ET, Lui A. The adult cervical spine: implications for airway management. Can J Anaesth 1990;37:77–93.
4. Stene JK, Grande CM, Giesecke AH. Shock resuscitation. In: Stene JK, Grande CM, eds. Trauma Anesthesia. Baltimore: Williams & Wilkins, 1991:107.
5. Rainey TG. Pharmacology of colloids and crystalloids. In: Chernow B, ed. The pharmacologic approach to the critically ill patient. Baltimore: Williams & Wilkins, 1983:188.

6. Dodge C. What to transfuse: blood, blood components, colloid or crystalloid? In: ASA Refresher Course 1987;165:2.
7. Szyfelbein SK, Martyn J, Cote CJ. Burns. In: Ryan JF, Cote CF, Todres ID, Goudsouzian N, eds. A Practice of Anesthesia for Infants and Children. Philadelphia: WB Saunders, 1986;229–241.
8. Martyn J. Clinical pharmacology and drug therapy in the burned patient. Anesthesiology 1986;65:67–75.

Chapter 17

Anesthetic Considerations in the Critically Ill

For the purposes of this chapter, a critically ill patient is defined as one who has a disease process with a propensity to cause or which has already caused significant organ dysfunction requiring observation, monitoring, and/or treatment in an intensive care unit (ICU). Examples of such patients include those having unstable angina, myocardial infarctions, serious burns, head injuries, trauma, respiratory insufficiency, gastrointestinal bleeding, sepsis, recent surgery, and multiple organ system failure (MOSF).

The preparation and administration of an anesthetic to a critically ill patient is, in many ways, similar to that for any other patient. The significant differences lie in the complexity of the patient's illness, the number and severity of the organ systems involved, the multitude of drugs administered, the invasive monitoring and life support systems utilized, and the obstacles that are often present in providing safe transportation of these patients to and from the operating room.

PREOPERATIVE CONSIDERATIONS

History

Ideally, patients should not be transported to the operating room (OR) until they have been evaluated by a member of the anesthetic team. (Depending on the nature of their illness, patients may not be able to give their own history.) The complexity of the illness, endotracheal intubation, altered mental status, or sedation may require that the history be elicited from chart, critical care nurse, and primary physician. Particular emphasis should be placed on the present illness leading to the ICU admission and the number and severity of the organ systems involved, particularly the cardiovascular, gastrointestinal, hematologic, neurologic, renal, and respiratory systems. A history of allergies should be noted, and the medication sheet reviewed. Special attention should be given to the administration of vasoactive drugs, other continuously infused medications, and paralyzing agents. If possible, an anesthetic history and a family history should be sought. Any previous anesthetic record or intubation note should be reviewed. Attention should be given to any significant past medical history and habits.

Physical Examination

The physical examination often gives limited information but is essential none the less.

Vital Signs

Vital signs include recent blood pressure (BP), pulse (P), noted spontaneous respiratory rate (RR), and temperature. Ranges and recent trends should be noted when possible.

Airway

Many critically ill patients may already be intubated. The type of artificial airway (orotracheal, nasotracheal, or tracheostomy), its size, and the indication for its placement should be noted. Endotracheal tubes should be well secured to prevent removal during patient movement. A previous intubation note should be reviewed.

The depth of placement of the orotracheal or nasotracheal tube should be examined. This placement may give information about the proper positioning of the tube and its security during transport. In adults, an orotracheal tube is generally in good position when the 20–22 cm mark is at the teeth; a nasotracheal tube at 25–26 cm at the entrance to the nostril. If an orotracheal tube is placed at less than 20 cm and a nasotracheal tube at less than 24 cm and an air leak is present or the cuff requires additional air placement, the tip of the tube *may* be at the level of the vocal cords or glottic opening. Inadvertent extubation is possible, and the tube should be repositioned prior to transport. If the orotracheal tube is placed greater than 22 cm or the nasotracheal tube is placed greater than 26 cm, the possibility of a right main stem intubation exists.

Prolonged nasotracheal intubation places the patient at risk for sinusitis. If a nasotracheal tube has been in place for more than 3 days, the patient will require intubation postoperatively, and there is no contraindication, then consideration should be given to changing the nasotracheal tube to an orotracheal tube in the operating room.

A patient with head injury (see chapter on trauma) requires evaluation for

1. Basilar skull fracture
2. Increased intracranial pressure
3. Facial fractures
4. Cervical spine injuries

For special problems such as burns, see chapter on trauma.

Chest Examination—Heart and Lungs

The examination of the chest should include observation of the chest wall during ventilation, palpation of the chest wall, and auscultation of the lungs and heart. While providing new information at times, this examination more importantly serves as a baseline for intraoperative care and a guide to the possible etiologies of intraoperative problems on inadequate oxygenation or ventilation.

The following observations of the chest wall during ventilation may suggest associated pulmonary, ventilatory, or chest wall pathology.

Observations	*Pathology*
1. Increased work of breathing	1. Decreased compliance, poor ventilatory reserve
2. Prolonged expiratory phase	2. Bronchospasm
3. Paradoxic ventilatory pattern	3. Spinal cord injury
4. Paradoxic chest wall movement	4. Flail chest
5. Absence of bilateral chest wall movement	5. Right main stem intubation, pneumothorax, effusion, or atelectasis

For those patients requiring artificial ventilatory support, palpation of the chest wall may reveal subcutaneous emphysema, which may be the first evidence of barotrauma.

Although difficult at times, an effort should be made to auscultate the lungs not only anteriorly but posteriorly and in the midaxillary line as well. This examination may reveal rales, wheezes, rhonchi, or decreased or absent breath sounds over one or both hemithoraces.

The cardiac examination provides information about the quality of the heart tones, the rate, the rhythm, and presence of a murmur or rub.

Abdominal Examination

Abdominal distention may adversely affect oxygenation and ventilation because of its effects on pulmonary mechanics and decreasing functional residual capacity (FRC). Rapid sequence induction or awake intubation should be used for patients at risk for pulmonary aspiration from abdominal distention.

Because the blood gas coefficient of nitrous oxide (N_2O) is 34 times greater than that of nitrogen, N_2O can leave the blood and enter an air-filled cavity more rapidly than nitrogen can leave the air-filled cavity and enter the blood. This results in expansion of a closed air space. To avoid further abdominal distention, N_2O should not be used.

Neurologic Examination

The neurologic examination should include an evaluation of the patient's mental status. The Glasgow Coma Scale (Chapter 8, Table 8.3) is a relatively simple and commonly used clinical grading system based on eye opening ability, motor response, and verbal response. Scores range from 3 to 15. A score of 3 indicates significant impairment. A score of 15 indicates patients who are oriented, move their extremities on command, and open their eyes spontaneously. However, the ability to use this scale in the critically ill is often hindered by sedatives, pain medication, and endotracheal intubation.

The neurologic examination should also include an assessment of reflexes, motor strength, and symmetry of these responses. The presence of a neck collar or cervical traction should alert one to the possibility of a spinal injury or an unstable neck fracture.

A more detailed neurologic examination is required if the patient's primary problem (e.g., spinal cord injury), the surgical procedure (e.g., excision of a brain tumor), or the anesthetic technique (e.g., spinal or epidural) is neurologic.

Intravenous Access, Monitoring, and Life Support Examination

After the brief examination of all systems, a second examination should be undertaken to assess intravenous access, monitoring, and other support devices already in place. An organ systems approach to this survey may be helpful. Note the presence, absence, and/or location of

Cardiovascular
> Peripheral intravenous lines (IVs)
> Arterial line (A-line)
> Central line
> Swan-Ganz catheter (SG catheter)
> Intraaortic balloon pump (IABP)
> Pacemaker—note type and setting

Gastrointestinal/nutrition
> Nasogastric tube (NG tube)
> Feeding tube
> Hyperalimentation—central IV access to which it is dedicated

Neurologic
> Intracranial pressure monitor (ICP)
> Ventricular drain
> Cervical collar/cervical traction

Renal
> Foley catheter
> Dialysis catheter
> Shunts, fistulas, grafts

Respiratory
> Endotracheal tube—oral vs. nasal
> Tracheostomy tube
> Chest tube—note the presence or absence of an air leak; note the application of suction or placement to water seal
> Ventilator

Flow Sheet

The flow sheet charted for each critically ill patient can be an invaluable source of information. As the course of these patients tends to be dynamic, the flow sheet can provide important trends and changes in the vital signs, hemodynamic profile, respiratory support, basic laboratory analysis, renal function, and fluid status.

Important parameters to note:
Vital signs including temperature and weight
Hemodynamic profile and urine output
Neurologic
    Intracranial pressure (ICP)
    Cerebral perfusion pressures (CPP)

$$CPP = \text{mean arterial pressure (MAP)} - \text{ICP}$$

    Glascow Coma Scale (GCS)
Respiratory profile
    Arterial blood gas (ABG)
    Fraction of inspired oxygen concentration (FIO_2)
    Mode of ventilation and settings
        Airway pressure release ventilation (APRV)
        Controlled mechanical ventilation (CMV)
        High frequency jet ventilation (HFJV)
        High frequency positive pressure ventilation (HFPPV)
        Intermittent mandatory ventilation (IMV)
        Pressure support ventilation (PSV)
        Synchronized intermittent mandatory ventilation (SIMV)
    Distending airway pressure
        Continuous positive airway pressure (CPAP)
        Positive and expiratory pressure (PEEP)
    Peak inspiratory pressure (PIP)

Laboratory/Radiology

Not all of the following tests will be available or necessary in all patients.

Cardiovascular
    Electrocardiogram (ECG)
    Cardiac enzymes (if indicated)

Mixed venous oxygen saturation (SvO_2)

Gastrointestinal

Liver function—SGOT, alkaline phosphatase, LDH, bilirubin, albumin

Hematologic

Hgb/Hct, WBC

Coagulation

PT, PTT, platelets, fibrinogen, fibrin split products, D-dimers

Blood product availability

Neurologic

Cervical spine films

CT of head

Renal

Electrolytes—Na^+, K^+, Cl^-, CO_2^-, Mg^{2+}, Ca^{2+}

BUN, Cr

Respiratory

Chest x-ray

Arterial blood gas (ABG)

Drug levels

Aminophylline, digoxin, Dilantin

Antiarrhythmics: lidocaine, procainamide

Antibiotics: vancomycin, gentamicin, tobramycin

ANESTHETIC PLAN AND CONSENT

After the patient has been examined and the flow sheet and chart reviewed, an anesthetic plan can be formulated. Provisions for transport, monitoring, anesthetic technique, possible postoperative ventilation, and postoperative analgesia should be included. When possible, these plans, especially the possibility of postoperative ventilation, should be discussed with the patient and/or family. Consent for procedures such as postoperative regional techniques for pain control should be obtained.

Preoperative Orders

NPO Status

Many ICU patients will be receiving enteral feedings through a nasogastric tube. These feedings should be discontinued 8 hours prior to surgery.

Premedication

No specific recommendations can be given for the premedication of critically ill patients. Patients and their particular underlying pathology must be considered separately. A few *general guidelines* may be helpful:

1. For patients with *cardiovascular compromise,* reduced doses of narcotics may be tolerated, but a combination of a narcotic and a benzodiazepine may cause hemodynamic instability.
2. In patients with *respiratory insufficiency and spontaneous ventilation,* narcotics or benzodiazepine may cause respiratory depression leading to hypoxemia or hypercarbia.
3. Many of these patients are already receiving narcotics and anxiolytics. Review their medication sheets and consult with their critical care nurses to see what and how much the patient needs and tolerates.
4. Almost all critically ill patients receive oxygen therapy in the setting of pulmonary or cardiovascular insufficiency. Patients should be given supplemental O_2 during transport, especially if sedated with a narcotic or benzodiazepine.
5. If a *difficult airway* is anticipated or a fiberoptic intubation planned, an antisialagogue should be given.
6. If there is a concern about *increased intracranial pressure,* respiratory depressants, which may lead to hypercarbia and resultant cerebral vasodilation, should be avoided.
7. Patients who are *hemodynamically unstable* may not tolerate any premedication.
8. If a *patient is intubated,* attempts should be made to sedate the patient prior to transport. If the patient is hemodynamically unstable or will not tolerate sufficient sedation and may be uncooperative during transport, paralysis prior to transfer may need to be considered.

Anesthetic Preparation

The anesthetic preparation for a critically ill patient begins with the routine preparation for any anesthetic. Additional preparation should be guided by the preoperative visit and resulting anesthetic plan.

Airway

Airway equipment including a variety of endotracheal tubes, a stylet, laryngoscope handle, a curved and straight blade, an oral airway, and suction should be prepared and available even if the patient is already intubated. A fiberoptic scope and light source should be readied as determined by the anesthetic plan.

Drugs

Drugs needed for the anesthetic will vary depending on the patient's condition and the anesthetic technique chosen. *Ketamine and/or etomidate* should be available for induction of a hemodynamically unstable or hypovolemic patient. The type of *muscle relaxant* chosen will depend on the need for rapid sequence induction (succinylcholine), the anticipated length of the procedure, and cardiovascular stability (vecuronium). *Resuscitation drugs,* including lidocaine, epinephrine, and atropine, should be readily accessible. The number and type of vasoactive drugs to be prepared should be guided by the preoperative evaluation and the planned surgical procedure. *Vasoactive drugs* that might be needed include dopamine, dobutamine, epinephrine, phenylephrine, nitroglycerin, and sodium nitroprusside. Use of an infusion pump will allow accurate delivery of these drugs. Because of their relative hemodynamic stability, narcotics are typically part of the anesthetic plan for critically ill patients.

Invasive Monitoring

Preparation for intraoperative monitoring should be guided by the preanesthetic visit, monitors previously placed, and the contemplated surgical procedure. *Basic invasive intraoperative monitoring* includes an arterial line and a central line for central venous pressure monitoring. *Special cardiovascular monitors* and support devices include a Swan-Ganz catheter, a left atrial line, and an intraaortic balloon pump. *Special neurologic monitors* include an intracranial pressure monitor and somatosensory evoked potential monitor. The monitoring systems should be prepared, zeroed, and calibrated before the patient arrives in the operating room.

Ventilatory Support

The ventilators attached to the anesthesia machine will provide adequate ventilatory support for most critically ill patients. However, special consideration must be given to meeting respiratory support requirements in some patients.

1. If the *peak inspiratory pressures* during positive pressure ventilation *exceed 60 cm H_2O,* most anesthesia ventilators may fail to provide the needed ventilation. In this situation, plans must be made to ventilate the patient in the operating room with the ventilator that is currently delivering the required level of support. This may require having a respiratory therapist present or readily available during the operative procedure.

2. If the patient requires *positive end expiratory support* (PEEP) to maintain adequate oxygenation, PEEP valves must be available if not installed on the anesthesia machine.

3. Some modes of ventilatory support require a specific type of ventilator. If the patient is receiving high-frequency jet ventilation or airway pressure release ventilation, provisions must be made to secure these particular ventilators for intraoperative care. The use of these ventilators may preclude the use of an inhalation anesthetic. In this situation, an intravenous anesthetic technique is commonly used.

Other

In the appropriate circumstances, a rapid fluid infusion system with warming capabilities and an external pacemaker/defibrillator must be available.

Anesthetic Technique

Because critically ill patients often have some pulmonary or cardiovascular embarrassment, a narcotic-based anesthetic technique is commonly used. However, any anesthetic technique can be used as long as the degree of organ system dysfunction is considered.

1. If *gastrointestinal dysfunction or a full stomach* is present, a rapid sequence induction should be used if there are not overriding cardiovascular concerns.

2. Because of its sympathomimetic effect, *ketamine* is often used as an induction agent in patients who are hypovolemic. Since it also is a direct myocardial depressant, it may produce hypotension in patients who have maximal sympathetic stimulation.

3. *Etomidate* is a short-acting induction agent that lacks cardiovascular effects. Its use should be considered for those with underlying cardiovascular disease.

4. If a *patient has been previously intubated,* narcotics and/or an inhalation agent can be slowly introduced for induction of anesthesia to assess hemodynamic effects.

5. The use of *nitrous oxide* is limited in patients requiring high FIO_2 and in those with intestinal obstruction. Care is required when using N_2O in the presence of a pneumothorax, even if decompressed.

6. *Air* can be added to oxygen to decrease the FIO_2 to a minimal level, guided by SaO_2 and arterial blood gases. This will reduce atelectasis and prevent O_2 toxicity in patients requiring high FIO_2 for prolonged periods.

7. *Inhalation agents* may be well tolerated by some patients. Others, because of hemodynamic instability or compromise, will not tolerate these agents. A narcotic-based technique is then often indicated.

8. If a *narcotic/muscle relaxant technique* is chosen, the possibility of intraoperative recall exists. Scopolamine or a benzodiazepine can be used to produce amnesia in patients who do not tolerate potent inhalation agents.

9. Patients with *third degree burns or spinal cord injuries* producing paraplegia are likely to develop hyperkalemia when succinylcholine is administered 24 hours or more after the injury. This occurs as a result of an increase in extrajunctional cholinergic receptors. The risk of hyperkalemia may persist for 2 years after the injury.

10. The anesthetic plan should incorporate techniques for *postoperative pain control.* Options for pain control include intravenous narcotics, central axis narcotics via the subarachnoid or epidural space, and local anesthetics administered in the epidural, axillary, femoral, pleural, or intercostal spaces. Patient-controlled analgesia may give effective postoperative analgesia in conscious, cooperative patients.

11. If a reinforced or double-lumen endotracheal tube is used for the operative procedure and the patient requires post-operative ventilation, the tube should be removed and replaced by a polyvinyl endotracheal tube prior to transfer to the ICU. If significant airway edema has developed, consider a tracheal tube exchanger or fiberoptic-assisted replacement. If a patient inadvertently bites on a reinforced tube, it may become irreversibly kinked and obstructed.

12. Prior to transporting a patient who requires postoperative ventilation to the ICU, the endotracheal tube should be securely taped in place around the neck, unless contraindicated, to prevent dislodgment.

13. If a patient is to be directly admitted to the ICU from the operating room, a *report* should be given to the admitting ICU nurse and responsible MD and include

    Brief history and operative procedure
    Intraoperative complications
    Postoperative monitoring requirements
    Cardiovascular support—vasoactive drugs
    Ventilatory support if needed
    Special postoperative pain control techniques

INTRAHOSPITAL TRANSPORTATION

Transporting a critically ill patient to and from the operating room can be one of the most dangerous times in the perioperative period. Critically ill patients deserve the same care and monitoring during transportation that they receive in the ICU. Careful planning is necessary to ensure proper patient monitoring and hemodynamic and respiratory support. Some of the most *commonly encountered problems* during transport of these patients include arrhythmias, hypotension, hypertension, hypoxemia, hypercarbia, and hypocarbia.

Transport Team

Ideally, a transport team should consist of

1. A member of the anesthesia team
2. A respiratory therapist
3. A critical care nurse

The anesthesiologist should always assume the position at the head of the bed to assist with airway and ventilatory management.

Monitoring

Monitors needed during transport will vary with the condition and stability of the patient but may include

1. Stethoscope—precordial or esophageal
2. ECG
3. Pulse oximeter
4. Blood pressure monitor—sphygmomanometer or arterial line
5. Pulmonary artery pressure monitoring if Swan-Ganz catheter is in place and if expected to change during transport.

Airway and Ventilatory Support

Airway equipment will vary with the conditions of the patient but may include

1. Full E cylinder of oxygen (2200 psi = 660 liters)
2. Nasal cannula or face mask
3. Nasal and oral airway
4. Bag, valve, mask
5. Self-inflating bag with reservoir tubing
6. PEEP valve (with same level of PEEP as on ventilator) and adaptor for resuscitation bag
7. Intubation equipment
    Styletted endotracheal tube
    Laryngoscope blade and handle
    Drugs
        Vasoactive (see below)
        Succinylcholine
8. Transport ventilator

Resuscitation Drugs

Drugs needed for resuscitation that should accompany the patient during the transport include

1. Atropine
2. Lidocaine
3. Epinephrine

Suggested Readings

Braman SS, Dunn SM, Amico CA, Millman RP. Complications of intrahospital transport in critically ill patients. Ann Intern Med 1987;107:469–473.

Capan LM, Miller SM, Turndorf H, eds. Trauma Anesthesia and Intensive Care. Philadelphia: JB Lippincott, 1991.

Civetta JM, Taylor RW, Kirby RR, eds. Critical Care. Philadelphia: JB Lippincott, 1988.

Gervais HW, Eberle B, Konietzke D, Hennes H, Dick W. Comparison of blood gases of ventilated patients during transport. Crit Care Med 1987;15:761–763.

Insel J, Weissman C, Kemper M, Askanazi J, Hyman Al. Cardiovascular changes during transport of critically ill and postoperative patients. Crit Care Med 1986;14:539–542.

Rosenthal J, Dunham CM. Intrahospital transport. Crit Care Rep 1990;1:380–388.

Shoemaker WC, Ayers S, Grenvik A, Holbrook PR, Thompson WL, eds. Textbook of Critical Care. 2nd ed. Philadelphia: WB Saunders, 1989.

Stene JK, Grande CM, eds. Trauma Anesthesia. Baltimore: Williams & Wilkins, 1991.

Chapter 18

Ambulatory Anesthesia

Even though Ralph Waters introduced the Downtown Anesthesia Clinic in 1919, ambulatory (or outpatient) surgery is a relatively new and rapidly expanding service, being accepted by the medical community only within the past 10 years. It has been estimated that more than 50% of all surgery performed in 1990 was performed on an outpatient basis. This number is certain to grow because of the changing patterns of health care administration as well as financial considerations.

Ambulatory anesthesia is an evolving specialty. The current criteria for selection of patients, choice of appropriate surgical procedures, techniques of anesthesia, and postoperative discharge criteria all differ from those of inpatient surgery and from standards of even 5 years ago.

PATIENT SELECTION AND EVALUATION

When ambulatory surgery began, service was limited to ASA class I and II patients. Now more class III patients are having surgery performed as outpatients. This is partially due to pressure from third-party payers who realize the increased expense of hospitalization.

Appropriate Patients for Outpatient Surgery

1. Healthy patients without systemic diseases
2. Patients with stable chronic diseases, including
   a. Insulin-dependent diabetes mellitus that is well controlled
   b. Chronic stable angina
   c. Chronic stable pulmonary disease

Contraindications for Outpatient Surgery

1. Patients with unstable chronic diseases, including
   a. Insulin-dependent diabetes that is poorly controlled (e.g., glucose > 250) and may require an insulin infusion intraoperatively
   b. Unstable angina pectoris or congestive heart failure
   c. Acute exacerbations of chronic lung disease
2. Patients who are morbidly obese
3. Patients with mediastinal masses
4. Patients taking MAO inhibitors
5. Patients with airway compression
6. Patients with a history of malignant hyperthermia

Any ASA class IV patient must be evaluated very carefully with appropriate consultations from specialists before they can be considered for outpatient surgery.

PROCEDURE SELECTION

Previously, procedures that could be done as outpatient were limited to a few, short peripheral procedures. Now, more extensive surgery is being performed on outpatients.

Acceptable procedures include

1. Gynecologic (tubal ligation, laparoscopies, mini laparotomies)
2. Orthopaedic (arthroscopy, hardware removal)
3. Plastics (facelifts, rhinoplasties, breast augmentations or reconstructions)
4. Urologic (cystoscopies, bladder biopsies)
5. General (excision of skin lesions, biopsies)
6. Ophthalmologic (cataracts, glaucoma procedures, corneal transplants)
7. Bone marrow harvest

Inappropriate procedures for outpatient surgery include procedures that

1. Might induce large fluid shifts and "third spacing" (most intraabdominal procedures)
2. May result in pain not controllable with oral pain medications
3. Require more invasive monitoring than an arterial line

PREOPERATIVE VISIT AND PREMEDICATIONS

The purpose of the preoperative visit is to evaluate the health of the patient and to educate the patient about what to expect on the day of surgery. Since most patients do not receive preoperative sedation, a thorough explanation about the operative experience is important in allaying anxiety.

Methods of preoperative evaluation for outpatient surgery include a visit to the facility and appointment with the anesthesiologist before surgery, a preoperative phone call by a nurse or anesthetist but no visit, a questionnaire to be completed by the patient with or without a meeting with the anesthesiologist, or being seen by the anesthesiologist the morning of surgery. This last method usually has the highest cancellation rate.

After being deemed appropriate for outpatient surgery, patients should be instructed not to eat or drink anything after midnight on the night before surgery. If they are taking medication on a regular basis, they should be told which medications, if any, they should take the night before and on the morning of surgery. Most patients are given a prescription for an H_2-blocker and metoclopramide and are instructed to take both the night before and the morning of surgery with a small sip of water. These agents are used to increase the pH of the gastric contents, to decrease any pulmonary damage from aspiration of gastric contents. Patients should be told that an intravenous catheter will be started before surgery, about any other painful procedures they might have, approximately how long they will be in the preoperative holding area, how long the procedure will take, how long they will be in the postanesthesia care unit, and how their postoperative discomfort will be managed.

During the preoperative visit, patients are informed of the risks of anesthesia, including dental damage and the remote possibility of unplanned admission. They are also told that they need a responsible adult to drive them home and preferably stay with them overnight.

At this time any indicated laboratory tests or other diagnostic procedures, including ECG and chest x-ray, are performed.

PREOPERATIVE HOLDING AREA

The patient is instructed to arrive approximately 2 hours before the scheduled time for surgery. The chart is reviewed, laboratory and other test results are checked, and the patient's NPO status is confirmed. After the patient has changed from street clothes into a hospital gown, an intravenous line is started in the preoperative area. If the patient is extremely nervous, IV anxiolytics can be given. Most commonly, midazolam is used for this purpose in 0.5- to 1-mg increments, up to a total dose of 3 mg. *Before amnesic drugs are administered,* patients should have the opportunity to speak to their surgeon and anesthesiologist, and all consent forms must be completed.

Patients are taken to the OR by wheelchair if they have received any sedatives, otherwise they may walk to the operating room, escorted by an operating room nurse.

INDUCTION AND MAINTENANCE

The anesthetic techniques (general, regional, local) and agents used in outpatient surgery are modifications of those used for inpatients, usually involving the shortest-acting drug within a class. Doses are carefully titrated to effect in outpatients, to allow the lowest possible dose to be given.

General anesthesia in outpatients is frequently induced with intravenously administered barbiturates (3–5 mg/kg) or propofol (2–3 mg/kg). Both produce rapid onset of unconsciousness and redistribute quickly for relatively rapid awakening. Unless patients require rapid sequence induction, the initial dose can be given slowly over 1–2 minutes and titrated to loss of lid reflex. Propofol has the advantage of rapid emergence with minimal "hangover" and is slowly replacing pentothal in many practices. Propofol may produce pain on injection, but this can be minimized by prior administration of IV lidocaine (10–40 mg) and by injecting into a rapidly running IV located in a proximal vein.

Since outpatient procedures are usually of very short duration (less than 45 minutes), many general anesthetics can be performed without endotracheal intubation. This avoids instrumentation of the airway and reduces postoperative sore throat.

Indications for Intubation

1. Full stomach (surgery should be done only in emergencies)
2. Symptomatic reflux or hiatal hernia

3. Difficult mask airway
4. Procedure lasting longer than 1 hour (this is simply for convenience of the anesthetist)
5. Position other than supine or lithotomy, where access to the airway might be difficult
6. Muscle relaxation required during the procedure

Muscle Relaxants

The most commonly used muscle relaxant for intubation in outpatients is succinylcholine, because of its short duration of action and since most outpatient procedures do not require additional muscle relaxants. If relaxation is required, a nondepolarizing agent can be used in doses near the ED_{95} of that drug. A peripheral nerve stimulator should be used to monitor all patients receiving relaxants. Neuromuscular blockade is reversed with an anticholinergic and an anticholinesterase, and sustained tetanus to 50 Hz stimulation should be documented in all patients to ensure adequate strength.

Narcotics

Parenteral narcotics may be used in small doses in outpatients. Fentanyl and alfentanil are the narcotics of choice because of their short durations of action. As adjuvants to general anesthesia, narcotics are administered in intermittent boluses or continuous low-dose infusions. Narcotics may increase the incidence of nausea and vomiting by up to 300%.

Miscellaneous Drugs

Antiemetics are used liberally in outpatients because postoperative nausea and vomiting is one of the most common causes for unplanned hospital admission. The incidence of nausea and vomiting has been reported to be from 15 to 80%, depending on surgical procedure and anesthetic technique. Droperidol 0.5–1.0 mg IV can be given prophylactically during the surgery, especially if narcotics are also being administered.

Long-acting sedatives such as lorazepam, pentobarbital, and secobarbital are avoided in outpatients. The preferred sedatives are midazolam and propofol because of their rapid redistribution and elimination.

EMERGENCE

To provide a more pleasant emergence from general anesthesia and to facilitate rapid turnover of the operating suite, patients are often extubated while still deeply anesthetized. Muscle relaxation should be reversed, sustained tetanus documented, and the patient should be breathing spontaneously with a regular respiratory pattern. To prevent laryngospasm after extubation, it is important to determine that the patient's airway reflexes are not intact. This is done by suctioning the pharynx and esophagus with a flexible catheter while watching the respiratory pattern for signs of coughing or breath holding. If the respiratory pattern remains regular, the N_2O is discontinued, and the patient is allowed to breathe >90% O_2 along with inhalational agent for approximately 60 seconds to wash out N_2O. Then the cuff of the endotracheal tube is deflated slowly, again watching for signs of airway reflexes. If the respiratory pattern remains regular, the endotracheal tube can be quickly removed, and the patient ventilated by mask. An oral airway may be used if necessary. Once adequate ventilation by mask is established, the N_2O may be reinstituted, depending on the time remaining in the procedure.

MONITORED ANESTHESIA CARE

Regional, topical, or local infiltration anesthesia supplemented by intravenous sedation are accepted alternatives to general anesthesia and may reduce recovery time in the postanesthesia care unit. Midazolam titrated in 0.5- to 1.0-mg increments to the endpoint of "sleepy yet arousable," provides calm operating conditions for the surgeon and nearly complete antegrade amnesia for the patient. Small amounts of narcotics (e.g., fentanyl 25–50 μg) potentiate the effect of midazolam without increasing the incidence of nausea.

Examples of common procedures appropriate for monitored anesthesia care

Cataract extraction	Dilatation and curettage
Corneal transplant	Cystoscopy
Glaucoma procedures	Myringotomy (adult)
Superficial biopsies	Diagnostic arthroscopy
Facial plastic surgery	Superficial orthopaedic procedures

Table 18.1
Regional Anesthesia Techniques

Technique	Duration of Action	Advantage/Disadvantage
IV Regional	½–1 ½ hours	Tourniquet pain
Spinal	¼–5 hours	Headache, urinary retention
Epidural	½ hour to indefinite	Long onset, delayed recovery, urinary retention

Major conduction anesthesia
    Brachial plexus
    Femoral-sciatic
    Ankle block
	½ hour to indefinite	Early discharge

REGIONAL ANESTHESIA

Regional anesthesia for outpatients requires careful attention to the selection of both the local anesthetic agent and the anesthetic technique. The block should provide adequate analgesia and its duration should approximate the length of the surgery (Table 18.1) so that return of function and subsequent discharge home will not be delayed. Otherwise, the same principles used in selection of regional anesthesia for inpatients apply.

Discharge criteria for patients who have had regional anesthesia are based upon the patient's ability to function with minimal assistance once discharged. The duration and type of regional anesthesia used will influence recovery time. With spinal and/or epidural anesthesia, it is necessary for the patient to have full motor function without orthostasis upon standing and be able to voluntarily urinate before being discharged.

POSTANESTHESIA CARE UNIT (PACU)

In the PACU, vital signs and recovery from anesthesia are monitored. Supplemental oxygen is administered, based on measured O_2 saturations.

Patients are moved to a recliner chair after they are awake, alert, and oriented; have been hemodynamically stable for 30 minutes; do not require oxygen to maintain oxygen saturations of 94% or greater; and do not have uncontrollable pain. If there is orthostasis when sitting, the chair should be reclined. After approximately 1 hour, patients are evaluated for discharge.

Discharge Criteria for Outpatients

1. Hemodynamic stability without orthostasis for at least 1 hour
2. Awake, alert, oriented, and returned to baseline mental status, although they can be a little drowsy
3. Adequate pain control with oral pain medications
4. Tolerate PO fluids without excessive nausea and vomiting
5. Ability to dress themselves
6. Ability to void
7. Have a responsible adult to take them home and assist them, preferably overnight
8. Understand written postoperative instructions including pain medications, wound appearance, dressing changes, and follow-up appointments.

Postoperative Follow-up

Patients should be called the day after surgery by outpatient personnel to inquire about any postoperative complications. If any anesthetic complications are documented, an anesthesiologist must provide appropriate continuing care until the anesthetic-related problem is resolved.

Suggested Readings

Apfelbaum J. Anesthetic management in the ambulatory surgery setting. Anesthesiol Rev 1990:17[suppl 2].

Wetchler B, ed. Anesthesia for Ambulatory Surgery. 2nd ed. Philadelphia: JB Lippencott, 1991.

White PF, ed. Outpatient Anesthesia. New York: Churchill Livingstone, 1990.

Chapter 19

Pediatric Anesthesia

Pediatric anesthesia offers many unique challenges because of the substantial differences between children and adults with respect to anatomy, physiology, and psychology, and the different surgical procedures done in pediatrics. Despite the differences, the principles of vigilance, safety, care, and attention to detail, which are the essentials of good practice of adult anesthesia, should also be applied to pediatric anesthesia.

Treat children with respect, remembering their developmental level. Prepare fully for each case, remembering the size of the child when choosing equipment and the special physiology of the child when choosing fluids and medications.

GROWTH AND DEVELOPMENT (Table 19.1)

Premature Infant

Premature infants are a heterogeneous group, ranging from 500 to 2500 grams in weight and from 26 to 36 weeks of gestation. Since conditions that predispose to premature birth often impair fetal growth, the relationship between age and weight is important. An infant may be large, appropriate, or small for its gestational age (LGA, AGA, SGA). The premature infant who is also SGA is in many ways more unprepared for surgery and anesthesia than an AGA infant. During the last trimester, many important maturational events occur that prepare the fetus for extrauterine life, and premature infants, to a greater or lesser degree, have not experienced them.

Respiratory Distress Syndrome

Respiratory distress syndrome (RDS) or hyaline membrane disease occurs mainly in premature infants and is due to inadequate and immature surfactant, which leads to progressive atel-

Table 19.1
Normal Values[a]

Age	Weight (kg)	BSA (M²)	HR, RR, BP	Blood Volume (ml/kg)	Hgb (g/100 ml)
Newborn	3.4	0.22	120, 40–60, 65/45	90–100	16.8 (14–20)
1 month	4.2	0.25	160, 30–40, 90/50	90–100	16.5 (13–20)
6 months	7.6	0.39	140, 25–35, 90/50	70–80	12.0 (10–14)
12 months	9.7	0.46	125, 30, 95/60	70	11.5 (9.8–13)
24 months	12.3	0.55	100, 25, 95/60	70	11.5 (9.8–13)
3 years	14.4	0.62	100, 25, 95/60	70	11.5 (9.8–13)
8 years	25	0.95	80, 22, 100/68	70	11.5 (9.8–13)
12 years	40	1.25	75, 22, 115/75	70	11.5 (9.8–13)

[a] Abbreviations: BSA, body surface area; HR, heart rate; RR, respiratory rate; BP, blood pressure; ( ) normal range for Hgb.

ectasis. When breathing spontaneously, infants with RDS have tachypnea, retractions, and an expiratory grunt. Hypoxemia due to a decrease in functional residual capacity (FRC) is present. Many infants with RDS are treated with continuous positive airway pressure (CPAP) or mechanical ventilation to support gas exchange. When infants with RDS come to the operating room, it is preferable to ventilate manually while listening to breath sounds with a precordial or esophageal stethoscope, or alternatively, to bring to the operating room the same ventilator used to ventilate the child in the intensive care nursery. This practice minimizes ventilatory changes that may result in drastic reductions in PaO_2 or increases in $PaCO_2$. Although most premature infants with RDS recover within 1 month, the illness may be quite severe and/or prolonged in a given patient.

Patent Ductus Arteriosus (PDA)

In fetal life, the ductus arteriosus carries most of the right ventricular output to the descending aorta, and it normally is functionally closed shortly after birth. The ductus arteriosus reopens or remains open in response to hypoxemia that accompanies RDS, with resulting left-to-right shunting of blood. As RDS resolves and pulmonary vascular resistance falls, the PDA allows an increased left-to-right shunt, leading to congestive heart failure.

There are several important implications for the anesthesiologist caring for a child with a PDA. Particular care must be taken with regard to bubbles in the intravenous fluids, since any air that enters through a peripheral IV can enter the arterial circulation. Also, since the ductus arteriosus may not functionally close in premature infants until several weeks, if not months, after birth, excessive fluid administration may precipitate congestive heart failure.

Retinopathy of Prematurity (ROP)

ROP primarily affects infants weighing less than 1700 grams at birth, and it has been reported in children with a postconceptual age of up to 44 weeks (postconceptual age = gestational age at birth + postnatal age). The incidence of ROP varies inversely with birth weight, so that prematurity is by far the most important etiologic factor. Environmental factors have been implicated as well, such as PaO_2, $PaCO_2$, pH, and anemia. Since high PaO_2 may play a role in the development of ROP, the oxygen saturation measured by a pulse oximeter should be kept between 93 and 96% for at-risk infants. The development of ROP should not come at the cost of systemic hypoxemia. Therefore, an FIO_2 of 1.0 should be used before tracheal intubation, as well as before and immediately after extubation. In those procedures where impaired O_2 delivery is likely (thoracotomy, tracheostomy, bronchoscopy), a higher FIO_2 is indicated.

Hypoglycemia

Premature infants are born without the usual glycogen stores of full-term infants (SGA infants have even less liver glycogen) and easily develop hypoglycemia if kept NPO too long or if given IV fluids without adequate glucose. Premature infants often require D10 via peripheral IV to maintain normal glucose when fasted prior to surgery. Typically, the infant arrives in the operating room with an infusion of glucose already running. It should be adjusted only after the glucose has been checked.

Neonate

An average newborn weighs 3.4 kg and has quite different body proportions than the adult, e.g., the head is relatively larger and the mandible smaller. At rest, newborns assume the position of partial flexion with somewhat increased muscle tone throughout. They may fixate on a light, but show a visual preference for the human face.

Temperature Maintenance

Newborns are particularly vulnerable to heat loss for a variety of reasons. They have little subcutaneous fat, a high surface area to volume ratio, and poor vasomotor control. Heat production, which occurs in the brown fat (nonshivering thermogenesis) when a newborn is exposed to cold, results in linear increase in oxygen consumption.

Steps that minimize the risk of hypothermia in newborns in the surgical suite include (a) warming the operating room (80°F), (b) the use of a warming mattress, (c) radiant heat lamps (kept at a safe distance to avoid skin burns), (d) wrapping the head and extremities with plastic wrap and/or cotton, and (e) heating and humidifying the inspired gases (breathing circuit temperature should be monitored near the patient when heating the inspired gases).

Transitional Circulation

A healthy full-term newborn has successfully made a transition from intrauterine life, in which the placenta is the organ of gas exchange and the lungs are filled with amniotic fluid, to extrauterine life, in which the lungs receive the entire output from the right ventricle and are responsible for gas exchange. This change, although necessarily sudden at birth, is neither functionally nor anatomically permanent until at least 7 days after birth. The pulmonary vasculature is very reactive to many stimuli, and pulmonary vascular resistance (PVR) may increase dramatically in response to hypoxemia, acidemia, hypercarbia, hypoglycemia, anemia, polycythemia, sepsis, and hypothermia.

Even in a healthy newborn, PVR is higher than in adults and children and only gradually decreases during the first few months of life. It may not reach adult levels for several years.

The transitional nature of the circulation in neonates is important to the anesthesiologist. If, during a surgical procedure a baby develops hypoxemia, hypercarbia, or acidemia and PVR increases, a decrease in pulmonary blood flow will result, gas exchange will be impaired, and a downward spiral may occur, resulting in a situation similar to that seen during fetal life. The foramen ovale opens, as will the PDA, and pulmonary blood flow will markedly decrease, except now there is no placenta. This condition, called either persistent fetal circulation (PFC) or persistent pulmonary hypertension of the newborn (PPHN), is very difficult to treat and often requires systemic catecholamine infusions and/or pulmonary vasodilators along with vigorous efforts to correct the underlying causes (i.e., hypoxemia, hypercarbia, acidemia). It is far better to prevent this condition with careful monitoring of arterial blood gases, pH, and body temperature and meticulous administrations of anesthetics to blunt the increased sympathetic response associated with surgery.

Infants

At 7 months, infants weigh approximately 8 kg, may have erupted lower incisors, and may be able to sit alone, leaning forward on the hands for support. They will transfer a rattle from hand to hand. At this age, infants are initially shy with strangers and may cling to caregivers in the presence of strangers. However, when left alone in the company of strangers, they usually warm to a soft voice and a friendly face.

Access/Airway

Infants are often quite chubby at this age, so placement of an intravenous catheter before the induction of anesthesia is very difficult. Additionally, the airway is often difficult to manage because of redundant tissue, large tongue, and often copious secretions. For this reason, performance of a "routine" inhalation induction in infants is a potentially dangerous situation, with the possibility of losing the airway part way through the induction without having obtained IV access.

ANESTHESIOLOGY

Stranger Anxiety

At this age, children will often cling tearfully to parents when a stranger approaches. Allow the child to remain with the parents while you are speaking with them. During the preoperative visit, the interviewer should occasionally speak to the child, using a friendly tone of voice and a big smile. Don't expect to make a friend while the parents are present, but if you have made a good impression, the child may come to you in the OR or the preoperative holding area, when yours is the only familiar friendly face.

Toddlers

At 3 1/2 years, children weigh approximately 15 kg and are just over 3 feet tall. They can dress themselves with supervision and can copy a circle or a cross. They can speak in simple sentences, know their full names, and can name colors, but have a limited understanding of temporal relationships. They may separate from their parents.

Cooperation

Children in this age range present quite a challenge to the anesthesiologist. They are old enough to experience fear and anxiety about surgery (an unknown), but not sophisticated enough to have their fears allayed with reason and explanation. Occasionally, if they are uncooperative, children of this age are strong enough to hurt themselves, either by wriggling off a stretcher or an OR table or by struggling enough during an inhalation induction to lose the airway. When a toddler arrives in the OR neither anxious nor fearful, but interested in the monitors and lights, the induction may be begun expeditiously if an inhalation induction is planned. The precordial stethoscope can be placed, the only necessary monitor with which to begin. As the child loses consciousness, the other monitors can be placed quickly by the OR team. The time necessary to place all the monitors before beginning an inhalation induction is not well spent if, during that period, the child becomes anxious, fearful, and combative.

School-Age Children (6–12 Years Old)

An 8 year old weighs approximately 25 kg and is 4–4 1/2 feet tall. Permanent teeth have begun to erupt, accompanied by the shedding of deciduous teeth. This will continue for 4–5 more years. Upper respiratory infections are frequent, and lymphoid tissue is prominent, especially in the pharynx and neck in children of this age. School-age children are increasingly independent, and although they can understand some abstract concepts, some of their thinking is still concrete.

Communication

Children of school age easily fool adults into treating them and speaking to them as though they were adults when this is hardly the case. Words should be chosen carefully when explaining what the experience of anesthesia, surgery, and recovery will be like. "Going to sleep" could bring to mind a family pet who was "put to sleep" or the thought that normal sleep will occur in the OR and that the child is expected not to awaken during the surgical procedure. Speak as little as possible to parents, instead make the anesthetic plan with the patient, allowing some choices with regard to premedication and method of induction, etc. Be sure to state clearly when the child will be reunited with the parents.

Adolescents

A 13-year-old young woman weighs 46 kg and is approximately 5 feet tall. Menarche probably has occurred, and her sexual maturation is nearing completion. A 13-year-old young man weighs 45 kg and is also nearly 5 feet tall. His sexual development is probably not as complete as that of a 13-year-old female, but his secondary sex characteristics have begun to appear. Adolescents can understand concepts related to anesthesia and surgery, even though their thinking has not reached adult level with regard to abstractions, but adolescents are also sophisticated enough to hide anxiety and fear behind bravado, silence, or humor. The tasks of adolescents—emotional separation from the family, development of a sexual identity, career choice, and achievement of a personal identity—are formidable and therefore occupy much of their energy.

Communication

Adolescence may be the period in life of best physical health, however the emotional and intellectual unrest that accompanies this developmental stage may present problems for the anesthesiologist. When interviewing adolescents, assume they are anxious and fearful. Specifically, the common fears that adolescents have regarding anesthesia and surgery are lack of control and/or dignity and fear of mutilation. During part of the interview, speak to them away from their parents, as a gesture of your respect for them as individuals. It is especially important to do this when interviewing young women, since truthful answers to questions about the possibility of pregnancy are very important before undertaking an elective anesthetic and operation.

SPECIAL CONSIDERATIONS

Airway

The airway of infants and children differs from that of adults in several important ways.

1. The **larynx** is higher in the neck, located at the level of C3 in premature infants and C3-4 in full-term infants.
2. In infants, the **tongue** is relatively larger and the mandible relatively smaller than that of the adult.
3. The **epiglottis** in infants is short and narrow in contrast to the epiglottis in adults.
4. The **epiglottis** in children is at a more acute angle to the glottis, which makes visualization of the glottis more difficult.
5. The **larynx** is cone-shaped in children until approximately 8 years of age. Hence, the subglottic area is the narrowest part of the airway in these children (Fig. 19.1).

In addition, the mucosa overlying the subglottic area is loosely applied, so that any edema in this area easily narrows the lumen in the subglottic area. Since the tracheal lumen is small in infants and children and resistance to gas flow varies with radius to the fourth power and cross-section of area varies with radius squared, what would be a small amount of edema

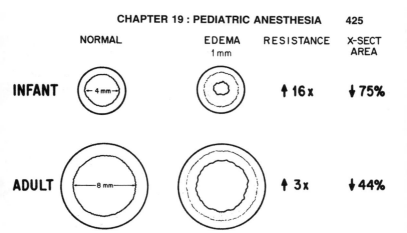

Figure 19.1.   Comparison of adult and child laryngeal anatomy.

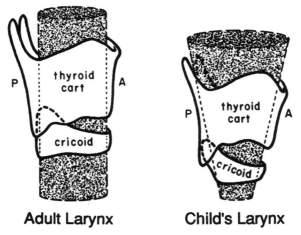

Adult Larynx   **Child's Larynx**

Figure 19.2.

(1–2 mm) in an adult trachea (10 mm) has considerably more impact on the neonate's airway (4 mm) and the dynamics of gas flow through that airway (Fig. 19.2).

Intubation of the Trachea

In preparation for intubation of the trachea, all needed equipment should be tested and at hand. The low oxygen reserves of newborns and children allow little time for intubation without having to stop and obtain equipment. The choice of laryngoscope blades depends upon personal preference. Anatomic considerations (i.e., the short neck and bulky tongue in infants) make use of straight blades generally more desirable in newborns and small children. Most premature and SGA infants require a Miller #0 or Goodell #1 blade; the Miller #1 is more suitable for term infants. At the age of 2 years, curved blades become an equally acceptable choice. In all cases, more than one size blade should be on hand should the primary choice be unsuitable.

Choice of appropriate endotracheal tube size and type should be based on the patient's age and size (Table 19.2). Other considerations, such as previous recent intubation, history of prolonged intubation, or previous surgery, may modify the selection of the expected endotracheal tube size. If a cuffed endotracheal tube is chosen, be aware that a deflated cuff adds one-half size to the external diameter of an endotracheal tube. For example, a 4.5-mm cuffed endotracheal tube with the cuff deflated has the same outside diameter as a 5.0-mm endotracheal tube.

Time plays a critical role in the safety of intubation in the infant and small child. These patients are at a disadvantage by having substantially increased oxygen demands over the adults and therefore proportionately lower oxygen stores in the functional residual capacity. The elapsed time between loss of oxygen supply or alveolar ventilation and the onset of hypoxemia is very short in children. When other pathology exists, such as congestive heart failure, pneumonia, or respiratory distress syndrome of the newborn, borderline hypoxemia already exists

Table 19.2
Endotracheal Tube Size

Age	Internal Diameter (mm)
Premature	2.5–3.0
Term newborn	3.0–3.5
1–6 months	3.0–4.0
12–24 months	4.0–5.0
>2 years	[16 + age (years)]/4

and can be dangerously exaggerated during intubation. Intubation techniques should include the following points.

1. *Stabilize the head.* The prominent occiput and relatively large head size of an infant causes it to be unstable and to roll easily on the table. The use of a foam rubber doughnut or similar device helps stabilize the head and place it in the sniffing position.

2. *Identify both esophagus and trachea during laryngoscopy.* The newborn and small child's vocal apparatus does not resemble that of an adult. Care is required to avoid inadvertent esophageal intubations.

3. *Visually assess endotracheal tube passage beyond the cords.* The short distance (4–6 cm in infants) between the vocal cords and the carina makes unintended passage into the right or left main stem bronchus relatively easy. This can be prevented by careful observation of the endotracheal tube as it is inserted. Auscultation after intubation is required to determine whether breath sounds are equal bilaterally. In children under 2 years of age, after equal breath sounds are heard, the right main stem bronchus may be deliberately intubated to determine the distance to the carina. While listening over the left chest, the endotracheal tube is gradually advanced until breath sounds diminish. The endotracheal tube is then carefully withdrawn, and when breath sounds heard on the left equal those on the right, the centimeter mark at the child's alveolar ridge or teeth is noted. This number corresponds to endotracheal tube position at the carina. The tube can then be withdrawn 2 additional centimeters and securely taped. This allows the greatest likelihood of midtracheal placement of the endotracheal tube without having x-ray confirmation of positioning.

4. *Avoid excessive manipulation of airway structures.* Multiple attempts at intubation result in tissue edema and bleeding, both of which may complicate extubation. Of all possible causes of postextubation croup, multiple attempts at intubation is perhaps one of the most important. The mucosa of the infant's larynx is very loosely applied to the cartilage of the subglottic area, and even a small amount of edema may significantly decrease the lumen size and adversely affect gas flow.

5. *Do not prolong attempts at intubation.* Infants and small children do not have the oxygen reserves of older children and adults. Although the use of the pulse oximeter is very helpful during intubation, remember that bradycardia may be an early sign of hypoxemia. *(If bradycardia occurs during laryngoscopy and attempted intubation, the treatment is not IV atropine, but ventilation with oxygen.)*

Fluids

Fluid administration in pediatrics requires more attention to detail than in adults. Three aspects of IV fluid therapy must be considered during anesthesia and surgery in children: mainte-

Table 19.3
Maintenance Water Requirements

Weight (kg)	ml/kg/day	ml/kg/hr
0–10	100	4
10–20	50	2
>20	20	1

Example: A 23-kg child has been NPO for 3 hours prior to surgery.

Maintenance Calculation:
0–10 kg   10 kg × 4 ml/kg/hr = 40 ml/hr
10–20 kg   10 kg × 2 ml/kg/hr = 20 ml/hr
>20 kg   3 kg × 1 ml/kg/hr = 3 ml/hr

Maintenance water, sodium, and glucose needs can be met with D_5 0.2% NS

Deficit Calculation: 3 hr × 63 ml/hr = 189 ml
The deficit should be replaced with isotonic fluid such as lactated Ringer's. One-half of the deficit is replaced during the first hour with one-fourth replaced in each of the next 2 hours.

Hour	Maintenance (ml)	Deficit Replaced (ml)
1	63	95
2	63	47
3	63	47
4	63	0

Replacement of surgical bleeding or evaporative losses is in addition to the above calculation.

Allowable Blood Loss

[Blood volume ×(patient's Hct − 30)]/patient's Hct

or

10–15% of estimated blood volume

Figure 19.3.   Calculation of maximum allowable blood loss to keep the Hct above 30%

nance, deficit replacement, and replacement of ongoing losses (evaporative and blood loss).

Maintenance fluid requirements are based on metabolic rate; therefore it is not surprising that maintenance requirements are higher on a ml/kg basis for children of lower mass (high surface area to volume ratio). The daily water requirement is 1 ml/cal/day. Using D_5 0.2% normal saline at the rate determined for maintenance will fulfill the requirements for glucose and sodium for infants and children. **Deficit replacement is done with solutions that do not contain glucose and which are isotonic, such as lactated Ringer's, not hypotonic as are maintenance fluids** (Table 19.3).

Ongoing losses are very variable and depend upon the procedure; evaporative loss can range from 10 ml/kg/hr when much bowel is exposed during a laparotomy to only 1–2 ml/kg/hr for minor urologic procedures. This loss should also be replaced with isotonic fluid.

Blood loss must be carefully monitored, especially in smaller children and infants, since the blood volume is so small. The maximum allowable blood loss should be calculated prior to the start of each case (Fig. 19.3).

When administering intravenous fluids to infants and children, a volume-limiting device should be used in the intravenous tubing. The amount of fluid to be administered over the subsequent 1 hour should be put into the soluset each hour. With this technique, inattention to the IV fluid will not lead to excessive administration to a very small child.

Monitoring

Routine monitoring for pediatric anesthesia includes

1. *Stethoscope*

     A precordial stethoscope is used for all inhalation inductions as well as IV inductions. It is the single most important monitor in pediatric anesthesia. Lightweight, low profile models are available for use with infants. An esophageal stethoscope may be placed after intubation if necessary.

2. *Electrocardiogram*

Used for rate and rhythm primarily, but not usually for the detection of ischemia as in adults. Since nodal rhythms are common with inhalation inductions, the leads should be placed so that the P wave is easily seen.

3. *Blood pressure cuff*

When monitoring blood pressure in children, proper cuff size is critical, as is awareness of the normal ranges for various ages.

4. *Oxygen monitor*

As in adult anesthesia, the FIO_2 must be monitored. In addition, pulse oximetry is a standard of care and is especially useful in the care of neonates when a high PaO_2 may lead to retinopathy of prematurity. The oximeter is also especially useful during induction of and emergence from anesthesia, when the risk of airway problems and resulting hypoxemia is greatest.

5. *Temperature*

Monitoring temperature is especially important in pediatric anesthesia since infants (children to a lesser degree) lose heat quite rapidly. Axillary temperature monitors have the advantage of being noninvasive; however, they are very easily moved and only monitor trends in temperature change. The rectum is a common site for temperature monitoring, especially in neonates and infants; however, the delicate rectal mucosa may be easily damaged if a probe is improperly placed or lubrication is not used prior to placement. A rectal probe may be inadvertently dislodged during surgery, when it is invisible to the anesthesiologist, and the temperature monitor lost. Midesophageal, nasopharyngeal, or tympanic temperature more closely reflects core body temperature, and probes are available for monitoring temperature in these locations. Liquid crystal temperature strips are available for skin placement in children, and these are often placed on the forehead for easy visibility.

6. *Exhaled carbon dioxide monitor*

Monitoring exhaled carbon dioxide concentration is very useful in pediatric anesthesia. Although the carbon dioxide concentration at end exhalation is most useful as a reflection of arterial carbon dioxide, the presence of carbon dioxide in exhaled gas after intubation is a reliable sign that the endotracheal tube is in the trachea. Also, a progressive and continuous rise in end-tidal carbon dioxide concentration under previously stable conditions during anesthesia may be the initial sign of the hypermetabolic state in malignant hyperthermia.

7. *Breathing circuit pressure measurement*

It is very useful to monitor inspiratory pressure, especially when ventilating neonates and infants, since measurement of delivered volume of gas is often inaccurate. These pressure gauges may be used to determine the leak around an endotracheal tube as well.

8. *Apnea monitors*

Ex-premature infants are at risk for prolonged apnea after anesthesia. This risk exists even in ex-premature infants who did not exhibit apnea before undergoing anesthesia and surgery. The likelihood of postoperative apnea is inversely related to an infant's postconceptual age but is a problem up to 52 weeks postconceptual age. For this reason, ex-premature infants younger than 52 weeks postconceptual age who have undergone anesthesia and surgery should be monitored for apnea for at least 12 hours after recovery from anesthesia. In almost all cases, this requires admission to the hospital overnight. This recommendation applies whether the child was anesthetized with general anesthesia, regional anesthesia, or a combination of both.

9. *Urinary catheter*

The rate of urine formation is a good indicator of glomerular filtration rate and thus of intravascular volume and cardiac output. This is especially true in children without intrinsic cardiac or renal disease. Some indications for placement of a urinary catheter are prolonged surgical procedure, procedures associated with large blood loss or fluid shifts, and administration of diuretics or radiologic contrast during a procedure. In general, and when diuretics have not been given, urine output in children should be 1/2–1 ml/kg/hr.

Regional Anesthesia and Pain Management

Any regional technique available for use in adults may be used with appropriate modification in children. However, the discussion here will be limited to caudal anesthesia, ilioinguinal and iliohypogastric nerve blocks, and the use of a patient-controlled analgesia device.

Regional anesthesia in children is commonly used as an adjunct to general anesthesia with two goals: to provide postoperative analgesia and to decrease the anesthetic requirement during the procedure.

Caudal anesthesia may be used for several surgical procedures done in children, such as herniorrhaphy, hydrocelectomy, orchiopexy, hypospadias repair, and circumcision, and it can provide excellent postoperative analgesia. Since the caudal block is placed after induction of general anesthesia, this may create several problems that are not commonly seen in adults when blocks are placed in an awake, conscious, communicating patient: accidental intrathecal or intravascular injections are more difficult to diagnose and the effectiveness of the block cannot be assessed until the child is awake. In children and young toddlers with whom communication is a problem, it will be difficult to distinguish suffering due to anxiety separation, etc. from suffering due to surgical pain. It is also difficult to explain any motor block that may be present in the child.

The *ilioinguinal and iliohypogastric* nerves may be blocked after induction of general anesthesia to provide analgesia during and after inguinal hernia repair. A B-beveled needle and 0.25% bupivicaine with or without epinephrine may be used. The most important landmark is the anterior-superior iliac spine. The needle pierces the skin approximately one patient-fingerbreadth medial and cephalad to this landmark. Two distinct pops are felt as the needle traverses both the external and internal oblique muscles. A dose of 0.5 ml/kg is used for each side (a total of 2.5 mg/kg of bupivicaine). Approximately two-thirds of the volume to be given is injected slowly as the needle is partly withdrawn. Without emerging from the skin, and with the needle beneath the skin, it is redirected toward the umbilicus, up to the hub, and the remainder of the local anesthetic is injected subcutaneously while slowly withdrawing the needle.

Patient-controlled analgesia (PCA) enjoys widespread use in adults for postoperative pain management and may be quite advantageous for older children. At our institution, children as young as 5 or 6 years of age have used PCA pumps effectively, as have older children and adolescents. Some teaching is necessary, preferably preoperatively, but this may be accomplished in the recovery room. Parental approval should be obtained for preadolescents. It is prudent to have standard orders prohibiting administration of sedatives and narcotics to children who have PCA pumps, as well as orders instructing the nursing staff who or when to call for problems or questions. A member of the anesthesia pain service should make daily visits to children who are using PCA pumps, to note the amount of narcotic administered, to assess the degree of analgesia, and to deal with problems or complications. Morphine is the drug most commonly used in PCA pumps, and the usual postoperative settings are as follows: loading dose, often given intraoperatively, is 0.1–0.15 mg/kg of morphine; the PCA dose is from 0.01 to 0.02 mg/kg of morphine; the lockout interval varies between 6 and 10 minutes, and the 4-hour limit is 0.25 mg/kg.

Pharmacology (Table 19.4)

Inhalational Agents

Inhalational agents are taken up more rapidly in children than in adults, so myocardial depression and hypotension are significant concerns during inhalational inductions in children. The minimum alveolar concentration (MAC) varies considerably with age. Neonates have a low MAC (premature infants even lower), while infants and teenagers have a relatively higher MAC. In pediatric anesthesia, isoflurane offers little advantage over halothane for maintenance of anesthesia, since both appear to decrease both heart rate and blood pressure in infants. For induction of anesthesia using an inhalational technique, when compared with halothane, isoflurane has the disadvantage of being irritating to the airway and therefore associated with a higher incidence of laryngospasm.

Nitrous oxide has the same advantages and disadvantages in adult anesthesia as in pediatric anesthesia. Low solubility is its major advantage; a rapid emergence results after discontinuing the drug. Its primary disadvantage is its rapid entry into closed spaces, which may produce an increase in size or pres-

Table 19.4
Medications

Medication	Dose	Comments
Inhalational Agents		
Halothane		Myocardial depression; bradycardia; vasodilation
Isoflurane		Myocardial depression; airway irritant, if used for inhalation induction
Nitrous Oxide		Good analgesic; weak anesthetic; causes expansion of gas-containing closed space
Barbiturates		
Thiopental	3–6 mg/kg IV	Vasodilation; myocardial depression
Pentobarbital	2–3 mg/kg p.o.	Premedication; syrup has unpleasant taste, capsules available
Methohexital	25 mg/kg PR	Premedication/induction agent for children 6 months to 6 years; may cause airway obstruction
Propofol	2–3 mg/kg IV	Induction dose
	6–10 mg/kg/hr	Maintenance dose
Analgesics		
Morphine[a]	0.1–0.15 mg/kg IV	0.05 mg/kg IV for children 6-12 months
Fentanyl[a]	1–3 μg/kg IV	May cause bradycardia
Acetaminophen	10–15 mg/kg p.o. 15–20 mg/kg PR	Dosing interval is q4h
Ketorolac	0.9–1.0 mg/kg IV, IM	Little experience with long-term use in children
Sedatives		
Midazolam	0.08–0.15 mg/kg IV 0.3–0.7 mg/kg p.o.	Acts synergistically as a respiratory depressant with narcotics
Diazepam	0.1–0.2 mg/kg IV	May cause pain when injected
Diphenhydramine	1 mg/kg p.o.	Antihistamine; mild sedative
Muscle Relaxants		
Pancuronium	0.09–0.1 mg/kg IV[b]	Vagolytic effect
Curare	0.3 mg/kg IV[b]	Histamine release may cause hypotension, bronchoconstriction
Atracurium	0.4–0.6 mg/kg IV[b]	Mild histamine release

Vecruronium	0.09–0.1 mg/kg IV[b]	Negliglible cardiovascular effects
Succinylcholine	1–2 mg/kg IV[b] 4 mg/kg IM	Depolarizing relaxant; dysrhythmias common; potassium release; malignant hyperthermia trigger
Reversal agents		
Neostigmine	0.06–0.07 mg/kg IV	
Edrophonium	1 mg/kg IV	
Naloxone	0.5–1.0 μg/kg IV, IM	Two formulations; neonate (0.02 mg/ml) or 0.4 mg/ml
Anticholinergics		
Atropine	0.01–0.02 mg/kg IV 0.02 mg/kg IM 0.04 mg/kg p.o.	May cause CNS side effects
Glycopyrrolate	0.005–0.01 mg/kg IV 0.01 mg/kg IM 0.02 mg/kg p.o.	Does not cross the blood-brain barrier
Resuscitation medications		
Oxygen		
Atropine	0.02 mg/kg IV, ET[c]	
Epinephrine	10 μg/kg IV, ET	
Calcium chloride 10%	5 mg/kg (0.05 ml/kg) IV	
Calcium gluconate 10%	15 mg/kg (0.15 ml/kg) IV	
Sodium bicarbonate	1–2 mEq/kg IV	
Lidocaine 2%	1 mg/kg IV, ET	
Glucose 25%	500 mg/kg IV	
Defibrillation	2–4 watt-sec/kg	
Cardioversion	0.2–1 watt-sec/kg	
Infusions		
Epinephrine Isoproterenol	0.1–1 μg/kg/min	Mix 0.6 mg in 100 ml D$_5$W; begin the infusion at the wt (kg) per hour for 0.1 μg/kg/min
Dopamine	3–20 μg/kg/min	Mix 30 mg in 100 ml D$_5$W; begin the infusion at the wt (kg) for 5 μg/kg/min
Lidocaine	20–50 μg/kg/min	Mix 120 mg in 100 ml D$_5$W; begin the infusion at wt (kg) per hour for 20 μg/kg/min

[a] All narcotics are respiratory depressants, exhibiting the same degree of respiratory depression in equianalgesic doses.
[b] Intubating dose.
[c] ET, via endotracheal tube.

sure in gas-containing closed spaces within the body. In pediatric anesthesia, these spaces include the middle ear (since the eustachian tube may be blocked), congenital lobar emphysema, and bowel obstruction. In certain cases, nitrous oxide should be avoided.

Narcotics

Narcotic analgesics are frequently useful in pediatric anesthesia, and their effects and side effects are similar to those seen in adults. Morphine may cause histamine release; fentanyl may lower the heart rate and may cause chest wall rigidity when given rapidly; and meperidine is more likely to cause abnormal behavior or dysphoria. The doses listed in Table 19.4 are those usually used for children above 1 year of age in our institution. For children between 6 and 12 months, a smaller dose should be used in selected, closely monitored patients. Narcotics should not be given to neonates and children under 6 months of age unless close monitoring is available to quickly detect and treat apnea or bradypnea.

Barbiturates

Methohexital may be used in pediatric anesthesia as a rectal premedication/induction agent for children 1–5 years of age. Some 80–90% of patients given a rectal dose of 25 mg/kg of a 10% solution become unconscious within 10 minutes of administration. Induction is enhanced if after administration of the drug, the child is returned to the arms of a parent and swaddled in a blanket in a darkened room. The anesthetist must not leave the patient once the methohexital has been given, since a small percentage of children may develop airway obstruction. For this reason, airway equipment, oxygen, suction, and emergency medications must be immediately available when this technique is used. Parents should be forewarned that the children lose head control once unconscious. In children given rectal methohexital in this dose, we have measured oxygen saturation (using pulse oximetry) while they are breathing room air and found no saturation below 94%, while end-tidal CO_2 was not significantly elevated.

The dose of thiopental necessary for induction of anesthesia in healthy, unpremedicated children is 5–6 mg/kg IV. Hypovolemic, debilitated patients as well as neonates should be given lower doses. Thiopental should not be used in premature infants.

Ketamine

Ketamine, a derivative of phencyclidine, is a dissociative anesthetic as well as a potent analgesic that may be given IV (1–2 mg/kg/dose) or IM (5–8 mg/kg/dose). Induction using IM ketamine is useful in very uncooperative pediatric patients. In children, ketamine may cause myocardial depression masked by sympathetic stimulation, increased secretions, increased airway irritability, and increased intracranial pressure. When ketamine is used as an IM induction agent, atropine may be mixed in the same syringe to minimize secretions.

Sedatives

Midazolam has gained popularity in pediatric anesthesia (and in pediatric emergency rooms) as an oral sedative. It has also been given via the rectal or intranasal routes as a premedication. When used as an oral premedication, its bitter taste may be masked with a fruit flavoring. The recommended dose for oral premedication is 0.3–0.7 mg/kg, with the higher per kilogram dose used in younger children. Children given this dose often arrive in the operating room or preoperative holding area rather alert but pleasant and cooperative. Diazepam is also an effective sedative premedicant in children and has been used orally and rectally.

Muscle Relaxants

It is a rare anesthetic that is done without muscle relaxants in pediatrics. Nevertheless, care must be exercised if they are used in children, since there are some important unique considerations. Neuromuscular transmission is immature at birth, and it is not until approximately 2 months of age that a normal response to train-of-four or tetanic stimulation can be expected in children. Clinical measures of neuromuscular function that require understanding and cooperation, such as head lift, are less reliable with children. Infants, however, often lift their hips when crying and upset, and this is useful in assessing the adequacy of reversal of neuromuscular blockade. Maximal inspiratory force may be measured, since this also does not require patient cooperation.

TECHNIQUE OF ANESTHESIA

Preanesthetic Evaluation

During the preanesthetic visit, the anesthesiologist should determine the child's general medical health and ASA classification of physical status, establish rapport with the child and parent(s), and gather other data necessary to plan the anesthetic.

For newborns, infants, and young children, **history** begins with *perinatal events* and includes *birth, birth weight, gestational age,* and *any unusual events that occurred immediately after birth,* such as a prolonged stay in the hospital for respiratory distress. Other important historical information includes *allergies, preexisting medical conditions* (asthma, tonsillitis, upper respiratory infection) and a list of any *medications* the patient is taking and why. It is always helpful, if the child has had *general anesthesia in the past,* to learn whether any unpleasant or untoward events occurred, as well as any *family history of unusual reactions to anesthesia.*

The **physical examination** of the child begins with *weight* and *vital signs,* noting the appropriate normal values for age when looking at the vital signs (Table 19.1). As with adults, *airway evaluation* is of paramount importance. In addition to the standard airway evaluation used for adults, *missing or loose teeth* should be noted. When examining the cardiovascular and respiratory systems, the normal values for age for heart rate and respiratory rate should be kept in mind (Table 19.1). Innocent *murmurs* are not infrequent during infancy and childhood, and the examiner should be familiar with the more common ones to avoid alarming a family about a normal finding. The extremities should be examined in children to note *potential sites for venous access.* During the examination, the anesthesiologist should be assessing the *child's level of anxiety,* as well as the likelihood of a successful or unsuccessful separation from the parent(s). This information is important in determining what premedication should be given, if any.

In healthy young children, few **laboratory data** are necessary. However, at our institution, a *hemoglobin* and *hematocrit* are

Table 19.5
NPO Times (hours)

Age	Clear Liquids	Solids or Milk
<6 months	2	4
6 months–3 years	2	6
>3 years	2	6

obtained on all children. Other laboratory tests may be necessary in specific instances, including *chest x-ray, arterial blood gases, electrolytes,* and *pulmonary function testing.* The necessity for these tests should be determined by the anesthesiologist in conjunction with the surgeon. NPO times are listed in Table 19.5.

It is important to establish good rapport with the family during the preanesthetic visit. When dealing with a developing young child, it is helpful to know the common fears usual at various ages regarding anesthesia and surgery and to address these without being asked by the child or family, who may be too anxious or embarrassed to ask about them. **Children between 6 months and 6 years** often have a great *fear of separation from the family.* At this age, children are not particularly concerned with the specifics of anesthesia and/or surgery but simply with the unfamiliar environment and the presence of strangers. When interviewing children between **1 and 6 years,** it is important to reassure them that they *will* be reunited with their family very soon after operation. **Children between 6 and 12 years** often are *afraid of mutilation occurring during surgery and/or of awakening during the operation itself.* Reassurance that this will not happen is often very consoling to these children. **Adolescents and preadolescents** fear *loss of control, loss of dignity,* or *death.* Patients in this age group are especially likely to keep these fears to themselves, even after direct questioning, so it is important for the anesthesiologist to mention them and to allay them with explanation and reassurance.

The anesthetic plan for any child should include fluid administration (outlined in the section on fluids) and calculation of the allowable blood loss. Equipment must be of the correct size for the child, including the pressure cuff, endotracheal tubes, laryngoscope blades and handles, pulse oximetry monitor, and temperature monitors.

Premedication

Premedication is useful in children to block vagal reflexes, to minimize oral secretions, to sedate and calm, and possibly to reduce intraoperative anesthetic and postoperative analgesic requirements. **Neonates** should receive *only atropine* as a premedication. The dose is 0.02 mg/kg p.o. or 0.01 mg/kg IV. **Infants** also should be given *atropine* and sometimes a *small amount of sedative or narcotic,* preferably given by the *oral route.* The emotional upset caused by an IM injection often more than offsets any possible sedative or anxiolytic effect produced by the medication in infants and young children. Premedication for **older children and adolescents** should be done in conjunction with the child's wishes. Often children in this age group prefer to remain awake and lucid during the separation from parents and the trip to the operating room. Therefore, within the bounds of safety and reason, the choice is left to the child. There are several useful alternatives if an oral premedication for children is chosen. Pentobarbital and secobarbital are two short-acting barbiturates that are frequently used and can be given orally. At our institution, we use a combination of meperidine, atropine, and diazepam suspended in a flavored syrup as an oral premedication. Midazolam has gained popularity recently as an oral premedication for children as well.

Induction Techniques

Inhalation induction is probably the most common method of induction of general anesthesia for all ages of pediatric patients. There are several important factors to consider, especially for anxious children, to promote a smooth inhalation induction. Induction should begin soon after bringing the child to the operating room, the precordial stethoscope being the only monitor used as the induction begins. All necessary equipment and drugs should be carefully prepared *before* the child enters the operating room. Use a smooth, calming, and monotonous voice to tell a story involving the child's interests. Aromatic oils, applied to the inside of the mask in small amounts, may be used to cover the odor of the anesthetic gases. Allow the child to have some control if possible, e.g., induction may begin in the sitting position with the child holding the mask. Alternatively, a cupped hand can be used for a child who refuses a mask or tries to push the mask away when the induction begins. Assistants may hold or stroke the child's hands but only the anesthesiologist performing the induction speaks to the child, to avoid confusion. Halothane is most often used, since this potent agent is associated with smooth inhalation induction. If there are no contraindications to its use, begin with 30–90 seconds of 70% nitrous oxide and 30% oxygen before gradually adding halothane, increasing the inspired concentration 0.5% every 2–3 breaths. It is important to allow the child to breathe spontaneously and not assist respiratory effort at first, since this may result in greater myocardial depression and hypotension. Once the child is unconscious, assistants should quickly apply the other monitors and start an intravenous line through which other medications, such as muscle relaxants and atropine, can be given.

Intravenous induction technique may be preferred for older children, including adolescents, since they will often accept placement of an IV catheter preoperatively. Rapid induction of anesthesia after IV injection of thiopental through a small needle is a good alternative to a struggling mask induction in a frightened child. Any child with a "full stomach" requires a rapid sequence (IV) induction.

Awake intubation may be used in neonates, especially if a "full stomach" is a consideration. An infant may breath-hold during laryngoscopy as the blade enters the vallecula, or bradycardia may occur abruptly. For these reasons, all routine monitors must be applied before beginning an awake intubation in a neonate.

IM induction with ketamine may be used for uncooperative, especially anxious, children to prevent excessive struggling, kicking, and perhaps harm to themselves.

Maintenance of Anesthesia

It is important to remember the effect of age on minimum alveolar concentration (MAC). Temperature maintenance is an important part of pediatric anesthesia. Measures to prevent heat loss should be a routine part of pediatric cases.

Emergence from Anesthesia

Laryngospasm occurring in stage II of anesthesia is a not uncommon problem in pediatric patients. Prior to extubation, 100% oxygen should always be administered via the endotracheal tube, and clinical signs assessed to be sure of emergence beyond stage II. After extubation, attention should be completely focused on the child's airway and respiratory effort. The use of the precordial stethoscope should be continued during transport to the postanesthesia recovery unit (PACU). In the PACU, supplemental oxygen should be administered and oxygenation monitored with a pulse oximeter. Infants at risk for postanesthetic apnea should be monitored appropriately (as described in the section on neonates). Children who have had airway procedures may benefit from longer periods of observation in the PACU before being discharged to less intensely monitored areas of the hospital. With infants, postoperatively administered narcotics should be used judiciously. Swaddling and a pacifier go a long way to soothing a crying 3 month old. For this age child, acetaminophen is often an effective analgesic.

Common Problems in PACU Patients

Hypoxemia after general anesthesia may manifest in children as restlessness and combativeness, rather than with visible cyanosis. Causes of hypoxemia after general anesthesia include decreased FRC, depressed peripheral chemoreceptor response to hypoxia, weakness secondary to residual neuromuscular blockade, atelectasis, pulmonary edema, pneumothorax, or aspiration.

Aspiration pneumonia is a constant worry to the anesthesiologist, and in children, cuffed endotracheal tubes are often not used. Some steps can be taken to minimize this risk, including emptying the stomach after intubation. Postanesthetic vomiting is common after strabismus repair, middle ear surgery, orchiopexy, and tonsillectomy/adenoidectomy. Vomiting is a concern, not only because of the possibility of aspiration when airway protection reflexes are not fully recovered, but also because it is one of the most common reasons for unplanned hospital admission for children having outpatient procedures. Adequate fluid administration intraoperatively is especially important in children likely to have postoperative vomiting.

Postintubation stridor, a complication primarily seen in the pediatric patient, has an incidence of approximately 1% in most centers. It is most common in 1–4 year olds and may present as hoarseness, stridor, or retractions. Postintubation stridor has a surprisingly low incidence in children under 1 year of age. Risk factors for the development of postintubation croup include *traumatic intubation, surgery on the head and neck, position change during surgery,* and the use of *an endotracheal tube that is too large.* (A proper size endotracheal tube should have an air leak at less than 40 cm H_2O pressure.) Most cases of postintubation stridor occur within 1 hour of extubation, reach their maximum intensity within 4 hours, and resolve within 24 hours. Nebulized racemic epinephrine is an effective treatment, but it is prudent to admit the child overnight to observe for the possibility of recurrence of airway obstruction and to repeat racemic epinephrine treatments as needed.

Chapter 20

Anesthesia and Analgesia for Obstetrics

Anesthesia for the parturient involves many challenges:

1. The anesthetic plan has to consider two individuals, mother and fetus.
2. The timing and need for management may begin and end abruptly.
3. Care plans may last over extended periods or may change as labor progresses.

MATERNAL PHYSIOLOGY

Physiologic changes of pregnancy that affect anesthetic management:

1. Decreased FRC and increased O_2 consumption lead to rapid deoxygenation during apnea.
2. Oral pharyngeal mucosal edema and swelling may lead to difficult intubation.
3. Enlarged breasts and gravid uterus may make external cardiac massage less effective.
4. Aortocaval compression decreases venous return; therefore, left uterine displacement (LUD) is essential to improve cardiac filling. Even brief periods of maternal hypotension can have detrimental effects in the maturing fetus.

Cardiovascular Changes That Occur in Pregnancy

Change	Percentage[a]	Comments
Blood cell mass	+20	
Plasma volume	+45	RBC volume increases but at a slower rate than plasma volume
Cardiac output*	+40	*Can increase up to 45% above pre-pregnancy level in the expulsive phase of labor
Stroke volume	+30	
Heart rate	+15	
TPR	−15	
Systolic BP MAP	−5 mm Hg	
Diastolic BP	−15–20 mm Hg	

[a]Symbols: +, increase; −, decrease.

Aortocaval Compression (Supine Hypotensive Syndrome)

Approximately 15% of parturients develop signs and symptoms of shock secondary to aortocaval compression (hypotension, pallor, sweating, nausea, and vomiting) in the supine position.

Left uterine displacement improves cardiac filling by relieving venocaval compression. Procedures that achieve LUD:

1. Lateral tilt of OR table
2. Manual or instrumental displacement
3. Wedge under right buttock

Cardiopulmonary resuscitation (CPR)

CPR in the obstetrical patient can be technically difficult because of the anatomic and physiologic changes of pregnancy listed above. Consequently, Trendelenberg position with or without LUD may *worsen* uterine blood flow.

Some etiologies of cardiopulmonary arrest in the obstetrical patient:

1. Preexisting cardiac or pulmonary disease
2. Acute embolic events—amniotic fluid, clot, air
3. Anesthetic complications—failed intubation, regional complications
4. Preeclampsia/eclampsia

5. Hemorrhage
6. Acute trauma

Perimortem cesarean may be performed for a viable fetus and may assist in resuscitation of the mother.

Hypotension secondary to blood loss, regional, or arrest requires treatment with vasopressors. General guidelines for treatment: *(a)* systolic pressures ≤90–100 mm Hg in symptomatic patients or *(b)* decreasing pressures and decreasing fetal heart rate. Ephedrine (5- to 10-mg increments IV) has primarily β-adrenergic effects leading to increased cardiac output without evidence of significant uterine artery vasoconstriction.

Respiratory

Airway evaluation before regional or general anesthesia is important. Examine for loose teeth, swelling, and adipose tissue in the head/neck area, in addition to the usual factors.

Changes in lung volumes and capacities during pregnancy:

Parameter	Percentage
Minute ventilation (MV)	+50
Alveolar ventilation	+70
Tidal volume	+40
Respiratory rate	+/−
O_2 stores	−
FRC	−20
ERV	−20
Residual volume	−20

The potential risk for complications in oxygenation during labor and GA occurs primarily because of *(a)* elevated O_2 consumption and *(b)* decreased FRC and lower maternal oxygen reserve.

Decreased FRC/MV leads to faster inhalational induction.

Gastrointestinal

The following GI changes increase the risk of aspiration in the pregnant patient (>18 weeks gestation).

1. Parturients are more prone to esophagitis and heartburn secondary to reduced esophageal sphincter tone.
2. Gastric motility is decreased and emptying prolonged in the pregnant patient; this is exacerbated by labor and opioids.
3. Gastrin production is increased (by the placenta), leading to increased acid content in the stomach, more marked with a multiple pregnancy.
4. Since these changes do not reverse in the immediate postpartum period, aspiration precautions are indicated for patients undergoing surgical procedures postdelivery (e.g., tubal ligation).

Renal

1. RPF/GFR are increased 30/60% over prepregnancy levels; hence BUN and creatinine decrease (normal levels: BUN 6–8 mg/ml, creatinine 0.4–0.6 mg/ml).
2. Plasma renin activity is increased along with the renin substrate, angiotensin.
3. Glucosuria/protenuria occur and may not be related to coexisting disease.
4. Anatomic changes include ureteral enlargement leading to an increased incidence of UTIs.

CNS

1. MAC is decreased; progesterone has been shown to have a potent sedative-like effect in the gravid patient.
2. Pregnant patients have a decreased requirement for local anesthetic for any given level of SAB (see SAB).
3. CSF pressures can increase in the expulsive phase to levels that could be significant in patients with CNS masses or pathology creating a mass effect.

Hematologic Changes

1. WBC increases during pregnancy and labor and returns to normal by 1st week postpartum.
2. Platelet count decreases for unknown reasons. If preeclampsia exists, remaining platelets may have functional abnormalities.
3. Circulating clotting factors (VII, VIII, X) along with fibrinogen, fibrin, and fibrin complexes increase, leading to a hypercoagulable state.

ANATOMY OF LABOR

Stages of labor

1st stage—Onset of contractions until cervix is fully dilated

2nd stage—Begins with complete cervical dilation and ends with delivery of infant

3rd stage—Delivery of fetus to delivery of placenta

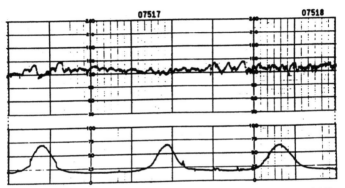

Figure 20.1. Fetal heart rate monitoring with normal rate and variability with uterine contractions. (Reproduced from Shnider SM, Levinson G, eds. Anesthesia for Obstetrics. 3rd ed. Baltimore: Williams & Wilkins, 1993.)

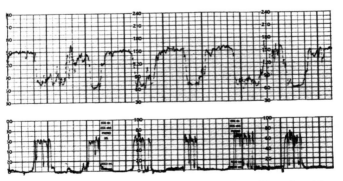

Figure 20.2 Variable decelerations with contractions. (Reproduced from Shnider SM, Levinson G, eds. Anesthesia for Obstetrics: 3rd ed. Baltimore: Williams & Wilkins, 1993.)

Fetal Monitoring

Fetal Heart Rate (FHR)

Normal HR 120–160 beats per minute

Patterns of deceleration
1. Early deceleration—head compression
2. Late deceleration—ureteroplacental insufficiency
3. Variable deceleration—cord compression
4. Systemic sedative drugs can affect FHR, leading to a decrease in variability of tracing. Concomitant maternal medications also affect FHR (e.g., β-blockers can lead to fetal bradycardia).

When possible, document FHR before and after regional anesthesia, elective operative procedures, and CPR.

Scalp pH

The scalp-sampling technique makes PO_2 difficult to obtain; however, pH, PCO_2, BE are useful in determining fetal well-being. Evaluation is done in conjunction with assessment of maternal acid base status.

pH $>$ 7.25, within normal limits
7.20–7.25, range of possible fetal distress
$<$ 7.20, indication of hypoxia or distress

SYSTEMIC MEDICATIONS IN OBSTETRICS

Opiods

Opioids are used for pain control during lst and 2nd stage of labor. They can cause a decrease in beat-to-beat variability of FHR.

Butorphanol
—Has both agonist and antagonist properties
—Crosses placenta
—Passes into breast milk
—No reports of congenital defects
Nalbuphine(Nubain)
—5-mg increments IV (analgesia equivalent to morphine)
—Agonist-antagonist properties

—Useful supplement to regional anesthesia after delivery of fetus
—Kappa action leads to maternal sedation

Meperidine
—Pure agonist analgesic
—Rapid placental transfer
—Can cause neonatal depression postdelivery up to 72 hours
—Active metabolite: normeperidine
—Often used in regional anesthesia for labor

Morphine
—Rarely used for preterm labor in modern obstetrics
—No reports of congenital defects
—Pure agonist
—Increased fetal respiratory depression
—Maternal and fetal addiction possible
—Epidural use does not give satisfactory analgesic results for second-stage labor
—Intrathecal use with SAB has been successful for supplementation of postoperative pain; usage requires monitoring for up to 24 hours after block and treatment of narcotic side effects (pruritus)

Fentanyl
—Synthetic opioid—pure agonist
—Given in 50–100 μg increments IV
—No reports of congenital defects
—Rapid redistribution limits fetal effect
—Like sufentanil, can be used in regional anesthesia for labor

Sedative Hypnotics

Benzodiazepines (midazolam, diazepam)
—Rapidly cross placenta
—Can cause decreased beat-to-beat variability in FHR
—Displaces lipid soluble bilirubin from albumin binding sites, possibly increasing infant kernicterus

Phenothiazines (Promethazine, Phenergan)

—Rapid placental transfer
—Frequently used with meperidine, produce significant hypotension, poor antiemetic, pronounced sedation

Dissociative (Amnestic) Drugs

Ketamine (low-dose 10-mg increments) 0.5–1 mg/kg maximum
—Provides intense analgesia
—May require benzodiazepines for prevention of undesirable side effects
—Has vasopressor effects
—Produces a dose-related oxytocic effect
—Crosses placenta rapidly
—Careful maternal assessment obligatory
Scopolamine (rarely used)
—Associated with maternal confusion, delirium, and amnesia

INHALATIONAL ANESTHETIC AGENTS

Despite studies indicating that inhalational anesthetic agents cause direct change at the cellular level (reversible decreases in mobility, prolongation of synthesis, cell division, inhibition of both cytoplasmic streaming and microtubule function) in clinical doses, anesthetic agents have no direct link with teratogenicity. Animal studies have, however, implicated a dose-related increase in fetal wastage with N_2O.

The anesthetic management goal during general anesthesia is to provide protection for mother and fetus during surgery (i.e., prevention of hypoperfusion, hypoxia, and hypothermia) and protection of airway (Table 20.1). Inhalational anesthesia

Table 20.1
Recommendation for Fetal Management with Nonobstetrical Surgery

1. Maintain high O_2 concentration
2. Use regional when possible, especially during 1st trimester
3. Avoid aortocaval compression
4. Use drugs with a proven record, e.g., morphine, fentanyl
5. Give adequate IV fluids
6. Use vasopressors as necessary but recognize their effect on placental perfusion
7. Avoid hypercapnia
8. Monitor fetus if possible
9. Use standard monitors as a minimum for the mother, and monitor for uterine contractions if possible

during labor has limited use, as it produces depression in both mother and fetus and increases the risk of maternal aspiration.

NATURAL CHILDBIRTH

Natural childbirth relies upon

1. Information—with comprehension
2. Education
3. Breathing techniques
4. Relaxation
5. Support

ACUPUNCTURE AND HYPNOSIS

Acupuncture and hypnosis have been used with some success. Cultural experiences and availability play an important role in these methods.

ANESTHESIA FOR CESAREAN SECTION AND COMPLICATED VAGINAL DELIVERY

Common Indications for Intervention

1. Fetal distress
2. Hemorrhage/coagulation disorders
3. Preeclampsia
4. Abnormal position
5. Fetal anomaly
   Size—macrosomia
   Preterm—to protect fetus through delivery
   Congenital disorders—e.g., hydrocephalus
6. Coexisting disease or infection
7. Failure to progress

Record and Preparation

1. History and physical examination, airway evaluation, allergies, last meal, and medications are important.
2. Type and screen for transfusion.
3. Insert large-bore IV (16 gauge); patients with previous cesarean sections may require two IV sites with large-bore catheters.
4. Use ultrasound to assess placental location in patients with previous c/section; increased blood loss can result from an

incision through the placental site (placenta previa/accreta can result in massive blood loss).

5. Premedicate with a nonparticulate antacid more than 30 minutes before surgery; if surgery is delayed more than 2 hours, antacid may be repeated.

6. Ensure operating room preparation; OR should be set up and available for emergency obstetrical cases at all times.
   a. Check machine, laryngoscope
   b. Suction (Yankauer) for rapid sequence induction
   c. Variety of endotracheal tube sizes: 6.0, 7.0, 7.5 mm (small tubes for edematous larynx)
   d. Drugs: thiopental, succinylcholine, atropine, pitocin, ephedrine, narcotics, β-blockers, hydralazine

Anesthetic Plan

Plan includes preoperative evaluation, antacid, 0_2, fetal monitoring, patient monitors, and LUD. Anesthetic technique is determined by the medical situation and obstetrician and patient preference/cooperation. Options include epidural, subarachnoid block, general, and local.

Local Anesthesia

1. Paracervical
   a. *Anatomy:* Frankenhauser's plexus, just within mucosa of fornix, can be blocked at base of broad ligament; block is usually performed by obstetrician
   b. *Indications:* 1st stage of labor—before 7-cm dilation
   c. *Risks:* Fetal injection; intravascular injection—maternal toxic effect of local anesthetic, fetal toxic effects if arterial injection or absorption, fetal level greater than maternal

2. Pudendal
   a. *Anatomy:* palpate ischial tuberosities; inject per vagina at, and beyond, tuberosity; pudendal nerve lies behind tuberosity; usually performed by obstetrician
   b. *Indications:* to block pain due to vaginal distension on incision (2nd and 3rd stages)
   c. *Risks:* Local anesthetic toxicity; high failure rate (up to 40%) because of aberrant innervation

Table 20.2
Dosing for Epidural Anesthesia during Labor

State	Radiation of Pain	Dose[a]	Complications and Treatment
1st stage	Mid/lower back pain T_{10}–L_2	Bupivacaine 0.125% or 0.25%, 5–10 ml intermittent dose; effective for 1–1½ hours; monitor vital signs and level of block	Patient must remain on side or with LUD; one-sided block may be treated by dosing patient with painful side down or catheter adjustment/replacement
2nd stage	Perineal pain; abdominal pain; pain postdelivery from lacerations $S_{1,2,3,4}$(T_{10}–L_2 for forceps delivery)	Bupivacaine 0.25% 5–10 ml sitting, 0.5% 5 ml 10–45 min, prior to delivery; for rapid effect 3% 2-chloroprocaine 5–10 ml	

[a]Each dose is a test dose, monitor accordingly.

3. Local infiltration field block can be done by obstetrician at surgical site for gravely ill patients or patchy regional anesthetic
4. Epidural analgesia (Table 20.2)
   a. Benefits in obstetrical patients
      i. Minimal interference with progress of labor
      ii. Give pain relief allowing for patient cooperation with intact motor function
      iii. Minimal impact on fetus/neonate
   b. Potential complications of epidural anesthesia: total spinal, postdural puncture headache, infection, hematoma, backache (most common complaint but difficult to differentiate from back pain related to pregnancy)

   Postdural puncture headache(PDPH)

   Conservative treatment: Hydration for 24 hr with bed rest. Encourage caffeine products, abdominal binder, and PO pain medications if required. Most headaches resolve spontaneously.

   Blood patch after 24 hours of conservative treatment. Discuss risks and benefits of patch. Use sterile skin preparation, sterile technique. Slowly inject 10–14 ml of patient's blood obtained under sterile conditions by an assistant. Ninety-five percent of headaches resolve with patch. If headache persists, continue conservative treatment; 98% of patients respond to a second patch.

Alternative: immediate blood patch (not as effective); a saline patch may reduce incidence of headache (use preservative-free saline).

Headaches have infrequently been associated with seizures both pre- and postdural puncture. A completely satisfactory explanation has not been given for these seizures, but low intracranial pressure may be involved.

5. Subarachnoid block
   a. Direct placement of local anesthetic into the CSF means that the anesthetic level can be rapidly achieved, but it may be associated with rapid onset of sympathectomy and hypotension.
   b. Spinal anesthesia is used for cesarean section, forceps delivery, or retained placenta.
   c. *Management* (Table 20.3)

   Prehydration using physiologic salt solution (10–15 ml/kg)

   Have resuscitation equipment available

   LUD

   Document fetal heart tones

   Use small-bore needle (25–27 gauge) to reduce incidence of post dural puncture headache

   After injecting spinal, displace uterus by inserting wedge under right buttock; check BP immediately, then at 3- to 5-minute intervals

   Check level and progression of block (by pinprick or alcohol wipe) for at least 20 min

Table 20.3
Local Anesthetic Doses for C-section under Spinal Anesthesia

Short (1 hr)	Intermediate (2 hr)	Long (2½ hr)
5% Lidocaine in dextrose 7.5% 60–100 mg	0.75% Bupivacaine in dextrose 8.25% 9–15 mg	1% Tetracaine in dextrose 5%, 7–10 mg; epinephrine 0.2 mg

Altering table position can lead to progression of block with hyperbaric agents; goal is T_2-T_4 anesthetic level

d. *Risks of subarachnoid block*

Hypotension

Postdural puncture headache

Infection

Hematoma

Neurologic deficits

6. **Management of local anesthetic toxicity** (remember basics of resuscitation: airway, breathing, and circulation); symptoms: perioral numbness, paresthesia, tinnitus, metallic taste, tachycardia from epinephrine; may be seen with epidural or local infiltration

   a. Decrease incidence by observing maximal dosage guidelines and using incremental doses of dilute concentration of local anesthetic

   b. Observe recommended maximum dosage by weight

   c. Aspirate prior to injection

   d. Check sensory level hourly when using infusions and at redosing

7. **Management of convulsions**

   a. Clear and maintain airway—intubation if necessary to prevent aspiration

   b. Oxygen

   c. Thiopental 50–100 mg (preferred) or diazepam/midazolam in low dosages

   d. Fluids and pressors to maintain blood pressure

   e. LUD to prevent aortocaval compression

   f. Monitor fetus

8. **Management of high spinal** (diagnosed by continuous assessment of anesthetic level); signs: yawning, nausea and vomiting, restlessness or disorientation, hypotension

   a. If respiratory compromise is imminent, secure airway, intubate if required, and assist or control ventilation with 100% oxygen

   b. Vasopressors to maintain adequate perfusion pressure

   c. Monitor fetus

   d. Remember LUD, as aortocaval compression can worsen hypotension

9. **Epidural and subarachnoid opiates in obstetrics**
    a. Fentanyl, alfentanil, sufentanil, and meperidine all have a low pKa and high lipid solubility, leading to rapid dural penetration and onset, with a short duration of action. Morphine has a slower onset with slow clearance from CSF. These agents, when used in epidural or subarachnoid block, potentiate local anesthetics for labor and delivery. Alone, they provide satisfactory analgesia during the first stage of labor and delivery with minimal side effects. Opioids work at their spinal receptor sites in conjunction with local anesthetics to lower total anesthetic dose requirement, providing better analgesia with minimal motor blockade.
    b. Opioids used in regional anesthesia
        i. Morphine (0.5 mg intrathecally) provides excellent analgesia but with slow onset 45–50 minutes.
        ii. Epidural fentanyl (50–100 μg bolus) or infusion with bupivacaine 0.5% for cesarean section enhances analgesia during surgery and for 2–3 hours after recovery; infusion of 0.125% bupivacaine and 1–2 μg/ml of fentanyl enhances analgesia for labor.
        iii. Sufentanil 1 μg/ml and bupivacaine 0.125–0.03125% analgesia provides more rapid onset of anesthesia and a better quality of analgesia; alfentanil 10 μg/kg/hr along with 0.125% bupivacaine at 10 ml/hr has been used in epidural infusions.
    c. *Side effects* of epidural or intrathecal opioids include pruritus, nausea and vomiting, urinary retention, respiratory depression, and drowsiness.

        Treatment of side effects can be symptom-directed (diphenhydramine for relief of pruritus) or through direct antagonism of the opioid at the receptor (naloxone, naltrexone, nalmephine, or nalbuphine intravenously).

GENERAL ANESTHESIA FOR CESAREAN SECTION

Indications for Emergency Surgical Intervention

1. Fetal distress, severe bradycardia
2. Shoulder dystocia
3. Umbilical cord prolapse
4. Hemorrhage, unstable cardiovascular status

5. Abruptio placenta/placenta previa
6. Head entrapment

Rapid Sequence—Assistance Required

1. Preoxygenation
2. Defasciculation with curare (3 mg) unless patient is receiving magnesium therapy
3. IV induction with thiopental (4–5 mg/kg) or ketamine (1–2 mg/kg) and succinylcholine (2 mg/kg)
4. Cricoid pressure, 3 fingers (equivalent to uncomfortable pressure on bridge of nose); do not release until cuff is inflated
5. $FIO_2 \geq 0.5$, N_2O, isoflurane or other inhalational agent 0.5 to 0.7 MAC
6. Add muscle relaxant as required; follow with nerve stimulator.
7. After delivery of infant, rapidly decrease inhalational anesthesia to avoid uterine relaxation; supplemental narcotics with low concentrations of inhalational agents provide for rapid awakening.
8. Use precautions for extubation to prevent aspiration: awake, return of airway reflexes; document reversal, strength, and arousability.

Supplemental Airway Equipment to Have Available

1. Variety of tube sizes
2. Choice of laryngoscope blades
3. Eschmann tube changer
4. 16-gauge catheter for insertion into the cricothyroid membrane and 3-ml syringe with size 6 endotrachial tube adapter (remove plunger, replace with adapter)—can provide oxygenation from high-pressure O_2 source but not ventilation
5. Emergency cricothyroidotomy tray/kit; ENT availability
6. Fiberoptic laryngoscope

HIGH-RISK PARTURIENTS

Malpresentation

1. *Breech* is the most common malpresentation. Fetus is at risk for cord compression, entanglement, placental separation,

hypoxia from inability to deliver head, shoulders, intracranial hemorrhage from too sudden decompression and force of delivery, fractures of limbs, clavicles, or neck. Delivery is by elective cesarean section for primipara; vaginal delivery can be done in multiparity. Consider an epidural for delivery (can convert to general, if necessary).

2. *Persistent occiput posterior* may require forceps or vacuum extraction. Regional can provide relief of painful contractions and anesthesia for surgical intervention.

3. *Face presentation* has a high incidence of prolonged labor and probably needs a cesarean section.

4. *Shoulder presentation* is more common in multiparas; it carries a high risk of uterine rupture, hemorrhage, prolonged labor, and lacerations.

5. *Prolapsed cord*
   —Emergency treatment requires general anesthesia (stat cesarian section)
   —elevated risk of perinatal mortality from cord compression

Multiple Births

1. High risk of prematurity
2. Lower birth weight infants
3. First twin often delivered without complication
4. Second twin more likely to have abnormal position with more depression
5. May want to prepare patients early with selective sensory epidural analgesia
6. Prepare for general with rapid sequence induction if required

Preeclampsia/Eclampsia

Pathophysiology

Risk groups: those with prior history, coexisting disease, previous hypertension, renal disease, diabetes, primi/multigravida, or multiparity, and members of the African-American population; the incidence is increased above 28 weeks but most common at 36 weeks; symptoms usually resolve within hours of delivery.

Classification

Mild
1. Hypertension—systolic BP > 140, diastolic BP > 90, or a 15–20 mm Hg rise from baseline
2. Edema—common in normal pregnancy

Severe
1. Hypertension—160/100 mm Hg or above
2. Cerebral disturbances with headache, intracranial hemorrhage, retinal changes, seizures
3. Proteinuria > 0.3 gm/liter, 2 random samples at least 6 hours apart
4. Epigastric pain (subcapsular hepatic hemorrhage)
5. Coagulation disorders (thrombocytopenia)
6. Liver dysfunction
7. Renal dysfunction, oliguria

Risks

Fetal: Hypoxia, intrauterine growth retardation, poor placental perfusion

Maternal: Intracranial hemorrhage and pulmonary edema (most common causes of death), chronic renal insufficiency, placental abruption, cardiac arrest, HELLP syndrome (hemolysis, elevated liver function tests (LFTS), low platelets); anesthetic risk significant

Management

1. Bed rest—quiet, nonstimulating environment
2. Monitoring

   Mild   BP, urinary output, proteinuria

   Severe   *Maternal*

           Coagulation studies (PT, PTT, platelets, bleeding time)

           Chemistry profile

           Foley catheter

           Arterial line

           CVP/PA catheter

       Fetal

           FHR by scalp electrode

           Fetal pH

3. *Medical management:*
   Blood pressure control should be directed toward preventing cerebral hemorrhage and cardiac failure. Goal of BP treatment is to reduce mean pressure by 33%.

   Magnesium increases muscle weakness by decreasing acetylcholine release from the motor nerve terminal and by decreased excitability of postjunctional membrane to reduce incidence of eclamptic seizures; it affects both nondepolarizing and depolarizing relaxants (ND > D).

   Other properties of magnesium:
   Anticonvulsant
   Tocolysis
   Negative inotrope
   Excreted by kidney
   Normal blood level: 1.5–2 mEq/liter
   Therapeutic: 4–6 mEq/liter
   Respiratory depression: 12 mEq/liter

   Labetalol used in incremental doses can blunt hypertension and tachycardia with endotracheal intubation (dosage: 5–10 mg) along with lidocaine 100 mg IV at induction.

   Hydralazine is an arteriolar vasodilator with onset 7–10 min and occasionally associated reflex tachycardia.

   Severe hypertension may necessitate use of a more potent agent such as nitroglycerin or sodium nitroprusside.
4. Fluid management: Severe preeclamptic patients tend to have intravascular volume depletion. Any parturient with a "normal" Hct (prepregnancy Hct) should have her volume status evaluated. An Hct of 38% indicates volume depletion. Hydrate with lactated Ringer's slowly, to prevent fluid overload in patients with limited cardiac reserve. Monitor CVP or PA pressures if in doubt.
5. Sedatives/anticonvulsants
   a. Benzodiazepines may be required despite known effects on the fetus (hypotonia, kernicterus, respiratory depression, temperature instability).
   b. Thiopental 50–150 mg IV for seizures (carefully observe for loss of protective airway reflexes), emergency airway, and resuscitation equipment must be available in the room.
6. Pain management
   a. Systemic opioids may be necessary in patients with coagulopathy. The systemic effect of progesterone in preg-

nancy can cause gravid patients to be very sensitive to any opioid/sedative.

b. Epidural advantages are good pain relief, vasodilation, and minimal neonatal depression.

    i. Give fluid preload, carefully; observe CVP or pulmonary arterial catheter for evidence of heart failure or renal failure.

    ii. Follow coagulation profiles with platelet counts; look for stable counts and measure bleeding time before epidural.

    iii. Do history/physical with airway assessment; observe for signs of pharyngeal/laryngeal edema.

    iv. Use continuous BP monitoring—arterial line in severe or progressive cases.

    v. Avoid aortocaval compression in patients with limited cardiac reserve and placental compromise.

    vi. Avoid epinephrine-containing solutions and test dose.

7. Coagulation:

Obtain bleeding time, PT, PTT, and platelet count as indicated. Evaluate for clinical signs of coagulopathy: bleeding, prolonged oozing at IV sites, petechiae.

a. Vaginal delivery (sedation, regional or GA). Contraindications to regional such as coagulation disorders may require supplementation with narcotics or superficial blocks (e.g.. pudendal).

b. Management under general anesthesia

    i. Monitor oxygen saturation, end-tidal CO_2, BP (arterial line), pulse, ECG, central venous pressure, and urine output.

    ii. Attenuate effects of laryngoscopy and intubation by giving antihypertensives: labetalol, lidocaine, hydralazine, esmolol, nitroprusside, nitroglycerin.

    iii. Oral pharyngeal edema and coagulopathy can make intubation difficult.

c. Postdelivery care may require ICU for monitoring.

NEUROLOGIC DISORDERS

1. Myasthenia gravis is an autoimmune disorder affecting motor endplates (incidence 1:15000). The disease affects mainly ocular motor, facial, laryngeal, and respiratory muscles. End-

plates are abnormally thin. Pregnancy may worsen the course of disease, with increasing muscle weakness or respiratory insufficiency.

2. Idiopathic epilepsy is most common type of epilepsy. Convulsions can be associated with preeclampsia or tumor. Status epilepticus, the most serious complication, is associated with a high mortality rate. Convulsions are treated with *(a)* oxygen, resuscitation equipment and *(b)* thiopental 50- to 100-mg increments (IV benzodiazepines: midazolam 1- to 2-mg increments with *airway protection*). *Note:* Seizures can occur in preeclamptic patients up to 48 hours postdelivery. Patients with seizures in pregnancy tend to become acidotic very rapidly.

3. Multiple sclerosis is a demyelinating disease, often leading to progressive deterioration. A low-dose epidural may be used; few recommend subarachnoid block. Some prefer to avoid potential complications by using alternatives that will not be confused with a deterioration of the disease state.

4. Neuromuscular diseases include muscular dystrophies (several categories): Duchenne (sex-linked to males but also occurs in females), limb girdle, ocular, etc. Avoid regional. Current recommendations include general anesthesia with possible postoperative ventilation. Patients are susceptible to changes in magnesium levels and muscle relaxants.

ANATOMIC ABNORMALITIES

1. For a patient with short stature with cephalopelvic disproportion, an epidural for labor may be converted for surgical use if trial of vaginal delivery is unsuccessful.

2. Scoliosis can make a regional technically difficult. Best approach for epidural or spinal is to use the convex side of curvature or paramedian approach.

3. Regional anesthesia has been used successfully in achondroplastic dwarfs (it may be technically difficult, however). Review previous x-rays if available. Evaluate these patients for unstable cervical spine. Large head/jaw make general anesthetic airway management more difficult.

MORBID OBESITY

Definition Using Body Mass Index (BMI)

$$BMI = weight (kg)/height (m^2)$$

$< 25 =$ normal
$25-29 =$ overweight
$> 30 =$ obese
$> 35 =$ morbid obesity

Complications Related to Obesity

1. Anatomic changes of obesity make positioning difficult.
2. There is increased incidence of coexisting disease (hypertension, diabetes mellitus)
3. Syndrome of hyper/hypoventilation in obese patients can lead to hypercapnia, hypoxemia, polycythemia, and somnolence. Use a pulse oximeter to monitor regional candidates.
4. FRC is further reduced, with the gravid uterus and large abdominal mass resulting in rapid desaturation during induction of general anesthesia.

Management

1. In positioning, elevate head, restrain breasts as required, suspend panniculus with tape for surgical exposure.
2. Regional anesthesia, while difficult, can decrease the likelihood of respiratory problems if the need for surgery arises. Epidural can allow for greater control of block by incremental dosing. (Patients are more sensitive to local anesthetic volume despite their massive size.)
3. Avoid oversedation; it may lead to respiratory depression.

SUBSTANCE ABUSE

Fetal Complications

There is an increased incidence of fetal wastage and perinatal mortality with cocaine use. Neonatal mortality is also increased because of a greater prevalence of meconium, low birth weight, sepsis, fetal distress, and spontaneous abortion.

Regional anesthesia in maternal addicts can limit narcotic analgesics that further depress newborn addict, premature infant, or infant in distress.

Maternal Complications

Concomitant medical and obstetrical disorders (e.g., infectious disease, poor nutritional status, toxemia, placenta previa, abruption, malpresentation) have a higher incidence in substance abuse patients. Abruptio placenta, placenta previa, and postpartum hemorrhage have been associated with cocaine abuse. Acute cocaine intoxication may be present, as some patients believe that the drug accelerates labor.

COEXISTING MATERNAL DISEASE

Endocrine/Diabetes Mellitus

1. Metabolic control during the intrapartum period may be difficult; blood glucose should be controlled with insulin infusions or intermittent boluses.
2. Vomiting during early pregnancy complicates management of metabolic status; patients may have gastroparesis.
3. Maternal acidosis has a direct effect on the fetus.
4. Hypertensive disorders occur more often in diabetic patients; autonomic dysfunction also occurs in many diabetics.
5. Risk of macrosomia, fetal distress, and fetal death increases in diabetic mothers
6. Risk of respiratory distress syndrome increases.
7. Metabolic derangements are more likely and will continue into the postpartum period, requiring continued electrolyte monitoring.

Respiratory

1. Asthmatic patients can generally continue prepregnancy medications; regional anesthesia represents best choice for patients with acute respiratory compromise.
2. Patients with lung resections tend to tolerate labor well if pulmonary compensation has taken place.
3. For pulmonary hypertension, optimize patient in controlled environment at term; use PA catheter to monitor hemodynamics; give O_2 to improve pulmonary vascular dilation.

Cardiovascular Disease

Heart disease occurs in 2% of parturients. Rheumatic heart disease is the predominant type; mitral stenosis and mitral insufficiency are the most common forms.

Patients who have undergone corrective procedures (valve replacement, valvotomy) are increasing in number in the childbearing population. These patients tend to tolerate labor well with continuous monitoring for signs of changing hemodynamic status. Patients with mild uncorrected lesions tend to tolerate medical management.

Note: SBE prophylaxis is usually required for valvular lesions and mitral valve prolapse with symptoms.

A well-managed regional anesthetic can be ideal for patients with some forms of valvular heart disease.

Specific Lesions

1. With *aortic stenosis,* hypotension cannot be corrected by increasing cardiac output; heart rate must increase. Therefore, avoid agents that induce bradycardia or hypotension. Avoid regional anesthesia, which may lower preload.

2. *Cyanotic heart disease* is generally caused by septal defects (atrial or ventricular). Left-to-right shunts can worsen with the stress of labor. Regional anesthesia can be used when there is no evidence of PVR $\geq$ SVR. In the latter circumstance, the shunt may reverse with a decrease in systemic pressure (e.g., regional anesthesia). In patients with progressive symptoms, a general anesthetic is preferred for hemodynamic control.

3. *Mitral stenosis* leads to an increase in left atrial pressures along with increased pulmonary venous and capillary pressures, increasing pulmonary congestion. The CV changes of pregnancy that worsen this condition are *(a)* increased heart rate—less diastolic filling time and *(b)* increased CO and blood volume through a narrow orifice, which can increase pulmonary blood volume. Regional anesthesia with peripheral vasodilation can decrease volume received by the pulmonary circulation in the expulsive phase of labor. Lumbar epidural anesthesia allows incremental dosing, thereby avoiding rapid hemodynamic changes.

4. *Mitral insufficiency* is a valvular defect that causes overloading of the left ventricle. Ventricular work may be decreased by afterload reduction with regional anesthesia.

5. *Mitral valve prolapse* can be mild and asymptomatic. These patients can be treated with either regional or general anesthesia without untoward sequelae.

INTRAPARTUM AND POSTPARTUM COMPLICATIONS

Obstetrical Hemorrhage

Patients with classical surgical incisions for previous cesarean section should have ultrasound localization of placenta and large-bore IV access for volume replacement.

Placental Abnormalities

1. *Placenta previa* is an abnormal implantation of placenta on the lower uterine segment. Patients often present with painless vaginal bleeding during third trimester. Management requires volume replacement through good IV access. Significant blood loss may lead to hysterectomy.
2. *Placenta accreta* is strongly associated with placenta previa. Placental villi are attached directly to myometrium, particularly over previous uterine incision. Treatment may require hysterectomy. Transient aortic clamping may be necessary.
3. *Abruptio placenta* is separation of the placenta from the uterine wall. Patients present with painful vaginal bleeding, fetal distress, coagulation disorders, or hypotonic uterus.
4. *Anterior placenta* if unrecognized can lead to intraoperative hemorrhage with surgical incision through placenta.

Embolic Events

1. Amniotic fluid embolus is a rare occurrence but 89% fatal.
   a. Clinical features include respiratory distress; hypotension with possible vascular collapse; derangements of oxygenation leading to cyanosis, seizures, or coma; hemorrhage; DIC; uterine atony; bronchospasm; and pulmonary edema.
   b. Differential diagnosis includes pulmonary embolus (a major cause of maternal mortality), aspiration, eclampsia, extracranial hemorrhage, and acute heart failure.
   c. Treatment involves supportive care and resuscitation, delivering fetus when possible, monitoring (CVP, PA catheter, A-line, obtaining right atrial sample to confirm diagnosis by fetal cells, etc.), and inotropes or vasopressors, which may be required for BP support.

2. Pulmonary embolus
   a. Risk factors are advanced maternal age, obesity, cesarean, prolonged bed rest, estrogen therapy, ABO group other than 0, and antithrombin III deficiency.
   b. Presentation includes pleuritic chest pain, acute dyspnea, hemoptysis, and ECG changes ($S_1Q_3T_3$).
   c. Treat with heparin/Coumadin, up to 36 weeks.

Preterm Labor

Incidence is higher in teenage parturients. Regional anesthesia is useful for instrumentation (e.g., forceps delivery for protection of preterm cranium). Often malpresentation occurs due to small size. Cesarean section is often required.

Drugs used in the interruption of labor and their side effects:

1. *Tocolytics:* Adrenergic agents (ritodrine) can cause hypotension, tachycardia, arrhythmias, fluid retention, pulmonary edema, anxiety, nausea, and vomiting.
2. *Magnesium*—important to monitor levels.
3. *ETOH* was used in past but rarely now, as it decreases CNS orientation, produces nausea and vomiting, and increases gastric acid secretion.

Uterine Rupture

Uterine rupture is diagnosed by fetal distress, abnormal labor, uterine shape, and pain/bleeding. Patients predisposed are those with prior cesarean section or previous myomectomy, trophoblastic invasion. Major volume replacement may be required.

Postpartum Hemorrhage:

1. Uterine atony is more common in grand multiparas patients.
   a. Treatment: volume replacement, uterine massage, ligation of blood supply vs. hysterectomy
   b. Additional treatment: Methergine (IV use may produce hypertensive responsive) or hemabat, prostaglandin E_2
2. Lacerations requiring surgical intervention need adequate anesthesia to aid in surgical repair (local, regional, general anesthesia, depending on hemodynamic status).

3. For retained placenta, use systemic analgesia or regional if patient is euvolemic and ≤12 weeks. For uterine sizes above 12 weeks, you may consider regional if patient is without cardiovascular instability. Uterine relaxation can be obtained with nitroglycerin in small increments (25–50 μg); use only with caution and vigilant monitoring. Too much traction on the umbilical cord may lead to uterine prolapse and severe blood loss.

Chapter 21

Postoperative Care

The immediate postoperative period demands the same level of medical care, nursing, and monitoring found in any intensive care unit. Immediate attention must be paid to problems that arise during the potentially unstable period resulting after general or regional anesthesia. Pain management is begun in the postanesthesia care unit (PACU) with small doses of opiates and other modalities.

Functions of Postanesthesia Care Unit (PACU)
- Intense nursing care at 1:1 nurse:patient ratio
- Early diagnosis of surgical bleeding
- Continuous or frequent vital sign observation (ECG, BP, pulse, urine flow, oximetry)
- Pain management
- X-ray verification of line placement or pulmonary assessment

Responsibility for nursing and medical care must be clearly delineated by procedures formulated by the hospital's nursing and anesthesiology representatives, approved by the hospital's governing body. When appropriate, medical and other consultations are obtained by the anesthesiologist, who maintains open communication with the patient's operating surgeon. Standards for postanesthesia care have been approved by the American Society of Anesthesiology; these standards include unit design and organization, patient transport and monitoring, transition of care to the unit, evaluation of the patient in the PACU, and discharge. A member of the anesthesia care team should not transfer responsibility for patient care until the full admission procedure has been completed, including a report that includes the patient's name, age, operative procedure, pre- and intraoperative drugs given and doses, allergies, medical

471

conditions, chronic medications, vital sign ranges, intraoperative fluid administration, estimated blood loss, evidence of renal function, initial plan for management, and physician responsible for care in the PACU.

NAUSEA AND VOMITING

Nausea and vomiting is more common in the younger female patient than in the older male patient. In addition to patient discomfort, vomiting can lead to incisional disruption or to compromise of the surgical outcome.

Conditions associated with nausea and vomiting
• Gastric distension or other visceral stimulation
• Blood in the stomach
• Recent chemotherapy
• Motion sickness
• Middle ear surgery
• Impairment of gastrointestinal motility
• Drugs (opiates)

Drugs Associated with Nausea and Vomiting

Opiates such as meperidine, fentanyl, alfentanil, and sufentanil are all associated with an increased incidence of nausea and vomiting, especially when used as the predominant form of anesthetic. No specific inhalation agent has been identified as an emetic agent. It is controversial whether nitrous oxide contributes to nausea and vomiting in the absence of gastric distention.

Drugs Used to Treat Nausea and Vomiting

Droperidol and metoclopramide have both been used most effectively in the prevention and treatment of nausea and vomiting in the PACU. Other drugs used for prevention and/or treatment of nausea and vomiting include scopolamine, benzquinamide, prochlorperazine, trimethobenzamide HCl, hydroxyzine, dimenhydrinate, and ondansetron.

Patients with a history of protracted vomiting after previous anesthetics or of motion sickness may benefit from preinduction placement of a scopolamine patch. Ondansetron (4 mg), administered IV before the induction of anesthesia, has been shown to be effective in preventing postoperative nausea and vomiting.

Mechanism of Action

Both **droperidol** and **metoclopramide** act by antagonizing dopaminergic receptors, blocking stimulation of the medullary chemoreceptor emetic trigger zone. Droperidol is a mild α-blocker and may cause hypotension as well as being associated with sedation and extrapyramidal symptoms, such as oculogyric crisis. Metoclopramide stimulates gastric motility by increasing resting tone of the lower esophageal sphincter and relaxation of the pyloric sphincter. Gastric emptying is thereby enhanced. **Ondansetron** is a serotonin ($5-HT_3$) receptor antagonist that acts at both the chemoreceptor trigger zone in the brainstem and in the proximal bowel.

Usual Doses

Droperidol is given intravenously in small doses (0.625–2.5 mg for the average adult; 25–75 $\mu g/kg$ for children). Metoclopramide is given in doses from 10 to 20 mg in adults, and this dose can be repeated in 2 hours. There is little or no sedation associated with the use of metoclopramide, but some patients may exhibit mild extrapyramidal symptoms. Extrapyramidal symptoms may be treated with small doses of benztropine, 1–2 mg or diphenhydramine 25–50 mg.

POSTOPERATIVE HYPERTENSION

Hypertension, a common problem in the recovery room, may require immediate treatment, especially in the patient at risk for myocardial ischemia or increased surgical bleeding. Hypertension is defined as a persistent diastolic pressure above 100 mm Hg or systolic pressures more than 30% of baseline resting values obtained on the ward. Patients with preexisting essential hypertension are especially likely to develop hypertension in the postoperative period, regardless of the anesthetic technique.

For the first 15 minutes, blood pressure should be taken and recorded at least every 5 minutes, and thereafter, blood pressure should be taken and recorded at least every 15 minutes, depending on the patient's condition. Direct intraarterial monitoring displays a continuous beat-to-beat wave form of arterial pressure. Automated devices (Dinamapp) have proven useful by allowing personnel to perform hands-on patient care instead of measuring vital signs. Even more important than the control of hypertension is the control of the patient's pulse rate, which is another determinant of myocardial oxygen supply. In general, the pulse rate should be treated when above 110 beats per minute in an adult patient. After assessment and treatment of specific causes of hypertension, vasoactive drug therapy might be initiated.

Causes of Hypertension

* Pain
* Hypercarbia (CO_2 retention from hypoventilation)
* Hypoxia
* Full urinary bladder
* Withdrawal of chronic antihypertensive drug
* Fluid overload
* Vasoconstriction from hypothermia
* Preexisting "essential" hypertension

Assessment of Patient Condition

Before any potent vasoactive drug is used, and after adequate pain therapy, hemodynamics should be assessed.

1. **Preload** can be assessed by measuring pulmonary artery catheter wedge pressure or simply by visual inspection of other direct and indirect signs of intravascular volume, such as superficial vein filling, deep neck vein pulsation, and urine flow. A review of surgical blood loss and intraoperative fluid replacement can help in assessing cardiac filling. The pulmonary capillary wedge (PCW) pressure is used to assess left ventricular preload. Normal PCW pressure is 10–18 mm Hg.
2. **Cardiac contractility** can be indirectly assessed by palpation of the pulse or by direct observation of the direct arterial pressure wave form upstroke. Contractility may be depressed by residual volatile anesthetic drugs, intrinsic heart disease, or hypothermia. When a pulmonary artery catheter is in place, thermodilution measurements of cardiac output are useful in assessing cardiac function.

3. **Vascular tone** can be grossly assessed by visually inspecting superficial veins, by feeling skin temperature, and by observing the upstroke of the arterial pressure wave form. If a pulmonary artery catheter is in place and cardiac output can be measured, systemic vascular resistance can be calculated.

Useful Drugs

Drugs used to control hypertension can be divided into categories that include α- and β-blockers, calcium channel blockers, α_2-agonists, ACE inhibitors and vasodilators.

Adrenergic receptors are classified as α-, β-, and dopaminergic; α- and α-receptors have been further subdivided. α_1-(Postsynaptic) receptors mediate vasoconstriction, mydriasis, gut relaxation, and gut and bladder sphincter constriction. α_2-(Presynaptic) receptors inhibit norepinephrine release. β-Receptors have been divided into β_1-receptors affecting cardiac contractility and β_2- receptors that cause peripheral vasodilation and bronchodilation. β-Blocking drugs can cause bronchoconstriction. No drug is entirely β_1-specific; all have some overlap in β_1- and β_2-blocking properties. Dopaminergic receptors affect renal blood flow.

Another class of drugs that is useful in controlling hypertension is angiotensin converting enzyme (ACE) inhibitors. An example is captopril (Capoten). Methyldopa (Aldomet), a sympatholytic drug, is useful in the intravenous and p.o. forms. Acute withdrawal of clonidine in patients who have been receiving chronic clonidine therapy for hypertension produces an especially troublesome withdrawal hypertension.

Other useful drugs to control hypertension are hydralazine, labetalol, metoprolol, nitroglycerin, and nitroprusside. Calcium channel blockers can be used to control heart rate and hypertension; these include nifedipine (Procardia), verapamil (Isoptin), diltiazem, and nadolol (Corgard). β-Blockers are more useful in controlling heart rate.

POSTOPERATIVE HYPOTENSION

Systolic blood pressures below 30% of resting preoperative baseline value or absolute values below 80 mm Hg are defined as hypotension and demand immediate assessment and intervention.

Causes of Hypotension

- Surgical bleeding, visible and occult
- Hypovolemia from inadequate fluid replacement
- Sympathetic block from conduction anesthetic or systemic drugs
- Vasodilator drug overdose (e.g., nitroglycerin)
- Arrhythmia
- Cariogenic shock
- Drug allergy, anaphylaxis
- Pneumothorax
- Pericardial tamponade
- Embolus (air, clot, etc.)

Postsurgical bleeding must be detected and treated. Some situations may require reexploration for surgical hemostasis. Blood should be available for transfusion if the blood loss is judged to be excessive. Having ruled out or treated surgical bleeding, the intravascular volume should be assessed by the same measures mentioned above (pulmonary capillary wedge pressures, deep superficial vein filling, urine flow, or arterial pressure wave form) and other causes of hypotension sought.

Treatment of Hypotension

Crystalloid or colloid solution should be used for immediate repletion of a contracted intravascular volume. While volume is being restored, the blood pressure can usually be immediately increased by using vasoconstrictors; phenylephrine and ephedrine are both useful drugs for the immediate correction of hypotension in the recovery room. Phenylephrine and ephedrine contract veins as well as arterial vascular beds and, since about 75% of the blood volume is contained in venous structures, redistribute blood from the venous to the arterial side and increase preload. Methoxamine is less useful because it is a pure α-agonist and can decrease cardiac output by arterial vasoconstriction.

After volume restoration and excluding sympathetic block, vasodilator drug overdose, or opiates as a cause of hypotension, cardiac contractility and the ECG should be assessed to detect myocardial ischemia. Other treatable causes of hypotension should be kept in mind. One useful approach is to clinically assess the CVP to separate causes associated with low CVP (hypovolemia, vasodilation) from those with increased filling pressures (pneumothorax, tamponade, embolus, cardiogenic shock).

EMERGENCE PHENOMENA

The patient emerging from a general anesthetic is frequently disoriented, in some pain, shivering, and partially responsive. Verbal communication with the emerging patient should be reassuring, to help the patient orient to time and place.

Emergence Delirium

Causes to be ruled out before nonspecific treatment is initiated include pain, a full bladder, hypoxemia, or noxious stimuli such as restraints. After the patient has been adequately treated for pain and it has been ascertained that the bladder is not full, the drugs used during the anesthesia care should be evaluated. Anticholinergics such as scopolamine and atropine can cause delirium, particularly in the presence of pain. Physostigmine (1–2 mg) is often effective in treating delirium caused by a variety of drugs including anticholinergics and ketamine or that from other, nonspecific causes. Flumazenil can be used to specifically reverse the sedative effects of benzodiazepines.

Prolonged Recovery

Residual Neuromuscular Blockade

The use of any neuromuscular blocker as part of the anesthetic technique may leave the recovering patient with residual blockade and muscle weakness, carrying with it the risk of inability to maintain a patent airway, clear secretions, take a deep breath, and cough. The use of a peripheral nerve stimulator is mandatory to measure the effect of neuromuscular blocking agents. The most sensitive clinical test of residual paralysis is the sustained head liftoff from the operating room table or stretcher for 5 seconds. In unconscious patients, a sustained tetanus using a peripheral nerve stimulator (PNS) can rule out neuromuscular block exceeding approximately 30–40% of the motor endplates. The patient who has significant neuromuscular paralysis will demonstrate a floppy, intermittent, "fish-out-of-water" movement pattern and may experience dyspnea. The partially paralyzed patient should be given ventilatory support using a bag-valve-mask or by reintubation and administering positive pressure ventilation while being treated. Residual neuromuscular blockade can be treated by additional doses of anticholinesterase. If the patient becomes stronger and the peripheral nerve stimulator indicates antagonism of the block, the patient may either be observed or be given additional anticholinesterase agent. Patients may require short-term sedation if they are being mechanically ventilated while awaiting resolution of neuromuscular blockade.

Residual Narcotic

Prolonged recovery may be due to residual narcotization. The pupils usually are small, the ventilatory rate is slow, and arterial blood gases usually demonstrate hypercarbia. A small dose of narcotic antagonist such as 20–40 μg of naloxone can be used as a therapeutic trial to determine whether ventilation increases and arousal occurs. This dose may need to be repeated in 10–20 minutes because the duration of effect of some narcotics may exceed that of naloxone. Large doses of naloxone should be avoided if possible because of undesirable side effects: pain, nausea, and hypertension.

Hypothermia

Extremely low temperature may prolong the effect of anesthetic agents. Warming is most rapid with warm forced air and warm ambient temperature. Rewarming may result in hypotension from vasodilation and in acidosis.

Neurologic Complications

Neurologic complications such as intracerebral hemorrhage must be considered in patients who fail to emerge from anesthesia in the expected amount of time. Neurologic examination for focal neurologic deficits should be performed. Diagnostic workup and neurologic consultation should be sought quickly if a significant neurologic event seems likely.

POSTOPERATIVE HYPOXEMIA

An arterial oxygen saturation in the immediate postanesthetic period of below 90% (corresponding to a PaO_2 of 60 mm Hg) is regarded as hypoxemia and should be treated and the cause sought. The routine use of pulse oximetry in the PACU has resulted in an increased awareness of postoperative hypoxemia and a greater use of supplemental oxygen. Some institutions require using supplemental oxygen during transport of all patients from the OR to PACU.

Causes of Hypoxemia

An increase in right-to-left intrapulmonary shunt is common in the immediate postanesthetic period because of a decrease in functional residual capacity (FRC), related to general anesthesia. The FRC returns to normal within 1–3 hours after general anesthesia. However, after a thoracotomy or with upper abdominal incisions, the patient may not take deep breaths, and intrapulmonary shunting is likely. Atelectasis is another cause of hypoxemia in the immediate postoperative period and may be caused by splinting, decreased respiratory drive, secretions plugging airways, previous endobronchial intubation, or residual lung compression after surgical retraction. Thoracotomy or upper abdominal surgery results in a 50% decrease in vital capacity.

Treatment of Hypoxemia

Deep breathing and coughing should be encouraged after adequate treatment of pain. The inspired oxygen can be increased to 35–40% using oxygen delivered by nasal prongs, a face mask, or shield. A close-fitting mask with a reservoir and a high fresh gas inflow can increase the inspired oxygen percentage to approximately 60%. Care should be taken to avoid increasing CO_2 rebreathing space when trying to increase inspired oxygen percentage. If coughing, deep breathing, and increase in the inspired oxygen percentage does not correct arterial desaturation, the patient may require intubation and ventilatory support provided by positive pressure. In cases of fluid overload and pulmonary edema, diuretics and vasodilators may improve oxygenation. Bronchodilators should be used to treat bronchospasm and wheezing. If upper airway obstruction is causing hypoventilation, a nasal or oral airway may be inserted as a temporary measure.

ASSESSMENT OF OTHER PROBLEMS THAT MAY ARISE IN THE POSTANESTHETIC PERIOD

Urinary Retention

The patient in the recovery room setting may have a full bladder and be unable to void. General anesthetics, opiates, and most forms of lower extremity conduction anesthesia (spinal/epidural) impair the normal voiding mechanism. If the operative site is near the urinary tract, muscle spasm may prevent normal voiding. If the patient cannot void spontaneously and complains of a full bladder, one-time catheterization may be necessary. Since some patients awakening from anesthesia may be unable to realize that the bladder is full, bladder size should be assessed by palpation. A distended bladder may cause agitation or hypertension.

Dental Damage

Dental damage may occur during anesthesia or during emergence. The most frequent injury to the teeth is abrasion of the upper incisors by the laryngoscope blade. Loose teeth may be dislodged during intubation or during emergence if the patient bites down on a hard oral airway. Dislodged teeth should be completely recovered to prevent aspiration of the tooth or tooth fragments. If there is a question of missing teeth, a chest x-ray should be performed.

Corneal Abrasions

Routine intraoperative anesthetic eye care includes taping the eyes shut with or without an ocular lubricant. Corneal abrasions can occur from objects touching the cornea, drying of the cornea if the eyes are left open, or foreign bodies under the lacrimal fold. Corneal abrasions may be diagnosed using fluorescein dye. Most corneal abrasions resolve spontaneously, but treatment including topical antibiotics and artificial eye closure may be required. An ophthalmology consultation should be obtained for diagnosis, treatment, and follow-up care.

Nerve Damage

Nerve damage can occur from stretch of upper extremity or lower extremity nerves or from direct pressure on superficial nerves. These injuries may first be apparent in the PACU but may not be evident until the patient is fully awake and beginning to move around. Brachial plexus injuries are most common, but other nerves can be injured by pressure or ischemia resulting from positioning. Most neuropathies resolve within weeks to months and are seldom permanent. A neurology consultation should be obtained, and EMG and nerve conduction studies are often performed to aid in the diagnosis of peripheral neuropathy that occurs during anesthesia.

Skin Burns or Abrasions

Skin burns or abrasions can occur from pulling sheets from underneath patients, removing adhesive pads, overheated warming mattresses, or other sources of heat or extreme cold. Precautions should be used in placing the electrical cautery grounding pad including application in a site remote from the operative field, good contact with the skin over a wide area of the grounding pad, and absence of electrical faults within the electric cautery. Elderly patients, those chronically taking steroids, and patients with skin disorders are most likely to have skin injuries. Patients undergoing long surgeries should be well padded to prevent pressure injuries. Local skin treatment should be started in the PACU when injuries are discovered and appropriate follow-up care should be arranged.

IV Extravasation

Drugs administered through the IV line may be injected into the subcutaneous tissue if the IV catheter is outside the vein lumen. Short-acting barbiturates have a pH of about 10.5 and may cause skin slough. Treatment including lidocaine, hyaluronidase (Wydase), heparin, or heat does not reliably prevent skin lesions or cellulitis after IV extravasation of drugs. Potent vasoconstrictors such as norepinephrine are particularly likely to cause skin slough, and if this occurs, a vasodilator (Regatine) or sympathetic block should be considered immediately after detection. Subcutaneous edema from an infiltrated intravenous catheter will quickly resolve if the extremity is elevated. Constricting dressings or identification bracelets should be removed to prevent a tourniquet effect.

Hoarseness

Hoarseness can occur after short-term intubation and usually resolves spontaneously within hours or a day. A sore throat may occur after intubation and may be treated by warm fluids or topical local anesthetics. If hoarseness persists beyond 48 hours, ENT consultation should be obtained to assess vocal cord function.

Aspiration

Risk factors for aspiration of gastric contents into the trachea include obesity, full stomach, hiatal hernia with reflux, pregnancy, intestinal tract obstruction or ileus, and extrinsic pressure on the epigastrium. Aspiration of acidic gastric contents is recognized by tachypnea, wheezing, hypoxemia, and infiltrate on chest x-ray. Intubation and tracheal suction is usually indicated for significant aspiration. Distending airway pressure with positive pressure ventilation is indicated to normalize arterial oxygen saturation. Antibiotics may be indicated, but steroids have not been found to be useful in the prevention or treatment of the acid aspiration syndrome.

Pulmonary acid aspiration should be treated rapidly because this complication is associated with high mortality.

Oliguria

Assuming normal preoperative renal function, the intraanesthetic urine flow should be 0.5–1.0 ml/kg/hr, and a urine flow below 0.5 ml/kg/hr is defined as oliguria.

When there is postoperative oliguria, assessment should include systemic blood pressure, cardiac preload, and possible obstruction of the urinary drainage system.

Hemodynamics should be optimized with fluid challenges, and if necessary, inotropic agents should be administered to increase cardiac output and renal perfusion. Invasive monitoring may be required for better assessment. If oliguria persists, a urine sample should be sent for urinalysis, sodium concentration, and osmolality to differentiate prerenal causes from acute tubular necrosis. A 2-hour creatinine clearance may be performed.

Hypothermia

The patient under anesthesia loses heat to the environment and may become hypothermic, with a 3–4°C heat loss not uncommon. As the patient emerges from general anesthesia, heat is produced by shivering, which increases oxygen consumption and may result in hypoxemia and metabolic acidosis. Cardiac output is increased to meet metabolic demands and may result in angina in patients with coronary artery disease. Most patients emerging from general anesthesia should be given additional oxygen, severe shivering should be treated, and cardiac output and oxygen-carrying capacity should be optimized. Shivering can be treated by warming the skin with warm blankets, forced air warmers, or warming lights. Small doses of opiates (meperidine) may be effective in treating shivering. In patients with limited cardiac reserve, intraoperative hypothermia is an indication for postoperative sedation and mechanical ventilation to allow gradual warming. Hypothermia is best prevented by intraoperative use of heated forced-air blankets.

CRITERIA FOR DISCHARGE FROM PACU

The anesthesiologist responsible for the patient's care should preferably be the person evaluating the patient for discharge from the PACU.

Assess both the patient's medical conditions and specifics relating to the surgery:

Sensorium and reflexes
Pain
Vital signs (BP, P, Resp, Temp, CVP, PCW, etc.)
Bleeding
Urine flow
Muscle relaxant reversal
Preexisting medical conditions (e.g., diabetes mellitus)
Laboratory assessment

Before patients are ready for discharge to either routine ward care or further intensive care, they should be alert, oriented, and possess normal cough and gag reflexes. (Some patients may be intentionally sedated to tolerate ventilatory support.) Pain should be adequately controlled. Blood pressure and pulse rate should be within acceptable limits: usually within 30% of the preinduction or resting systolic blood pressure, and generally the pulse rate should be below 100/min. There should be no evidence of surgical bleeding, urine flow should be adequate, and there should be no evidence of residual muscle paralysis if neuromuscular blocking drugs were used. Supplemental oxygen should be ordered for patients who have inadequate oxygen saturation measured on room air. For patients who have had significant blood loss, postoperative Hct and possibly coagulation tests should be checked, and the patient treated if necessary. ECG should be performed if indicated in patients with ischemic heart disease or if there was intraoperative evidence of ischemia. Chest x-ray should be evaluated in patients who have had placement of a central venous catheter, will retain an endotracheal tube, or have had a surgical procedure that may produce pulmonary pathology such as pneumothorax. Appropriate laboratory tests should be performed based on the patient's medical and surgical condition.

If the patient has received regional anesthesia as a primary anesthetic technique, the sensory block should be receding, there should be no evidence of hypotension from autonomic blockade, and there should be evidence of returning voluntary muscle function. Patients who had spinal or epidural anesthesia should be warned to stay in bed until full return of motor and autonomic function, and an order should be written requesting that an assistant be present the first time the patient gets out of bed.

WHAT TO DO FOR THE PATIENT WHO DOES NOT AWAKEN

Three general areas should be investigated for the patient who does not emerge from general anesthesia as expected. Residual volatile anesthetics, residual narcotization from opiates, and prolonged paralysis from neuromuscular blockers should be excluded as soon as possible. The patient who is narcotized has small pupils and ventilatory depression with a low respiratory rate. Arterial blood gases may show hypercarbia. If the patient is suspected of having residual narcotic effect, titration of small doses of naloxone can be used as a diagnostic and therapeutic intervention. A blockade monitor can be used to assess the presence and degree of residual neuromuscular blockade. A sustained tetanus at 100 Hz is strong evidence for excluding residual muscle paralysis. If there is a fade on tetanic stimulation, an additional dose of anticholinesterase may be given. If other sedatives such as scopolamine have been used, a trial of edrophonium should be considered, and benzodiazepines can be reversed with flumazenil. Hypoglycemia can be detected by blood glucose measurement.

When these causes have been ruled out, more serious neurologic complications such as intracerebral hemorrhage or ischemia must be considered. Neurologic examination for localizing signs should be performed, and neurologic consultation obtained. Rapid diagnosis by CT scan or MRI should be performed to look for treatable complications. Routine use of continuous pulse oximetry has improved recognition of hypoxic events, but prolonged hypoxemia is another possible cause of failure to awaken.

Suggested Readings

Bevan DR, Donati F, Kopman AF. Reversal of neuromuscular blockade. Anesthesiology 1992;77:785–805.

Kovac AL. Use of serotonin receptor antagonists in the prevention and treatment of nausea and vomiting. Hosp Formul 1993;28:988–998.

Marshall BE, Wyche MQ. Hypoxemia during and after anesthesia. Anesthesiology 1972;37:178–209.

Martin JT. Compartment syndromes: concepts and perspectives for the anesthesiologist. Anesth Analg 1992;75:275–283.

Shapiro G. Postanesthesia care unit problems. Anesth Clin North Am 1990;8:2.

Watcha MF, White PF. Postoperative nausea and vomiting: its etiology, treatment, and prevention. Anesthesiology 1992;77:162–184.

Woolf CJ, Chong MS. Preemptive analgesia—treating postoperative pain by preventing the establishment of central sensitization. Anesth Analg 1993;77:362–379.

Chapter 22

Postoperative Pain Management

Recent advances in pharmacologic agents and delivery systems for postoperative analgesia have improved patient outcome (1, 2) and potentially lowered overall surgical costs (3). This increase in sophistication and demand for greater technical skills has led to the explosive growth of postoperative pain management as a subspecialty in anesthesiology.

SYSTEMIC OPIOIDS

Systemic opioid administration remains the cornerstone of postoperative analgesic therapy. Familiarity, efficacy, ease of administration, and the relative safety record of systemic opioids have made them the most commonly used analgesic drugs. While new agonist-antagonists have proliferated in recent years, pure narcotic receptor agonists, such as morphine, are still the standard for comparison.

Practitioners who use narcotics for postoperative pain management should know the pharmacokinetic differences between drugs, including half-life ($t_{1/2}$), relative potency, and oral bioavailability (Table 22.1). Historically, anesthesiologists administered intravenous opioids in the operating room, using an understanding of IV pharmacokinetics. While easily titrated and advantageous to use in the operating room, opioids with short half-lives, such as alfentanil, are not appropriate for postoperative analgesia. Lipophilic opioids, such as fentanyl and sufentanil, cross the blood-brain barrier quickly and have short onset times. However, these opioids are redistributed quickly into a large volume-of-distribution, and their clinical effects are brief unless steady-state is reached. Opioids with intermediate half-

487

Table 22.1.
**Selective Pharmacokinetic Data of Narcotic Agents Commonly
Used for Postoperative Pain Management**

Narcotic	Onset (min)	$T_{1/2}$ (hr)	Equianalgesic Dose (mg)	Approximate Oral Bioavailability
Morphine	15–60	2–3	10	30–40%
Meperidine	10–45	3–4	100	40–60%
Hydromorphone	15–30	2–3	1.5	20%
Codeine	15–30	3	40	60%
Fentanyl citrate	7–8	1.5	0.1	ND
Methadone	30–60	15–30	10	80%
Pentazocine	15–60	2–4	60	20%
Propoxyphene	30–60	8–24	ND	40%
Buprenorphine	15–30	3	0.3	60%[a]

[a]Sublingual administration; ND, not determined.

lives, such as morphine, meperidine, and hydromorphone, are most commonly used for postoperative analgesia. While onset time is slower than that of more lipophilic opioids, their intermediate half-life permits maintenance of adequate plasma levels without frequent boluses or risk of accumulation.

The goal of opioid therapy is to balance analgesia against sedation and respiratory depression. A therapeutic window exists for opioid blood levels, below which pain relief is inadequate and above which undesirable effects occur. Minimum effective analgesic concentration (MEAC) is the minimum plasma concentration of an opioid that provides analgesia. The curve describing the relationship between analgesic response and blood levels becomes quite steep. Thus, as MEAC is approached, very small increases in drug level result in large decreases in pain scores. Although MEAC is remarkably constant for a particular individual, the levels required for different patients are quite variable. In Austin's study, a fourfold difference in MEAC was found between patients, emphasizing the need for individualization of analgesic therapy (4).

Problems of traditional intramuscular (IM) drug administration include pain from administration, accidental intravenous or intraneural injection, long delays between patient request and medication delivery, and a labor-intensive burden on the nursing staff. In addition, parenteral opioids, such as morphine or meperidine, administered every 3–4 hours, result in drug levels exceeding the MEAC during only 15–75% of the dosing interval (5). During periods of peak drug levels, the patient is often oversedated, and during periods when drug levels fall below MEAC, the patient has inadequate analgesia (Fig. 22.1.).

The unpredictability associated with IM opioids stems from both variability in absorption and the narrow range of therapeutic blood levels within a single patient.

Intravenous administration of opioids prevents the absorption problems seen with IM administration and allows careful titration to effect; however, after a single IV bolus, blood levels quickly fall below MEAC, making frequent dosing necessary. Continuous intravenous infusion (CII) of opioids relieves postoperative pain quite effectively (6–8). CII of meperidine at 0.3 mg/kg/hour results in sufficient analgesia for 80% of patients (6). The remaining 20% required adjustment of the CII rate to achieve adequate analgesia. A loading dose should be given at the start of a CII and with each increase in infusion rate, so that steady-state plasma levels are quickly achieved (9).

Patient-controlled Analgesia

Recent advances in infusion pump technology have resulted in devices that can deliver preset doses of IV opioids at patient request. In patient-controlled analgesia (PCA), the prescribing physician sets the amount of opioid to be given with each dose,

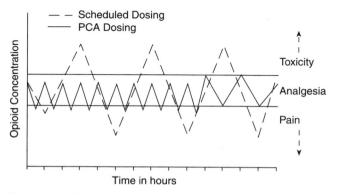

Figure 22.1 Opioid concentration with periodic parenteral dosing compared with PCA dosing (see text).

a minimum delay interval between doses, and an hourly allowable limit. Some devices also allow administration of a continuous background infusion.

A small amount of opioid per dose is usually chosen to allow for optimal incremental titration. Typically, morphine (1–1.5 mg/dose) or meperidine (10–15 mg/dose) is chosen. The delay interval, or "lock-out" period, commonly ranges from 5 to 15 minutes. This interval is long enough to allow patient evaluation of the drug effect, yet short enough to allow redosing, if necessary. The usual PCA settings for various opioids are shown in Table 22.2.

The hourly dosage limit is purposely set high to permit peak usage during especially painful periods, such as physical therapy, dressing changes, or ambulation. In actual practice, these hourly limits are rarely reached, since most patients prefer some pain to excessive sedation. A published report by Graves et al. confirms that postoperative patients tend not to overuse or abuse narcotics in a self-dosing situation (10).

Although clinically significant respiratory depression related to operator error has occurred (11), it is rare with PCA. This is because patients become sedated (and so unable to administer subsequent doses) before ventilation is impaired.

PCA remains extremely popular because it allows patients to participate in their own care, overcoming the inherent pharmacokinetic and pharmacodynamic differences that exist among patients (12). Studies comparing the use of PCA with conventional IM opioid therapy have shown that PCA results in greater pain relief and/or a higher degree of patient satisfaction. This improvement in pain relief is seen with less sedation (13), and it requires either the same (14) or slightly lower doses

Table 22.2.
Suggested PCA Settings

Drug	Conc (mg/ml)	Dose (mg)	Lockout (min)	Basal (mg/hr)
Morphine	1	1–1.5	5–15	0–1
Meperidine	10	10–15	5–15	0–10
Hydromorphone	0.25	0.25–0.375	5–15	0–0.25
Fentanyl	0.01	0.010–.020	5–8	0–0.020
Buprenorphine	0.03	0.03–0.045	5–15	0–0.03

of opioid than would have been given IM (15, 16). However, patients using the PCA technique show little or no improvement in postoperative pulmonary function, compared with using intermittent IM opioid administration (17, 18).

Other opioid delivery systems that appear to hold promise include transdermal and slow-release oral, buccal, sublingual, transnasal, and subcutaneous routes of administration (12). Therapeutic plasma fentanyl concentrations can be achieved with a transcutaneous delivery system. The prolonged time required to achieve stable analgesic levels (5–15 hours) and the slow decline in drug levels after patch removal (owing to skin drug depot) have raised concerns about this technique (19–21). Transdermal delivery does not allow rapid titration to achieve patient analgesia. Iontophoretic control of transdermal delivery is under investigation. The application of electric current to the transdermal system may allow rapid titration to patient response.

Fentanyl, methadone, and buprenorphine all have good transmucosal bioavailability (22). Regardless of the site of administration, transmucosal delivery provides a nonpainful route of delivery that avoids gastrointestinal degradation and first-pass hepatic metabolism (23). An oral fentanyl preparation (oralet) appears to have excellent bioavailability and titratability. Unfortunately, the issues of narcotic control and disposal (to prevent abuse) and side effects (nausea and vomiting) have limited its use.

LOCAL ANESTHETICS/PERIPHERAL NERVE BLOCKS

Local anesthetic nerve blocks can provide postoperative analgesia in certain circumstances, and historically, they are how anesthesiologists entered the area of postoperative pain management. Some of the more common peripheral nerve blocks for postoperative analgesia are listed in Table 22.3.

These blocks are easy, quick, and safe to perform, but their use is limited by the short duration of analgesia in relation to the duration of postoperative pain. For intermittent injection, 0.5% bupivacaine with epinephrine 1:2000,000 is the commonly used local anesthetic. When injected around a peripheral nerve, this agent produces a dense sensory block that provides pain relief for 12–24 hours.

Table 22.3
Common Peripheral Nerve Blocks for
Postoperative Analgesia

Surgical Site	Nerve Block
Shoulder/arm	Brachial plexus
Thoracic	Intercostal
Flank	Intercostal
Abdomen	Intercostal
Groin	Ilioiuguinal/iliohypogastric
Knee	Femoral

In an attempt to achieve prolonged analgesia, catheters may be placed in both the brachial plexus and femoral nerve sheaths. New catheters are available with "B" bevel needles or a rounded obturator, which help minimize potential nerve damage. For continuous infusion through an indwelling catheter, a dose of 0.15–0.25% bupivacaine usually provides a dense sensory block. The infusion rate differs for each type of block.

Many techniques have been described for placement of a catheter in the femoral sheath. The following procedure has been used very successfully in our practice. Using a peripheral nerve stimulator (Stimuplex-S-Burron), a Contiplex (Burron) needle/catheter is advanced one finger-breadth lateral to the femoral artery in the inguinal crease until quadriceps contraction is obtained with less than 0.5 mAmp. After withdrawal of the needle, a 20-gauge polyamide catheter is inserted 5–10 cm through the 18-gauge Teflon catheter and is secured with adhesive strips and a transparent dressing. Postoperatively, 10 ml of bupivacaine 0.25% with epinephrine 1:200,000 is injected through the femoral catheter, followed by a continuous infusion of bupivacaine 0.25% at 7 ml/hr. For inadequate analgesia, a 10-ml bolus of bupivacaine 0.25% is administered, and the infusion rate is increased by 2–4 ml/hr.

In a study of 22 patients following total knee arthroplasty, we found that patients with femoral nerve analgesia (FNA) had less pain than a control group during the first 24 hours following surgery and that passive range of motion progressed more quickly with FNA (24). Because the knee is innervated by the sciatic, lateral femoral cutaneous, and obturator nerves in addition to the femoral nerve, patients continue to have pain that requires treatment with potent systemic analgesics.

Infusion of local anesthetics into the pleural space of the thoracic cavity has received attention since Reiestad and Stromskog published this technique in 1986 (25). The use of intrapleural local anesthetics was reported to provide pain relief after cholecystectomy and renal and breast surgery in which there was a unilateral incision involving thoracic dermatomes. Also,it has been used for analgesia following thoracotomy and for the treatment of postherpetic neuralgia, reflex sympathetic dystrophy, and pancreatitis.

For prolonged postoperative analgesia, a catheter is placed in the interpleural space, with the patient in a 450 or full lateral position. The rib (5th or 8th) is palpated 8–10 cm lateral to the posterior midline. Following local infiltration, an epidural needle is directed slightly toward the midline and is advanced over the rib with a well-lubricated, air-filled, glass syringe attached. When the parietal pleura is penetrated, the plunger of the syringe falls because of the negative interpleural pressure. The syringe is removed, an epidural catheter is placed through the needle, and the needle is removed. A catheter can also be placed under direct vision during thoracotomy. Bupivacaine 0.5% with epinephrine 20 ml is injected as needed for pain. Although analgesia may last up to 12 hours, most patients require redosing at 4–6 hours.

The mechanism of action of the interpleural analgesic technique has yet to be proven, but it is postulated that the local anesthetic diffuses through the parietal pleura and endothoracic fascia to anesthetize the intercostal nerves. However, a sensory deficit to pinprick in the distribution of the intercostal nerves is not reliably obtained.

The initial enthusiasm for this technique has been tempered by the requirement for intermittent injections of local anesthetic every 4–8 hours and relatively poor results following thoracotomy. High peak plasma concentrations of local anesthetic may occur following bolus injection, and cases of local anesthetic toxicity have been reported in patients with pleural effusions. Infusion techniques have been uniformly disappointing (26).

INTRASPINAL OPIOIDS

After Wang reported profound and prolonged relief of cancer pain after intrathecal injections of morphine, intrathecal and epidural opioids began to be frequently applied for postoperative pain (27, 28). Analgesia is mediated by opioid receptors located in the substantia gelatinosa of the dorsal horn region of the spinal cord. Opioid binding to the receptors selectively inhibits the transmission of ascending pain signals in the spinal cord (29).

The major advantage of intraspinal (epidural or intrathecal) administration of opioids over systemic administration is that patients experience more complete pain relief with less sedation. This in turn results in improved postoperative pulmonary function. Intravenous morphine analgesia relief was shown by Bromage et al. to increase FEV_1 above the value obtained while the patient was in pain (30) (Fig. 22.2); however, the FEV_1 was only 44.5% of the preoperative value. When analgesia was obtained via epidural administration of morphine or local anesthetic, patients had an increase in FEV_1 to 68% of the preoperative value. Shulman et al. also found that epidural morphine was more effective than IV morphine in preventing a decrease in FEV_1 after thoracotomy (31). Although it is difficult to show a relationship between improved FEV_1 and prevention of pulmonary complications, Rawal et al. demonstrated that morbidly obese patients who received epidural morphine had fewer pulmonary complications after gastroplasty than those who received IM morphine (1).

In a randomized, prospective comparison of epidural anesthesia and analgesia (EAA) with general anesthesia and postoperative systemic opioids, Yeager et al. found a decreased incidence of pulmonary failure, cardiovascular failure, and major infection in the group of patients who received EAA (2). In addition, the patients in the group receiving EAA had a shorter period of postoperative intubation and lower hospitalization costs. Unfortunately, it is impossible to separate the effects of the combined epidural/general anesthetic received by the patients in the treatment group from their method of analgesia. Most patients in the control group had a high-dose opioid general anesthetic and remained intubated postoperatively. However, analgesia may affect outcome by avoiding the need for postoperative intubation in high-risk patients.

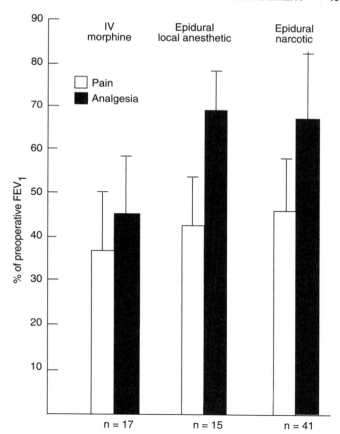

Figure 22.2.   FEV$_1$ values as percentage of preoperative values after upper abdominal surgery, before and after relief of pain with intravenous morphine, epidural local anesthetic, and epidural narcotic (means ± SD). FEV$_1$ is significantly improved after epidural local anesthetic or narcotic. (From Bromage PR, Camporesi E, Chestnut D. Epidural narcotics for postoperative analgesia. Anesth Analg 1980;59:473–480. With permission from the International Anesthesia Research Society.)

The cost-effectiveness of intraspinal opioids was confirmed by Isaacson et al. in patients undergoing aortic reconstructive surgery (3). Patients who received intrathecal morphine had shorter intubation times, length of ICU care, and total hospital days, as well as significantly reduced hospitalization costs.

INTRATHECAL OPIOIDS

Morphine is the most commonly used drug for intrathecal administration, because its low lipid solubility gives it a longer duration of action than that of other opioids. Preservative-free opioids should always be used for intraspinal administration to prevent direct neurotoxicity from formaldehyde, phenol, or chlorobutanol, which may be used as preservatives in multidose preparations. Although as little as 0.2 mg of morphine is an effective intrathecal dose, doses of 0.5–1.0 mg are commonly used to extend the duration of action. Since there is no significant difference between the half-lives of morphine in plasma and cerebrospinal fluid (CSF), prolonged analgesia from intrathecal morphine relies heavily on achieving extremely high peak CSF morphine levels so that effective analgesic levels are maintained for 16–24 hours.

Intrathecal morphine has a slow onset time (the time to maximum analgesia may be 30–60 minutes) and is usually given before the operation so that the patient is comfortable immediately after surgery. Intrathecal administration of morphine is associated with a relatively high incidence of nausea, itching, urinary retention, and respiratory depression caused by cephalad migration in the CSF, so most practitioners limit use of intrathecal morphine to patients who will be observed in an ICU for the first 24 hours. These side effects are all reversible with naloxone (32, 33).

EPIDURAL OPIOIDS

Epidural catheter placement allows the use of either repeated bolus doses or continuous infusion of opioids. The placement of lumbar and thoracic epidural catheters requires special technical training but is easy and safe to perform. The risk of infection or neurologic damage from prolonged infusion is minimal when proper techniques are used. The placement of an epidural catheter provides dosing flexibility and permits using the minimum effective dose, thereby decreasing the incidence of side effects.

Epidural administration of opioids is associated with plasma levels that are equivalent to an IM-administered dose; however, for hydrophilic opioids, the analgesia is more profound. The improved analgesia is produced by epidural opioids that reach the CSF by diffusion directly through the dura (34). Once in the CSF, the opioid bathes the spinal cord and penetrates to reach opioid receptors in the dorsal horn. Lipid-soluble opioids, such as fentanyl and sufentanil, penetrate the dura and spinal cord tissue rapidly but are also quickly absorbed or redistributed into the plasma from both the epidural space and CSF. This necessitates epidural dosage requirements that are similar to doses administered systemically. In contrast, hydrophilic opioids, such as morphine, penetrate the dura more slowly and have a longer duration of action and slower CSF clearance. The greater spread of hydrophilic opioids in the CSF provides a wider area of analgesia but increases the risk of rostral spread and respiratory depression.

Many opioids have been used for epidural analgesia. Recommended doses are listed in Table 22.4. Continuous infusion of opioids is usually preferable, because peak and trough CSF levels are avoided, and side effects are minimized (Table 22.5).

Table 22.4
Intermittent Bolus Dose, Onset, and Duration of Epidural Opioids

Narcotic	Dose (mg)	Onset (min)	Duration (hr)
Morphine	4–10	20–30	16–24
Meperidine	50–100	4–6	4–6
Fentanyl citrate	0.05–0.1	5–10	4–6
Methadone	4–6	10	6–8
Hydromorphone	1	15–20	8–10

Table 22.5
Average Concentrations of Epidural Opioids Used for Continuous Infusion

Narcotic	Average Concentration[a] (mg/ml)	Dose/Hour	
		Average	Range
Morphine	0.05	0.5 mg	0.25–1.5
Meperidine	1.0	10 mg	5–20
Methadone	0.05	0.5 mg	0.25–1.5
Fentanyl citrate	0.005	50 μg	25–150

[a]Mixed with preservative-free normal saline.

Epidural morphine has been extensively studied and is highly effective for thoracic pain, even when administered in the lumbar region (35). The most troublesome side effect of epidurally administered morphine is pruritus, which is not related to histamine release. Severe pruritus occasionally responds to diphenhydramine but usually requires treatment with naloxone (1 mg/kg/hr) or nalbuphine (5–10 mg q 4 hr). Respiratory depression has also been occasionally described, occurring up to 6 hours after a bolus dose of epidural morphine. This "late respiratory depression" is due to cephalad migration of morphine in the CSF, resulting from its low lipid solubility. In many hospitals, the risk of late respiratory depression has limited the use of epidural morphine to the ICU.

Meperidine, which has intermediate lipid solubility, appears to be an effective epidural analgesic with an effective epidural dose that is approximately 30% of that required for analgesia when given systemically. The incidence of both nausea and pruritus is extremely low. Meperidine also has a weak local anesthetic effect and appears to be synergistic with other local anesthetics.

Fentanyl and sufentanil are commonly used for epidural infusion, and some evidence suggests that these opioids are effective when given as bolus doses. However, fentanyl appears to be no more effective when given by the lumbar epidural route than when given intravenously, since steady-state plasma concentrations and dose requirements are identical (36–38). Although postoperative analgesia can be obtained by an epidural infusion of fentanyl, the need for placement of an epidural catheter for the administration of this drug may not be warranted. More studies on fentanyl are needed to determine whether thoracic epidural administration is more effective than lumbar. Although sufentanil is highly lipophilic, it has high receptor affinity, which may affect its intraspinal efficacy.

EPIDURAL LOCAL ANESTHETICS

Local anesthetics are much more effective in the prevention of pain than opioids. Epidural local anesthetics have long been used for surgical and obstetric anesthesia but, until recently, were rarely used outside the operating room. A comparison of epidural bupivacaine with epidural morphine revealed that better postoperative pain relief was achieved with the local anes-

Table 22.6
**Epidural Placement for Local
Anesthestic Infusions**

Procedure	Level
Thoracotomy	T6
Upper abdominal	T8
Lower abdominal	T10
Lower extremity	L3

thetic, but accompanying motor weakness and urinary retention were distressful to the patients (39). By using continuous infusion techniques, these side effects can be almost totally avoided, and the risk of tachyphylaxis minimized. Extensive motor and sensory blockade is prevented by placing the epidural catheter at the appropriate dermatomal level (Table 22.6) and by using a dilute local anesthetic solution (bupivacaine 0.1–0.15%). Prevention of motor blockade to the legs is important so that patients can be out of bed early in the postoperative period. The addition of an opioid improves analgesia (40).

Hypotension from sympathetic nerve blockade is the most troublesome problem with epidural administration of local anesthetics. Hypotension can usually be prevented by adequate hydration with IV fluids and titration of local anesthetic to the lowest effective volume and concentration. However, in some patients, these precautions will not prevent hypotension. In this situation, an epidural opioid without local anesthetic can be used to prevent sympathetic blockade and hypotension.

NONOPIOID ANALGESICS

While local anesthetics and opioid analgesics have traditionally been used for postoperative pain management, other modalities are useful adjuvants. Nonsteroidal antiinflammatory drugs (NSAIDs) reduce pain, swelling, and inflammation that develop after surgery. Ketorolac, a potent prostaglandin inhibitor, has profound analgesic and opioid-sparing effects. Opioid-related side effects such as postoperative ventilatory depression, nausea, and sedation are avoided (41). The usual dose of ketorolac is 30–60 mg given by IM injection every 6 hours. The absorption of ketorolac from the gut is nearly complete.

α_2-Agonists (i.e., clonidine, dexmedetomidine) and the enkephalinase inhibitors may prove effective in modulating post-operative pain. Nonpharmacologic approaches to decreasing postoperative pain that are potentially efficacious include trans-cutaneous electrical nerve stimulation (TENS), cryoanalgesia, acupuncture, and hypnosis (12).

SUMMARY

Using modern anesthetic principles and techniques, surgical morbidity has become mainly a postoperative occurrence, even in the most moribund patient. The anesthesiologist's role in creating a more favorable surgical outcome through the use of postoperative analgesia is becoming firmly established. By low-ering morbidity and mortality, increasing patient satisfaction, and decreasing medical expenses, anesthesiologists are ex-tending their expertise into pain management in the postopera-tive period.

References

1. Rawal N, Sjostrand U, Christoffersson E, et al. Comparison of intra-muscular and epidural morphine for postoperative analgesia in the grossly obese: influence on postoperative ambulation and pulmo-nary function. Anesth Analg 1984;63:583–592.

2. Yeager MP, Glass DD, Neff RK, et al. Epidural anesthesia and anal-gesia in high-risk surgical patients. Anesthesiology 1987;66:729–736.

3. Isaacson IJ, Weitz FI, Berry AJ, et al. Intrathecal morphine's effect on the postoperative course of patients undergoing abdominal aor-tic surgery. Anesth Analg 1987;66:S86.

4. Austin KL, Stapleton JV, Mather LE. Relationship between blood meperidine concentrations and analgesic response: a preliminary report. Anesthesiology 1980;53:460–466.

5. Austin KL, Stapleton JV, Mather LE. Multiple intramuscular injec-tions: a major source of variability in analgesic response to meperi-dine. Pain 1980;8:47–62.

6. Church JJ. Continuous narcotic infusions for relief of postoperative pain. Br Med J 1979:1:977–979.

7. Rutter PC, Murphy F, Dudley HA. Morphine: controlled trial of different methods of administration for postoperative pain relief. Br Med J 1980;1:12–3.

8. Nimmo WS, Todd JG. Fentanyl by constant rate infusion for postop-erative analgesia. Br J Anaesth 1985;57:250–254.

9. Portenoy RK. Continuous intravenous infusion of opioid drugs. Med Clin North Am 1987;71(2):233–241.

10. Graves DA, Arrigo JM, Foster TS, et al. Relationship between plasma morphine concentrations and pharmacologic effects in postoperative patients using patient-controlled analgesia. Clin Pharm 1985;4:41–47.

11. White PF. Mishaps with patient-controlled analgesia. Anesthesiology 1987;66(1);81–83.

12. White PF. Current and future trends in acute pain management. Clin J Pain 1989;5(suppl 1):551–558.

13. Bennett RL, Batenhorst RL, Bivins BA, et al. Patient-controlled analgesia: a new concept of postoperative pain relief. Ann Surg 1982;195(6):700–705.

14. Bollish SJ, Collins CL, Kirking DM, et al. Efficacy of patient-controlled versus conventional analgesia for postoperative pain. Clin Pharm 1985;4:48–52.

15. Robinson JO, Rosen M, Evans JM, et al. Self-administered intravenous and intramuscular pethidine: a controlled trial in labour. Anaesthesia 1980;35:763–770.

16. Bennett RL, Batenhorst RL, Bivins BA, et al. Drug use pattern in patient-controlled analgesia. Anesthesiology 1982;57(3):A210.

17. Bennett R, Batenhorst RL, Foster TS, et al. Postoperative pulmonary function with patient-controlled analgesia. Anesth Analg 1982;61(2):171.

18. Rosenberg PH, Heino A, Scheinin B. Comparison of intramuscular analgesia, intercostal block, epidural morphine and on-demand IV fentanyl in the control of pain after upper abdominal surgery. Acta Anaesthesiol Scand 1984;28:603–607.

19. Caplan RA, Ready LB, Olsson GL, Nessly ML. Transdermal delivery of fentanyl for postoperative pain control. Anesthesiology 1986;65:A196.

20. Duthie DJR, Rowbotham DJ, Wyld R, Henderson PD, Nimmo WS. Plasma fentanyl concentrations during transdermal delivery of fentanyl to surgical patients. Br J Anaesth 1988;60:614–618.

21. Holley FO, Van Steenis C. Postoperative analgesia with fentanyl: pharmacokinetics and pharmacodynamics of constant-rate I.V. and transdermal delivery. Br J Anaesth 1988;60:608–613.

22. Weinberg DS, Inturrisi CE, Reidenberg B, et al. Sublingual absorption of selected opioid analgesics. Clin Pharm Ther 1988;44:335–342.

23. Striesand JB, Stanley TH. Opiods: new techniques in routes of administration. Curr Opinions Anesth 1989;2:456–462.

24. Hord AH, Roberson JR, Thompson WF, et al. Evaluation of continuous femoral nerve analgesia after primary total knee arthroplasty. Anesth Analg 1990;70:S164.

25. Reiestad F, Stromskag KE. Intrapleural catheter in the management of postoperative pain: a preliminary report. Reg Anaesth 1986;11:89–91.

26. Covino BG. Intrapleural regional analgesia. Anesth Analg 1988;67:427–429.

27. Wang JK. Analgesic effect of intrathecally administered morphine. Reg Anaesth 1977;2:3–8.

28. Wang JK, Nauss LA, Thomas JE. Pain relief by intrathecally applied morphine in man. Anesthesiology 1979;50:149–151.

29. Zieglansberger W. Opioid actions on mammalian spinal neurons. Int Rev Neurobiol 1984;25:243.

30. Bromage PR, Camporesi E, Chestnut D. Epidural narcotics for post-operative analgesia. Anesth Analg 1980;59:473–480.

31. Shulman M, Sandler AN, Bradley JW, et al. Post-thoracotomy pain and pulmonary function following epidural and systemic morphine. Anesthesiology 1984;61:569–575.

32. Rawal N, Wattwil M. Respiratory depression after epidural morphine—an experimental and clinical study. Anesth Analg 1984;63:8–14.

33. Rawal N, Mollefors K, Axelsson K, et al. An experimental study of urodynamic effects of epidural morphine and of naloxone reversal. Anesth Analg 1983;62:641–647.

34. Sjostrom S, Tamsen A, Persson MP, et al. Pharmacokinetics of intrathecal morphine and meperidine in humans. Anesthesiology 1987;67:889–895.

35. Fromme GA, Steidl LJ, Danielson DR. Comparison of lumbar and thoracic epidural morphine for relief of post-thoracotomy pain. Anesth Analg 1985;64:454–455.

36. Loper KA, Ready LB, Sandler AN, et al. Epidural and intravenous fentanyl infusions are clinically equivalent following knee surgery. Anesth 1989;71:A1149.

37. Ellis DJ, Millar WL, Reisner LS. Comparison of epidural and intravenous fentanyl infusions after cesarean section. Anesthesiology 1989;71:A1153.

38. Badner NH, Sadler AN, et al. Lumbar epidural fentanyl infusions for post-thoracotomy patients: analgesic, respiratory and pharmacokinetic effects. J Cardiothorac Anesth 1990;4:543–551.

39. Modig J, Paalzow L. A comparison of epidural morphine and epidural bupivacaine for postoperative pain relief. Acta Anaesthesiol Scand 1981;25:437–441.

40. Logas WG, El-Baz N, El-Ganzouri A, et al. Continuous thoracic epidural and analgesia for postoperative pain relief following thoracotomy: a randomized prospective study. Anesthesiology 1987;67:787–791.

41. Gillies GW, Kenny GNC, et al. The morphine sparing effects of ketorolac tromethamine. Anaesth 1987;42:727–731.

Chapter 23

Chronic Pain Management

Chronic pain is a major health problem afflicting an estimated 65,000,000 people in the United States (1). In addition to the physical consequences of pain, there are social, psychic, and economic consequences. Pain leads to an impaired quality of life, disability, lost productivity, increased insurance and health care costs, depression, and invalidism. Bonica said, in the first edition of his book *The Management of Pain,* **"The proper management of pain remains, after all, the most important obligation, the main objective, and the crowning achievement of every physician"** (2). Anesthesiologists are the medical specialists who most commonly are involved in pain management and usually occupy leadership positions in pain treatment facilities.

POSTHERPETIC NEURALGIA

Postherpetic neuralgia (PHN) follows herpes zoster (HZ) in approximately 10% of all patients afflicted with this varicella virus infection. It is rare in younger patients with HZ, but more than half of the elderly afflicted develop PHN. PHN has been variously defined as pain following HZ that persists beyond 1, 3, 6, or 12 months. I arbitrarily define PHN as pain that persists more than 3 months after the eruption of the HZ rash. In 1965, Colding advocated sympathetic nerve blocks for treatment of HZ pain (3). He also made the poorly supported claim that if sympathetic nerve blocks were done within the first 14 days after the appearance of the rash, the incidence of PHN as reduced. Recent research has cast doubt on this finding (4, 5).

Mechanism of Pain

The herpesvirus preferentially destroys large myelinated fibers in peripheral nerves. In the gate control theory of pain, large fiber input to the dorsal horn of the spinal cord is believed to modulate nociception (6). A decrease in the population of large fibers impairs the central nervous system's ability to modulate pain.

Treatment for HZ Pain

Treatment for pain in patients with HZ (onset of rash less than 3 months), includes the following:

1. **Sympathetic or somatic nerve blocks** often relieve the neuralgic pain. This pain relief lasts longer than the expected duration of the local anesthetic. The blocks do not hasten resolution of the rash and probably do not prevent the development of the PHN.
2. **Oral analgesics,** such as nonsteroidal antiinflammatory analgesics or narcotic analgesics, are often often necessary to keep the patient comfortable.
3. The patient should receive **informative reassurance** about the natural history of HZ.

Treatment for PHN

Treatment for pain in patients with PHN (onset of rash more than 3 months ago) includes the following:

1. The first line of treatment is **tricyclic antidepressant** drugs. Amitriptyline is the most commonly used antidepressant, and its effectiveness is supported by randomized, double-blind studies (7, 8). Therapy should be started with a small dose, given once daily at bedtime, and increased until side effects (most commonly dry mouth, increased appetite, and drowsiness) interfere with compliance. If side effects limit the patient's willingness to take this medication, a different tricyclic antidepressant should be tried.
2. **Topical capsaicin,** 0.025%, has proven effective in relieving the pain of PHN in randomized double-blind studies (9). Burning or itching of the skin to which capsaicin has been applied may produce a lack of patient compliance. **Topical**

lidocaine is said to reduce the cutaneous burning and might, through its own action, benefit the patient with PHN.

LOW BACK PAIN

The most common cause of pain and disability is low back pain. The *Nuprin Pain Report* (10) indicated that 56% of Americans suffered from back pain in the year before the survey. All patients with back pain should have a careful medical history and a through physical examination. A careful evaluation helps to determine the origin and significance of the pain, and only then can rational treatment be undertaken.

Mechanisms of Low Back Pain

Mechanisms proposed to explain low back pain include the following:

1. Nerve root compression
2. Inflammation of nerve roots
3. Abnormal protein/polysaccharide bathing the nerve roots
4. Abnormal pH of tissue around the nerve root
5. Autoimmune process at the annulus fibrosis
6. Muscle spasm

Musculoskeletal Pain

The most common origin of back pain is the musculoskeletal system. The following **treatment modalities** have been useful:

1. **Tricyclic antidepressants** exert analgesic effects in some patients. Analgesia does not seem to be related to the presence or absence of depression.
2. **Trigger point injections** are useful in patients with myofascial pain syndrome in whom sensitive nodules in skeletal muscle can be found on physical examination. Trigger points are usually located in taut bands of skeletal muscle, and pressure on these points causes pain and/or autonomic changes in adjacent and sometimes distant sites.
3. **Stretching exercises** reduce muscle tension and increase range of motion. Conditioning gained by stretching exercises increases muscle strength and enables the muscle to withstand stress.

4. **Nonsteroidal antiinflammatory analgesics** are useful if the patient is carefully monitored for side effects. The most common side effect is gastric irritation; rarely, renal impairment is a problem. Their use is consistent with the philosophy of avoiding narcotic analgesics in the chronic pain patient.

5. **Teaching back care and lifting techniques** has decreased back injuries in both the industrial and clinic settings.

6. **Correcting postural defects** is an important tool in preventing back pain. Poor posture can lead to low back pain by causing "wear and tear" on the supporting bony structure. Corrections can be made by stretching and strengthening exercises.

Neurologic System

The neurologic system is less commonly the site of origin of low back pain than the musculoskeletal system and can be treated with the following modalities:

1. Following the pioneering work of Mixter and Barr (11), **surgery** to cure lumbosacral pain was developed and refined. Although long-term results with conservative therapy are better than results with surgery for patients with herniated disc, there are advantages in the first 4 years for the patient treated surgically (12). Therefore, it is prudent to identify patients who have acute pain related to a herniated disc and refer them for surgical evaluation. Initial identification is made by the description of the pain, which is often recurrent, and the medical history, which will usually include previous episodes. The pain is often increased by sitting and relieved in the supine or standing position. When considering surgical consultation, remember that pain relief following surgery is rare in the patient who has had previous back surgery.

2. **The injection of a steroid preparation into the epidural space** is a popular but unproven remedy for radicular pain. Although used since the early 1960s, widespread use of the technique dates to the report by Winnie et al. (13) in 1972. This report described the technique and claimed that 80% of patients improved. Like many other medical writings of this era, the work did not contain a control group, and evaluation of improvement was subjective. The best randomized,

controlled, double-blind study available to date is Cuckler's (14) 1985 study in which epidural steroids did not yield better pain relief than placebo.

Epidural steroid administration is overused. Many physicians use it for a variety of conditions, including PHN, painful diabetic neuropathy, and degenerative joint disease of the hips and knees. There is no evidence of benefit in any of these conditions.

Technique: Methylprednisolone acetate (Depo-Medrol) is the steroid preparation used most often; triamcinolone diacetate (Aristocort) is sometimes used. Eighty milligrams of methylprednisolone acetate (or 50 mg of triamcinolone diacetate) is suspended in 10 ml of 0.25% or 0.125% bupivacaine. The needle is placed in the epidural space as close as possible to the origin of the nerve responsible for the radicular pain. The block is usually repeated every 2 weeks, with a maximum of 3 times.

Side effects of epidural steroid administration are soreness and pain at the site of the epidural placement and accidental dural puncture. Side effects of the steroid preparation are water retention, Cushing's syndrome, hypertension, and rash. Patients who have had previous back surgery and those dependent on narcotic analgesics almost never benefit from epidural steroid treatment.

3. **Bed rest** for 2–3 weeks is a time-honored treatment for neurogenic pain of the low back. The patient is often more comfortable in the supine position, which reinforces compliance with bed rest. Deyo et al. (15) demonstrated that briefer periods of bed rest were associated with earlier return to work.

4. **Treatments of unproven value** are facet blocks, dorsal column stimulation, manipulation, and transcutaneous electrical nerve stimulation (TENS).

Other Physical Causes

Many other medical problems can manifest as back pain. Tumors, both primary and metastatic, can have back pain as a presenting symptom. Rheumatic diseases can cause back pain. Pain can be referred to the low back from pelvic viscera or from major blood vessels.

Psychologic/Social/Economic Causes

Psychogic/social/economic factors are universally involved in back pain, probably as contributing factors. Those who treat patients with chronic pain must be prepared to intervene or make appropriate referrals so that the impact of psychologic/social/economic factors on the patient's recovery is lessened.

SYMPATHETICALLY MAINTAINED PAIN

Sympathetically maintained pain (SMP) is a generic term that includes pain syndromes caused by sympathetic nervous system dysfunction.

Mechanisms of SMP

No completely satisfactory mechanism to explain SMP has been put forth; however, proposed mechanisms include the following:

Central nervous system mechanisms promote the belief that activity in neurons of the spinal cord can become self-perpetuating and lead to pain. Livingston (16) advanced the theory that afferent impulses from a painful locus in the periphery are carried to the central nervous system by somatic or sympathetic fibers. In the central nervous system, they activate the internuncial pool of neurons in the lateral and anterior horn of the spinal cord. He theorized that this activity caused increased reflex sympathetic efferent fiber activity. The increased efferent activity in turn caused muscle spasm, excess elaboration of products of metabolism, and vasoconstriction, all of which increase the original painful stimuli. Increased pain increases afferent impulses and sets up a "vicious circle" of pain. In this theory, sympathetic nerve blocks decrease pain by breaking the cycle.

Peripheral nervous system mechanisms seek to explain SMP on the basis of peripheral events. The artificial synapse theory (17) proposed that trauma or nerve damage in the periphery causes a synapse between sympathetic efferent fibers and afferent sensory fibers. This synapse allows sympathetic efferent activity to produce not only peripheral effects but also afferent impulses interpreted as pain.

Another peripheral nervous system theory proposes that SMP is the result of hypersensitivity of $A\delta$ and C fibers to circulating norepinephrine. Because of the rich vascular supply to peripheral nerves and the close association of sympathetic innervation with the vascular structures, there is ample opportunity for peripheral nerves to come in contact with circulating norepinephrine. Increased norepinephrine-stimulated peripheral nerve activity activates dorsal horn circuits and is interpreted as pain.

Causalgia

Approximately 1–2% of patients with partial nerve injury will develop causalgia. Causalgia was first reported after the Civil War, and there have been periodic increases in the incidence following wars since then. It often begins as a consequence of missile or bullet wounds. The incidence was lower in nerve-injured patients after the Vietnam War than after World War II. More rapid access to treatment is cited as the reason for the difference. This pain syndrome is identified by

1. Burning pain, usually in the distal portion of an extremity, beginning within days of the injury
2. Sympathetic nervous system dysfunction
3. Origin after injury to a major nerve
4. Allodynia—pain caused by a stimulus that does not normally cause pain
5. Hyperalgesia—markedly increased pain to a stimulus that normally causes pain
6. Hyperpathia—pain that begins with an increased reaction to a stimulus and persists or increases after the stimulus has been removed
7. Aggravation by emotional or environmental factors
8. Vasomotor and sudomotor changes such as vasodilation, vasoconstriction, and increased perspiration occurring during the course of the syndrome
9. Trophic changes including thin glossy skin, thick stiff nails, coarse hair on the extremity, and as a late change, joint contracture

Some have suggested that pain relief following a sympathetic block is necessary to establish the diagnosis of causalgia. However, there are typical cases of causalgia that do not respond to sympathetic blockade, especially if it is done late in the course of the syndrome.

Reflex Sympathetic Dystrophy (RSD)

RSD is a general term used to include pain, usually in the limb, that follows injury to bone and soft tissue.

Injuries associated with RSD include

Fractures
Traumatic injuries
Minor traumatic injuries
Laceration
Surgery
Frostbite
Burns
Myocardial or cerebral infarction (occasionally)

The pain of RSD has the same characteristics as the pain of causalgia.

Three Stages of RSD

The **acute stage** typically begins with the onset of pain several days after injury. During this stage the limb is warm, dry, and red, and there is edema. Growth of nails and hair increases. Toward the end of this stage, the limb becomes cold, pale, and wet with perspiration. The first stage lasts 1–3 months.

The **dystrophic stage** starts after approximately 3 months. The edema of the acute stage develops into a brawny edema. The hand or foot is pale, cool, and cyanotic. Hair growth diminishes, and ridging of the nails develops.

The **atrophic stage** is characterized by atrophy of skin, subcutaneous tissue, muscle, and bone. There are contractures of the joints. The skin is dry, cool, shiny, and smooth. In most patients, these changes are irreversible.

Treatment

The treatment outlined here applies to both RSD and causalgia.

1. Sympathetic interruption accomplished by sympathetic nervous system blocks is a time-honored treatment for SMP. Stellate ganglion block is used for pain of the upper extremities, and lumbar sympathetic block for pain of the lower extremities. Bupivacaine (0.25%) provides blockade lasting 3–

4 hours, but pain relief often lasts much longer. Wang et al. (18) compared the long-term effects of sympathetic nerve blocks in patients with RSD with those of conservative treatment and found that 75% of patients receiving sympathetic blocks had complete or good pain relief, while 45% of patients who had conservative treatment had comparable improvement.

2. Surgical sympathectomy and neurolytic block sympathectomy with 6% aqueous phenol and 50% ethyl alcohol have been used. The long-term success with sympathectomy is unpredictable. Postsympathectomy pain may occur in up to 44% of patients, especially after lumbar sympathectomy (19). In men, impotence can be a side effect of surgical or chemical lumbar sympathectomy.

3. Pharmacologic sympathectomy has been produced with the following oral drugs: phenoxybenzamine, guanethidine, propranolol, and prazosin. Case reports have indicated good results with phenoxybenzamine (20). Hypotension is the most serious side effect.

4. Intravenous regional sympathetic blockade (IRSB) was first reported as a successful treatment for causalgia by Hannington-Kiff (21). He used guanethidine, which is not commercially available now. Bretylium tosylate is an adrenergic-blocking agent that decreases norepinephrine release. It has been used to accomplish IRSB in doses of 1 mg/kg and is often combined with 0.5% lidocaine. Ford has reported good-to-excellent pain relief for up to 7 months after treatment with bretylium (22).

5. Transcutaneous electrical nerve stimulation (TENS) has been reported to be effective for causalgia (23) and RSD (24). The benefits, however, are usually transient, and TENS has not become a widespread treatment.

6. Physical therapy is an important part of all treatment programs for RSD and causalgia. Milder cases of causalgia have been treated successfully with physical therapy alone (25). More commonly, physical therapy is used in combination with sympathetic nerve blocks, IRSB, or TENS. Almost all patients can benefit from physical therapy as an adjunctive treatment.

MYOFASCIAL PAIN SYNDROME (MPS)

The *Nuprin Pain Report* (10) suggests that 53% of Americans suffer from muscle pain. The muscular system is vulnerable to traumatic injury, overexertion, and the microtraumas of everyday life. Sedentary individuals have a higher incidence of myofascial pain than those who are well-conditioned. Myofascial pain originates from trigger points in skeletal muscles. **Trigger points** are small hypersensitive sites located in tight bands of muscle.

Mechanism of MPS

The mechanism of myofascial pain syndrome is incompletely understood, and at the present time, the disease is described in clinical terms. Possible causes include

1. Traumatic injury to muscles
2. Scarring and unabsorbed cellular debris in muscles
3. Microtraumas of everyday life
4. Muscle overuse
5. Emotional stress, which may lead to increased muscle tension, and after a long period, myofascial trigger points

Treatment of MPS

Pain can be relieved and patients can be returned to a higher level of function by effective treatment of the myofascial pain syndrome.

1. Trigger point injections have been done with local anesthetics, saline, or dry needles. Injection with local anesthetic is believed to provide the best and longest-lasting relief. Bupivacaine (0.5%), without epinephrine, is frequently used. The total volume used should be limited to the maximum safe dose or less, calculated on a mg/kg basis.
2. Stretching exercises help reduce muscle tension and decrease tight muscle bands. Stretching serves as maintenance therapy to prevent reformation of tight muscles and trigger points.
3. Education to reduce muscle injury or postural stresses is an important adjunct to therapy.
4. Nonsteroidal antiinflammatory analgesics are useful in controlling the pain, especially in the early stages of treatment.

PHANTOM LIMB PAIN

Phantom limb pain is pain that is perceived as existing in a missing extremity. It should be distinguished from stump pain, which is localized in the stump of the amputated limb, and from phantom sensation. **Phantom sensation** or "normal phantom sensation" is a nonpainful, almost universal sensation that the missing limb is still present. The prevalence of phantom limb pain in amputees has been estimated to be as low as 2% and as high as 85%. The wide range of estimates of prevalence is due to a variety of factors including interview technique, confusion about what phantom limb pain is, and reluctance of patients to admit that they have pain in a missing limb.

Mechanism of Phantom Limb Pain

The mechanism of phantom limb pain is felt to be defective pain modulation in the central nervous system, related to incomplete neural afferent input from the missing extremity. Stump pain, on the other hand, is probably related to bone, muscle, tendon, or nerve abnormality in the periphery.

Treatment of Phantom Limb Pain

Sherman et al. (26) surveyed treatment of phantom limb pain and concluded that conservative therapy alone had statistically better results than either conservative therapy with surgery or surgery alone.

I usually recommend the following:

1. Injection of painful trigger zones in the stump of the painful limbs
2. Tricyclic antidepressants
3. Nonnarcotic analgesics
4. Carbamazepine—sometimes useful if the pain is episodic and lancinating
5. TENS—beneficial to a minority of patients. A therapeutic trial of TENS is a worthwhile intervention and has no potential side effects except skin irritation from the electrode adhesive.
6. Wearing the prosthesis everyday—the most beneficial intervention. In most patients, this decreases the pain experienced. This simple intervention is felt to work by recruit-

ment of large nerve fiber input to the spinal cord, subsequently activating the "gate" modulation system.

Traditional "block clinic" modalities including sympathetic nerve blocks, epidural blocks with local anesthetic, and/or corticosteroids, and major somatic nerve blocks have not been helpful in my experience.

Prevention

While "nerve block" interventions do not seem to play a role in the treatment of phantom limb pain, they might be an important component of prevention. Bach et al. (27) showed that patients with painful extremities who were scheduled for amputation had significantly lower incidence of phantom limb pain if they were kept pain-free for 72 hours before surgery, using local anesthetic, narcotics, or a combination of these drugs applied epidurally.

Phantom limb pain is, in many ways, a microcosm of all chronic pain. Its mechanism is unknown, conservative treatments are more successful than surgical treatments, and emotional or behavioral factors may play a role in perpetuating the pain.

CONCLUSION

Chronic pain is not "curable" in the traditional medical sense, but with proper management, most patients can lead full and normal lives. The hallmarks of the well-managed chronic pain patient do not always include complete freedom from pain, but do include a normal level of physical activity, freedom from depression, and freedom from excessive dependence on the medical care system.

References

1. Raj PP. Practical management of pain. Chicago: Year Book Medical Publishers, 1986:14.
2. Bonica JJ. The management of pain. Philadelphia: Lea & Febiger, 1953:25.
3. Colding A. The effect of regional sympathetic blocks in the treatment of herpes zoster. Acta Anaesth Scand 1969;13:133–141.
4. Yanagida H, Suwa K, Corssen G. No prophylactic effect of early

sympathetic blockage on postherpetic neuralgia. Anesthesiology 1987;66:73–76.

5. Riopelle JM, Naraghi M, Grush KP. Chronic neuralgia incidence following local anesthetic therapy for herpes zoster. Arch Dermatol 1984;120:747–750.

6. Melzack R, Wall PD. Pain mechanism: a new theory. Science 1965;150:971.

7. Watson CP, Evans RJ, Reed K, Merskey H, Goldsmith L, Warch J. Amitriptyline versus placebo in postherpetic neuralgia. Neurology 1982;32:671–673.

8. Max MB, Schafer SC, Culnane M, Smoller B, Dubner R, Gracely RH. Amitriptyline, but not lorazepam, relieves postherpetic neuralgia. Neurology 1988;38:1427–1432.

9. Bernstein JE, Korman NJ, Bickers DR, Dahl MV, Millikan LE. Topical capsaicin treatment of chronic postherpetic neuralgia. J Am Acad Dermatol 1989;21(2):265–270.

10. Taylor H, Curran NM. The Nuprin pain report. New York: Louis Harris and Associates, 1985.

11. Mixter WJ, Barr JS. Rupture of the intervertebral disc with involvement of the spinal canal. N Engl J Med 1934;211(5):210–215.

12. Weber H. Lumbar disc herniation: a controlled prospective study with ten years of observation. Spine 1983;8:131–140.

13. Winnie AP, Hartman JT, Meyers HL Jr, Ramamurthy S, Barangan V. Pain clinic II: intradural and extradural corticosteroids for sciatica. Anesth Analg 1972;51:990–1003.

14. Cuckler JM, Bernini PA, Wiesel SW, Booth RE Jr, Rothman RH, Pickens GT. The use of epidural steroids in the treatment of lumbar radicular pain. J Bone Joint Surg Am 1985;67-A(1):63–66.

15. Deyo RA, Diehl AK, Rosenthal M. How many days of bed rest for acute low back pain? N Engl J Med 1986;315:1064–1070.

16. Livingston WK. Pain mechanisms. New York: Macmillan, 1943.

17. Doupe J, Cullen CH, Chance GQ. Posttraumatic pain and causalgic syndrome. J Neurol Neurosurg Psychiatry 1944;7:33.

18. Wang JK, Erickson RP, Ilstrup DM. Repeated stellate ganglion block for upper-extremity reflex sympathetic dystrophy. Reg Anesth 1985;10:125.

19. Raskin NH, Levinson SA, Hoffman PM, Pickett JBE, Field HL. Post sympathectomy neuralgia: amelioration with diphenylhydantoin and carbamazepine. Am J Surg 1974;128:75–78.

20. Ghostine SY, Comair YG, Turner DM, Kassell NF, Azor CG. Phenoxybenzamine in the treatment of causalgia. J Neurosurg 1984;60:1263–1268.

21. Hannington-Kiff JE. Intravenous regional sympathetic block with guanethidine. Lancet 1974;1:1019.

22. Ford SR, Forrest WH, Eltherington L. The treatment of reflex sympathetic dystrophy with intravenous regional bretylium. Anesthesiology 1988;68:137–140.
23. Ruggeri SB. Reflex sympathetic dystrophy in children. Clin Orthop 1982;183:225.
24. Meyer GA, Fields HL. Causalgia treated by selective large fiber stimulation of peripheral nerve. Brain 1972;95:163.
25. Bunker RH. Causalgia and transthoracic sympathectomy. Am J Surg 1972;124:724.
26. Sherman RA, Sherman CJ, Grall NG. A survey of current phantom limb treatment in the United States. Pain 1980;8:85–99.
27. Bach S, Noreng MF, Tjellden NU. Phantom limb pain in amputees during the first 12 months following limb amputation after preoperative lumbar epidural blockade. Pain 1988;33:297–301.

Appendix 1

American Society of Anesthesiologists
Standards for Basic Intra-Operative Monitoring

(amended on October 13, 1993)

These standards apply to all anesthesia care although, in emergency circumstances appropriate life support measures take precedence. These standards may be exceeded at any time based on the judgement of the responsible anesthesiologists. They are intended to encourage high quality patient care, but observing them cannot guarantee any specific patient outcome. They are subject to revision from time to time, as warranted by the evolution of technology and practice. They apply to all general anesthetics, regional anesthetics and monitored anesthesia care. This set of standards addresses only the issue of basic anesthetic monitoring, which is one component of anesthesia care. In certain rare or unusual circumstances, 1) some of these methods of monitoring may be clinically impractical, and 2) appropriate use of the described monitoring methods may fail to detect untoward clinical developments. Brief interruptions of continual[1] monitoring may be unavoidable. *Under extenuating circumstances, the responsible anesthesiologist may waive the requirements marked with an asterisk (*): it is recommended that when this is done, it should be so stated (including the reasons) in a note in the patient's medical record.* These standards are not intended for application to the care of the obstetrical patient in labor or in the conduct of pain management.

---

[1] Note that "continual" is defined as "repeated regularly and frequently in steady rapid succession" whereas "continuous" means "prolonged without any interruption at any time."

STANDARD I

Qualified anesthesia personnel shall be present in the room throughout the conduct of all general anesthetics, regional anesthetics and monitored anesthesia care.

Objective

Because of the rapid changes in patient status during anesthesia, qualified anesthesia personnel shall be continuously present to monitor the patient and provide anesthesia care. In the event there is a direct known hazard, e.g., radiation, to the anesthesia personnel which might require intermittent remote observation of the patient, some provision for monitoring the patient must be made. In the event that an emergency requires the temporary absence of the person primarily responsible for the anesthetic, the best judgement of the anesthesiologist will be exercised in comparing the emergency with the anesthetized patient's condition and in the selection of the person left responsible for the anesthetic during the temporary absence.

STANDARD II

During all anesthetics, the patient's oxygenation, ventilation, circulation and temperature shall be continually evaluated.

Oxygenation

Objective

To ensure adequate oxygen concentration in the inspired gas and the blood during all anesthetics.

Methods

1. Inspired gas: During every administration of general anesthesia using an anesthesia machine, the concentration of oxygen in the patient breathing system shall be measured by an oxygen analyzer with a low oxygen concentration limit alarm in use.*
2. Blood oxygenation: During all anesthetics, a quantitative method of assessing oxygenation such as pulse oximetry shall be employed.* Adequate illumination and exposure of the patient is necessary to assess color.*

Ventilation

Objective

To ensure adequate ventilation of the patient during all anesthetics.

Methods

1. Every patient receiving general anesthesia shall have the adequacy of ventilation continually evaluated. While qualitative clinical signs such as chest excursion, observation of the reservoir breathing bag and auscultation of breath sounds may be adequate, quantitative monitoring of the CO_2 content and/or volume of expired gas is encouraged.

2. When an endotracheal tube is inserted, its correct positioning in the trachea must be verified by clinical assessment and by identification of carbon dioxide in the expired gas.* Endtidal CO_2 analysis, in use from the time of endotracheal tube placement, is encouraged.

3. When ventilation is controlled by a mechanical ventilator, there shall be in continuous use a device that is capable of detecting disconnection of components of the breathing system. The device must give an audible signal when its alarm threshold is exceeded.

4. During regional anesthesia and monitored anesthesia care, the adequacy of ventilation shall be evaluated, at least, by continual observation of qualitative clinical signs.

Circulation

Objective

To ensure the adequacy of the patient's circulatory function during all anesthetics.

Methods

1. Every patient receiving anesthesia shall have the electrocardiogram continuously displayed from the beginning of anesthesia until preparing to leave the anesthetizing location.*

2. Every patient receiving anesthesia shall have arterial blood pressure and heart rate determined and evaluated at least every five minutes.*

3. Every patient receiving general anesthesia shall have, in addition to the above, circulatory function continually evaluated by at least one of the following: palpation of a pulse, auscultation of heart sounds, monitoring of a tracing of intra-arterial pressure, ultrasound peripheral pulse monitoring, or pulse plethysmography or oximetry.

Body Temperature

Objective

To aid in the maintenance of appropriate body temperature during all anesthetics.

Methods

There shall be readily available a means to continuously measure the patient's temperature. When changes in body temperature are intended, anticipated or suspected, the temperature shall be measured.

Reprinted with permission of the American Society of Anesthesiologists from the ASA Directory of Members 1994:735.

Anesthesia Apparatus Checkout Recommendations, 1993

(from Revision of FDA Recommendations)

This checkout, or a reasonable equivalent, should be conducted before administration of anesthesia. These recommendations are only valid for an anesthesia system that conforms to current and relevant standards and includes an ascending bellows ventilator and at least the following monitors: capnograph, pulse oximeter, oxygen analyzer, respiratory volume monitor (spirometer) and breathing system pressure monitor with high and low pressure alarms. This is a guideline which users are encouraged to modify to accommodate differences in equipment design and variations in local clinical practice. Such local modifications should have appropriate peer review. Users should refer to the operator's manual for the manufacturer's specific procedures and precautions, especially the manufacturer's low pressure leak test (step #5).

Emergency Ventilation Equipment

*[1] 1. **Verify Backup Ventilation Equipment is Available & Functioning**

High Pressure Systems

*2. **Check Oxygen Cylinder Supply**
   a. Open O_2 cylinder and verify at least half full (about 1000 psi).
   b. Close cylinder.
*3. **Check Central Pipeline Supplies**
   a. Check that hoses are connected and pipeline gauges read about 50 psi.

---

[1]*If an anesthesia provider uses the same machine in successive cases, these steps need not be repeated or may be abbreviated after the initial checkout.

Low Pressure System

* 4. **Check Initial Status of Low Pressure System**

    a. Close flow control valves and turn vaporizers off.

    b. Check fill level and tighten vaporizers' filler caps.

* 5. **Perform Leak Check of Machine Low Pressure System**

    a. Verify that the machine master switch and flow control valves are OFF.

    b. Attach "Suction Bulb" to common (fresh) gas outlet.

    c. Squeeze bulb repeatedly until fully collapsed.

    d. Verify bulb stays fully collapsed for at least 10 seconds.

    e. Open one vaporizer at a time and repeat 'c' and 'd' as above.

    f. Remove suction bulb, and reconnect fresh gas hose.

* 6. **Turn On Machine Master Switch** and all other necessary electrical equipment.

* 7. **Test Flowmeters**

    a. Adjust flow of all gases through their full range, checking for smooth operation of floats and undamaged flowtubes.

    b. Attempt to create a hypoxic O_2/N_2O mixture and verify correct changes in flow and/or alarm.

Scavenging System

* 8. **Adjust and Check Scavenging System**

    a. Ensure proper connections between the scavenging system and both APL (pop-off) valve and ventilator relief valve.

    b. Adjust waste gas vacuum (if possible).

    c. Fully open APL valve and occlude Y-piece.

    d. With minimum O_2 flow, allow scavenger reservoir bag to collapse completely and verify that absorber pressure gauge reads about zero.

        With the O_2 flush activated, allow the scavenger reservoir bag to distend fully, and then verify that absorber pressure gauge reads < 10 cm H_2O.

Breathing System

* 9. **Calibrate O_2 Monitor**

    a. Ensure monitor reads 21% in room air.

    b. Verify low O_2 alarm is enabled and functioning.

    c. Reinstall sensor in circuit and flush breathing system with O_2.

    d. Verify that monitor now reads greater than 90%.

10. **Check Initial Status of Breathing System**
    a. Set selector switch to "Bag" mode.
    b. Check that breathing circuit is complete, undamaged and unobstructed.
    c. Verify that CO_2 absorbent is adequate.
    d. Install breathing circuit accessory equipment (e.g. humidifier, PEEP valve) to be used during the case.
11. **Perform Leak Check of the Breathing System**
    a. Set all gas flows to zero (or minimum).
    b. Close APL (pop-off) valve and occlude Y-piece.
    c. Pressurize breathing system to about 30 cm H_2O with O_2 flush.
    d. Ensure that pressure remains fixed for at least 10 seconds.
    e. Open APL (Pop-off) valve and ensure that pressure decreases.

    Manual and Automatic Ventilation Systems
12. **Test Ventilation Systems and Unidirectional Valves**
    a. Place a second breathing bag on Y-piece.
    b. Set appropriate ventilator parameters for next patient.
    c. Switch to automatic ventilation (Ventilator) mode.
    d. Turn ventilator ON and fill bellows and breathing bag with O_2 flush.
    e. Set O_2 flow to minimum, other gas flows to zero.
    f. Verify that during inspiration bellows delivers appropriate tidal volume and that during expiration bellows fills completely.
    g. Set fresh gas flow to about 5 L/min.
    h. Verify that the ventilator bellows and simulated lungs fill *and empty* appropriately without sustained pressure at end expiration.
    i. *Check for proper action of unidirectional valves.*
    j. Exercise breathing circuit accessories to ensure proper function.
    k. Turn ventilator OFF and switch to manual ventilation (Bag/APL) mode.
    l. Ventilate manually and assure inflation and deflation of artificial lungs and appropriate feel of system resistance and compliance.
    m. Remove second breathing bag from Y-piece.

Monitors

13. **Check, Calibrate and/or Set Alarm Limits of all Monitors**

Capnometer   Pulse Oximeter

Oxygen Analyzer   Respiratory Volume Mon-
                                  itor (Spirometer)

Pressure Monitor with High
  and Low Airway Alarms

14. **Check Final Status of Machine**

a. Vaporizers off
b. APL valve open
c. Selector switch to "Bag"
d. All flowmeters to zero
e. Patient suction level adequate
f. Breathing system ready to use

American Society of Anesthesiologists Difficult Airway Algorithm

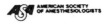

DIFFICULT AIRWAY ALGORITHM

1. Assess the likelihood and clinical impact of basic management problems:

   A. Difficult Intubation

   B. Difficult Ventilation

   C. Difficulty with Patient Cooperation or Consent

2. Consider the relative merits and feasibility of basic management choices:

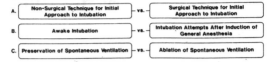

3. Develop primary and alternative strategies:

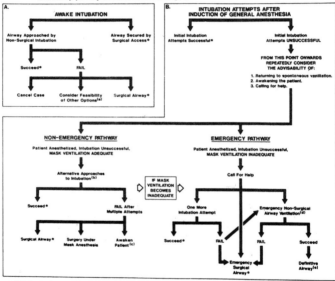

* CONFIRM INTUBATION WITH EXHALED CO_2

(a) Other options include (but are not limited to): surgery under mask anesthesia, surgery under local anesthesia infiltration or regional nerve blockade, or intubation attempts after induction of general anesthesia.

(b) Alternative approaches to difficult intubation include (but are not limited to): use of different laryngoscope blades, awake intubation, blind oral or nasal intubation, fiberoptic intubation, intubating stylet or tube changer, light wand, retrograde intubation, and surgical airway access.

(c) See awake intubation.

(d) Options for emergency non-surgical airway ventilation include (but are not limited to): transtracheal jet ventilation, laryngeal mask ventilation, or esophageal-tracheal combitube ventilation.

(e) Options for establishing a definitive airway include (but are not limited to): returning to awake state with spontaneous ventilation, tracheotomy, or endotracheal intubation.

Figure A3.1. Published with the permission of the American Society of Anesthesiologists, Park Ridge, IL. Anesthesiology 1993;78:600.

Adult Advanced Cardiac Life Support

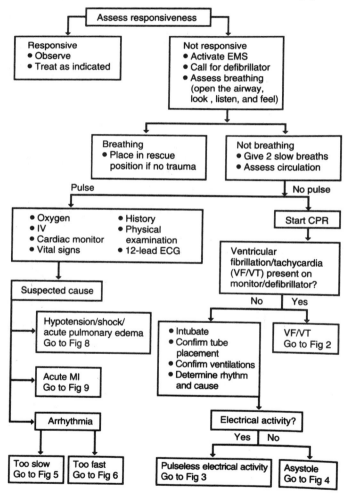

Figure A4.1. Universal algorithm for adult cardiac care. (Reproduced with permission of the American Medical Association from JAMA 1992;268:2171–2295.)

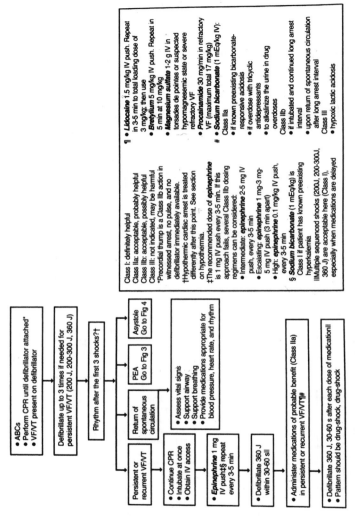

Figure A4.2. Algorithm for ventricular fibrillation and pulseless ventricular tachycardia (VF/VT). (Reproduced with permission of the American Medical Association from JAMA 1992;268:2171–2295.)

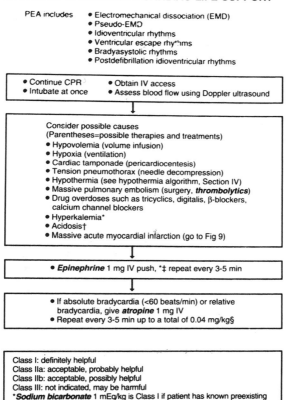

PEA includes
- Electromechanical dissociation (EMD)
- Pseudo-EMD
- Idioventricular rhythms
- Ventricular escape rhythms
- Bradyasystolic rhythms
- Postdefibrillation idioventricular rhythms

- Continue CPR
- Intubate at once
- Obtain IV access
- Assess blood flow using Doppler ultrasound

↓

Consider possible causes
(Parentheses=possible therapies and treatments)
- Hypovolemia (volume infusion)
- Hypoxia (ventilation)
- Cardiac tamponade (pericardiocentesis)
- Tension pneumothorax (needle decompression)
- Hypothermia (see hypothermia algorithm, Section IV)
- Massive pulmonary embolism (surgery, **thrombolytics**)
- Drug overdoses such as tricyclics, digitalis, β-blockers, calcium channel blockers
- Hyperkalemia*
- Acidosis†
- Massive acute myocardial infarction (go to Fig 9)

↓

- **Epinephrine** 1 mg IV push, *‡ repeat every 3-5 min

↓

- If absolute bradycardia (<60 beats/min) or relative bradycardia, give **atropine** 1 mg IV
- Repeat every 3-5 min up to a total of 0.04 mg/kg§

Class I: definitely helpful
Class IIa: acceptable, probably helpful
Class IIb: acceptable, possibly helpful
Class III: not indicated, may be harmful
***Sodium bicarbonate** 1 mEq/kg is Class I if patient has known preexisting hyperkalemia.
†**Sodium bicarbonate** 1 mEq/kg:
   Class IIa
   - if known preexisting bicarbonate-responsive acidosis
   - if overdose with tricyclic antidepressants
   - to alkalinize the urine in drug overdoses
   Class IIb
   - if intubated and long arrest interval
   - upon return of spontaneous circulation after long arrest interval
   Class III
   - hypoxic lactic acidosis
‡The recommended dose of **epinephrine** is 1 mg IV push every 3-5 min. If this approach fails, several Class IIb dosing regimens can be considered.
   - Intermediate: **epinephrine** 2-5 mg IV push, every 3-5 min
   - Escalating: **epinephrine** 1 mg-3 mg-5 mg IV push (3 min apart)
   - High: **epinephrine** 0.1 mg/kg IV push, every 3-5 min
§ Shorter **atropine** dosing intervals are possibly helpful in cardiac arrest (Class IIb).

Figure A4.3. Algorithm for pulseless electrical activity (PEA) (electromechanical dissociation [EMD]). (Reproduced with permission of the American Medical Association from JAMA 1992;268:2171–2295.)

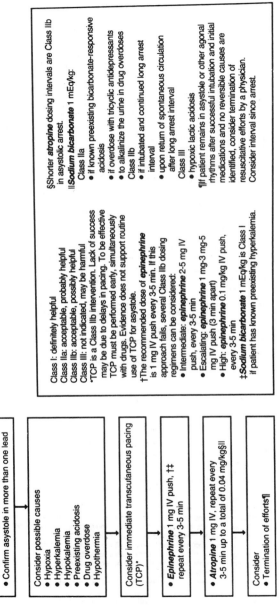

Class I: definitely helpful
Class IIa: acceptable, probably helpful
Class IIb: acceptable, possibly helpful
Class III: not indicated, may be harmful

*TCP is a Class IIb intervention. Lack of success may be due to delays in pacing. To be effective TCP must be performed early, simultaneously with drugs. Evidence does not support routine use of TCP for asystole.

†The recommended dose of *epinephrine* is 1 mg IV push every 3-5 min. If this approach fails, several Class IIb dosing regimens can be considered:
- Intermediate: *epinephrine* 2-5 mg IV push, every 3-5 min
- Escalating: *epinephrine* 1 mg-3 mg-5 mg IV push (3 min apart)
- High: *epinephrine* 0.1 mg/kg IV push, every 3-5 min

‡*Sodium bicarbonate* 1 mEq/kg is Class I if patient has known preexisting hyperkalemia.

§Shorter *atropine* dosing intervals are Class IIb in asystolic arrest.

||*Sodium bicarbonate* 1 mEq/kg:
Class IIa
- if known preexisting bicarbonate-responsive acidosis
- if overdose with tricyclic antidepressants
- to alkalinize the urine in drug overdoses
Class IIb
- if intubated and continued long arrest interval
- upon return of spontaneous circulation after long arrest interval
Class III
- hypoxic lactic acidosis

¶If patient remains in asystole or other agonal rhythms after successful intubation and initial medications and no reversible causes are identified, consider termination of resuscitative efforts by a physician. Consider interval since arrest.

- Continue CPR
- Intubate at once
- Obtain IV access
- Confirm asystole in more than one lead

Consider possible causes
- Hypoxia
- Hyperkalemia
- Hypokalemia
- Preexisting acidosis
- Drug overdose
- Hypothermia

Consider immediate transcutaneous pacing (TCP)*

- *Epinephrine* 1 mg IV push, †‡ repeat every 3-5 min

- *Atropine* 1 mg IV, repeat every 3-5 min up to a total of 0.04 mg/kg§||

Consider
- Termination of efforts¶

Figure A4.4. Asystole treatment algorithm. (Reproduced with permission of the American Medical Association from JAMA 1992;268:2171–2295.)

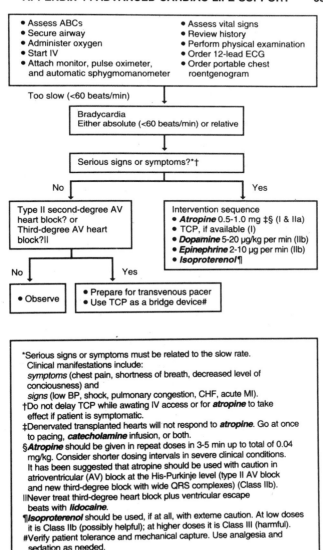

- Assess ABCs
- Secure airway
- Administer oxygen
- Start IV
- Attach monitor, pulse oximeter, and automatic sphygmomanometer

- Assess vital signs
- Review history
- Perform physical examination
- Order 12-lead ECG
- Order portable chest roentgenogram

Too slow (<60 beats/min)

Bradycardia
Either absolute (<60 beats/min) or relative

Serious signs or symptoms?*†

No   Yes

Type II second-degree AV heart block? or
Third-degree AV heart block?‖

Intervention sequence
- *Atropine* 0.5-1.0 mg ‡§ (I & IIa)
- TCP, if available (I)
- *Dopamine* 5-20 µg/kg per min (IIb)
- *Epinephrine* 2-10 µg per min (IIb)
- *Isoproterenol*¶

No   Yes

- Observe

- Prepare for transvenous pacer
- Use TCP as a bridge device#

*Serious signs or symptoms must be related to the slow rate.
  Clinical manifestations include:
  symptoms (chest pain, shortness of breath, decreased level of conciousness) and
  signs (low BP, shock, pulmonary congestion, CHF, acute MI).
†Do not delay TCP while awating IV access or for *atropine* to take effect if patient is symptomatic.
‡Denervated transplanted hearts will not respond to *atropine*. Go at once to pacing, *catecholamine* infusion, or both.
§*Atropine* should be given in repeat doses in 3-5 min up to total of 0.04 mg/kg. Consider shorter dosing intervals in severe clinical conditions. It has been suggested that atropine should be used with caution in atrioventricular (AV) block at the His-Purkinje level (type II AV block and new third-degree block with wide QRS complexes) (Class IIb).
‖Never treat third-degree heart block plus ventricular escape beats with *lidocaine*.
¶*Isoproterenol* should be used, if at all, with exteme caution. At low doses it is Class IIb (possibly helpful); at higher doses it is Class III (harmful).
#Verify patient tolerance and mechanical capture. Use analgesia and sedation as needed.

Figure A4.5. Bradycardia algorithm (with the patient not in cardiac arrest). (Reproduced with permission of the American Medical Association from JAMA 1992;268:2171–2295.)

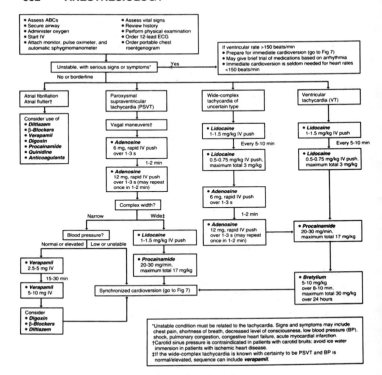

Figure A4.6. Tachycardia algorithm. (Reproduced with permission of the American Medical Association from JAMA 1992;268:2171–2295.)

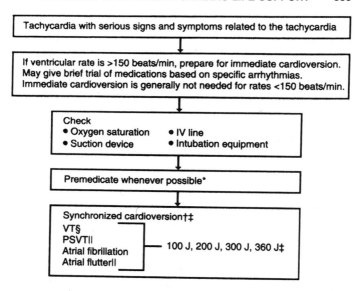

Tachycardia with serious signs and symptoms related to the tachycardia

If ventricular rate is >150 beats/min, prepare for immediate cardioversion.
May give brief trial of medications based on specific arrhythmias.
Immediate cardioversion is generally not needed for rates <150 beats/min.

Check
• Oxygen saturation   • IV line
• Suction device   • Intubation equipment

Premedicate whenever possible*

Synchronized cardioversion†‡
VT§
PSVTǁ
Atrial fibrillation   — 100 J, 200 J, 300 J, 360 J‡
Atrial flutterǁ

*Effective regimens have included a sedative (eg, *diazepam,
midazolam, barbiturates, etomidate, ketamine, methohexital*) with
or without an analgesic agent (eg, *fentanyl, morphine, meperidine*).
Many experts recommend anesthesia if service is readily available.
†Note possible need to resynchronize after each cardioversion.
‡If delays in synchronization occur and clinical conditions are critical,
go to immediate unsynchronized shocks.
§Treat polymorphic VT (irregular form and rate) like VF:
200 J, 200-300 J, 360 J.
ǁPSVT and atrial flutter often respond to lower energy levels
(start with 50 J).

Figure A4.7.   Electrical cardioversion algorithm(with the patient not in cardiac arrest). (Reproduced with permission of the American Medical Association from JAMA 1992;268:2171-2295.)

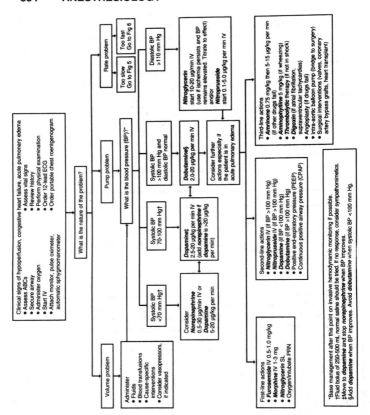

Figure A4.8. Algorithm for hypotension, shock, and acute pulmonary edema. (Reproduced with permission of the American Medical Association from JAMA 1992;268:2171–2295.)

Community
- Community emphasis on "call first/call fast, call 911"
- National Heart Attack Alert Program

EMS System
EMS system approach that should address
- Oxygen-IV-cardiac monitor-vital signs
- *Nitroglycerin*
- Pain relief with narcotics
- Notification of emergency department
- Rapid transport to emergency department
- Prehospital screening for *thrombolytic* therapy*
- 12-lead ECG, computer analysis, transmission to emergency department*
- Initiation of *thrombolytic* therapy*

Emergency Department
"Door-to-drug" team protocol approach
- Rapid triage of patients with chest pain
- Clinical decision maker established (emergency physician, cardiologist, or other)

Time interval in emergency department

Assessment
Immediate:
- Vital signs with automatic BP
- Oxygen saturation
- Start IV
- 12-lead ECG (MD review)
- Brief, targeted history and physical
- Decide on eligibility for *thrombolytic* therapy
Soon:
- Chest roentgenogram
- Blood studies (electrolytes, enzymes, coagulation studies)
- Consult as needed

Treatments to consider if there is evidence of coronary thrombosis plus no reasons for exclusion (some but not all may be appropriate)
- Oxygen at 4 L/min
- *Nitroglycerin* SL, paste or spray (if systolic blood pressure >90 mm Hg)
- *Morphine* IV
- *Aspirin* PO
- *Thrombolytic* agents
- *Nitroglycerin* IV (limit systolic BP drop to 10% if normotensive; 30% drop if hypertensive; never drop below 90 mm Hg systolic)
- β-*Blockers* IV
- *Heparin* IV
- Percutaneous transluminal coronary angioplasty
- Routine *lidocaine* administration is not recommended for all patients with AMI

30-60 min to *thrombolytic* therapy

*Optional guidelines

Figure A4.9. Acute myocardial infarction (AMI) algorithm. Recommendations for early treatment of patients with chest pain and possible AMI. (Reproduced with permission of the American Medical Association from JAMA 1992;268:2171–2295.

Appendix 5

Pediatric Advanced Life Support

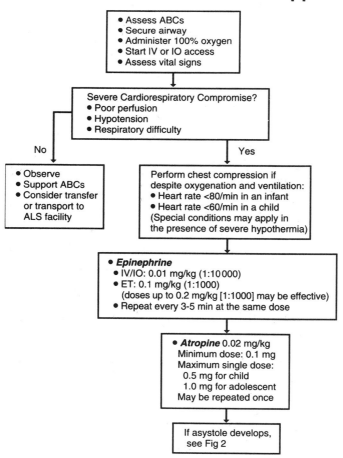

Figure A5.1. Bradycardia decision tree. *ABCs* indicates airway, breathing, and circulation; *ALS,* advanced life support; *ET,* endotracheal; *IO,* intraosseus; and *IV,* intravenous. (Reproduced with permission of the American Medical Association from JAMA 1992;268:2171–2295.)

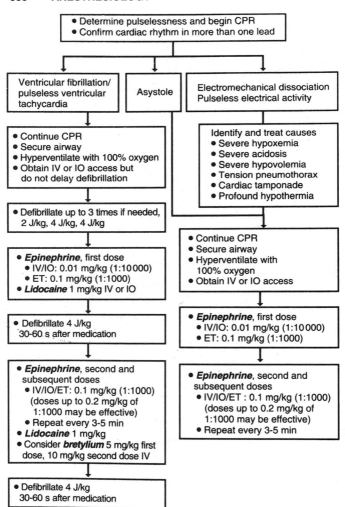

Figure A5.2. Asystole and pulseless arrest decision tree. *CPR* indicates cardiopulmonary resuscitation; *ET*, entotracheal; *IO*, intraosseous; and *IV*, intravenous. (Reproduced with permission of the American Medical Association from JAMA 1992;268:2171–2295.)

Appendix 6

Drugs Used in the Perioperative Period

List of Abbreviations

AV, atrioventricular
CHF, congestive heart failure
DOA, duration of action
IM, intramuscular
IN, intranasal
IV, intravenous
MAC, minimum alveolar concentration
MAO, monoamine oxydase
NS, normal saline
NSAIDs, nonsteroidal antiinflammatory drugs
p.o., by mouth
p.r., per rectum
PSVT, paroxysmal supraventricular tachycardia
SA, sinoatrial
s.c., subcutaneous
s.l., sublingual
t.d., transdermal
VF, ventricular fibrillation
VT, ventricular tachycardia
WPW, Wolff-Parkinson-White syndrome

Note: drug doses given are for adult patients unless otherwise noted.

Acetylcysteine (Mucomyst)

Effects: reduces viscosity of pulmonary secretions and increases mucociliary clearance
Use: reduction of viscous respiratory secretions

Adenosine (Adenocard)

Effect: slows AV conduction

Use: antidysrhythmic (PVST)

Dose: bolus IV, 6 mg; 12-mg bolus in 1–2 min if not converted

Onset: IV, less than 20 sec

DOA: IV, 3–7 sec

Metabolism: enzymatic in blood and vascular endothelial cells

Adverse effects: heart block, hypotension, dyspnea, flushing, transient heart block

Drug interactions: heart block increased with carbamazepine, potentiated by dipyridamole, antagonized by methylxanthenes

Alfentanil (Alfenta)

Effect: short-acting opioid analgesia

Uses: analgesic adjunct or primary anesthetic with N_2O/O_2, 750 μg equipotent to 10 mg morphine

Dose: general anesthesia, bolus IV (for induction), 50–150 μg/kg; infusion IV, 0.1–1.5 μg/kg/min

Onset: IV, 1–2 min

DOA: IV, 10–15 min

Metabolism: liver

Adverse effects: truncal muscle rigidity, respiratory depression

Drug interactions: hypotension with diazepam, decreased clearance with erythromycin

Aminocaproic Acid (Amicar)

Effect: enhances hemostasis in bleeding due to fibrinolysis

Uses: treatment of life-threatening bleeding disorder from fibrinolysis

Dose: IV/p.o., 4–5 g in 1 hr, then 1–1.25 g/hr

Amiodarone (Cordarone)

Effect: SA node depression and prolonged PR, QRS, and QT intervals

Use: p.o. medication for refractory or recurrent VT or VF

Aminophylline (Theophylline, Ethylenediamine)

Effect: bronchodilation, positive inotropic and chronotropic effects

Uses: left ventricular failure, increased diaphragmatic contractility, bronchial asthma

Dose: p.o. 3–6 mg/kg; IV (bolus 5 mg/kg; infusion 0.5–1 mg/kg/hr)

Onset: IV, rapid; p.o., within 30 min

DOA: 6–12 hr

Metabolism: liver (85–90%), kidney

Adverse effects: tachyarrhythmias, seizures, fetal toxicity via placental transfer

Drug interactions: benzodiazepines and β-blockers antagonized, seizures with ketamine, potentiation of nitroprusside, cardiac arrhythmias with halothane

Amrinone Lactate (Inocor)

Effect: phosphodiesterase inhibition leading to increased intracellular cyclic AMP, causing potentiated delivery of calcium ions to the myocardial contractile system, causing increased inotropy with arterial vasodilation to increase cardiac output

Uses: CHF short-term management, inotropic agent

Dose: IV bolus, 0.75 mg/kg over 2–5 min

Infusion: 5–10 μg/kg/min

Onset: less than 5 min

DOA: 30 min–2 hr

Elimination: renal, hepatic

Adverse effects: hypotension, arrhythmias, thrombocytopenia, hepatic dysfunction

Drug interactions: marked hypotension with disopyramide, potentiates arrhythmogenic response to catecholamines and theophylline, incompatible with dextrose solutions

Atenolol (Tenormin)

Effects: cardioselective β-blocking agent without intrinsic sympathomimetic activities; decreases myocardial contractility, heart rate and blood pressure

Uses: hypertension, angina, myocardial infarction, migraine prophylaxis

Dose: IV, 5 mg over 5 min, then 5 mg 10 min later; p.o., 50–
200 mg qd
Onset: p.o., <1 hr
DOA: p.o., 24 hr
Elimination: renal
Adverse effects: hypotension, bradycardia, bronchospasm, depression, disorientation, nausea/vomiting, thrombocytopenia
purpura
Drug interactions: hypotension with volatile anesthetics, catecholamine-depleting drugs and calcium channel blockers;
may unmask negative inotropic effects of ketamine

Atracurium Besylate (Tracrium)

Effects: nondepolarizing blockade of nerve impulses at neuro-
muscular junction
Uses: surgical relaxation
Dose: IV bolus, 0.4 mg/kg; infusion: 6–8 μg/kg/min
Onset: IV, 3–5 min
DOA: IV, 20–64 min
Metabolism: ester hydrolysis, Hofmann elimination; hepatic
Adverse effects: histamine release with bolus > 0.6 mg/kg
Drug interactions: enhanced by volatile anesthetics, prolonged
by aminoglycosides

Atropine Sulfate

Effects: blockade of acetylcholine at muscarinic receptors;
tachycardia; smooth muscle relaxation; inhibited salivary, gas-
tric and respiratory tract secretions; decreased airway resis-
tance
Uses: bradycardia, vagolysis, antisialogogue, antagonism of cho-
linesterase inhibitor effects (neostigmine and pyridostig-
mine)
Dose: bradycardia, 0.01–0.02 mg/kg IV/IM; antisialogogue
(adult), 0.4–0.6 mg IV/IM/s.q./p.o.
Onset: IV, rapid
DOA: IV, 1–2 hr
Metabolism: minimal
Elimination: kidney (mostly), liver
Adverse effects: tachycardia (high doses), bradycardia (low

doses), respiratory depression, confusion, hallucinations, urinary retention, increased intraocular pressure

Drug interactions: additive anticholinergic effects with antihistamines, phenothiazines, triyclic antidepressants, MAO inhibitors; potentiates sympathomimetics

Bicarbonate, Sodium (NaHCO₃)

Effects: buffers excess H^+ concentration, increases plasma carbonate

Uses: metabolic acidosis, urinary alkalinization, hyperkalemia, bicarbonate loss (diarrhea), cardiac arrest

Dose: bolus IV, mEq $NaHCO_3$ = (base deficit × wt (kg) × 0.2–0.3) or 1–2 mEq/kg

Onset: IV, rapid

DOA: IV, 30–60 min

Metabolism: blood

Elimination: lungs (CO_2), renal (1%)

Adverse effects: alkalosis, hypercarbia, hyperosmolality, IV extravasation can cause chemical cellulitis with tissue sloughing

Drug interactions: corticosteroids (sodium retention), urinary alkalinization increases $t_{1/2}$ and DOA of amphetamines, ephedrine, flecainide, quinidine, quinine, pseudoephedrine; Decreased $t_{1/2}$ for chlorpropamide, lithium, salicylates, tetracyclines; precipitation with calcium

Bretylium Tosylate (Bretylol)

Effects (inital): norepinephrine release from postganglionic sympathetic nerve endings

Effects (later): inhibition of norepinephrine release; direct increased myocardial contractility

Uses: prophylaxis and therapy for ventricular tachycardia and ventricular fibrillation refractory to lidocaine

Doses: bolus IV, 5 mg/kg initial (double if no response); IV infusion, 1–2 mg/min

Onset: IV, minutes

DOA: IV, 6–24 hr

Metabolism: minimal

Elimination: renal (70% in 24 hr)

Adverse effects: orthostatic hypotension, hypotension, bradycardia, increased PVCs, angina, nausea, and vomiting

Drug interactions: aggravated digoxin toxicity, enhanced catecholamine effects

Bupivacaine (Marcaine, Sensorcaine)

Effect: neural blockade
Uses: local and regional anesthesia (not IV regional)
Dose: maximum safe dose: without epinephrine, 2 mg/kg; with
epinephrine, 2–3 mg/kg
Onset: infiltration, 2–10 min; epidural, 4–27 min
DOA: infiltration/epidural, 120–400 min
Elimination: hepatic, pulmonary
Adverse effects: hypotension, arrhythmias, cardiac arrest, respi-
ratory arrest, seizures, tinnitus, anaphylactoid symptoms, an-
gioneurotic edema
Drug interactions: β-blocking agents and cimetidine reduce
clearance; duration of action increased by vasoconstrictor
agents

Buprenorphine (Buprenex)

Effects: agonist-antagonist opioid analgesic; 0.3 mg IM equals
10 mg morphine
Use: analgesia
Dose: IM, 0.3 mg
Onset: 30 min
DOA: 8 hr
Metabolism: liver
Elimination: kidney
Adverse effects: drowsiness, nausea and vomiting, respiratory
depression (may be prolonged and resistant to naloxone);
may produce withdrawal in patients dependent on narcotics
Drug interactions: high lipid solubility

Butorphanol Tartrate (Stadol)

Effect: potent opioid agonist/antagonist; κ-receptor agonist; 1
mg IV equal to 10 mg morphine sulfate, 2–3 mg IM equal to
10 mg morphine sulfate
Uses: analgesia, sedation, "ceiling" effect on MAC reduction
(10–15%) and respiratory depression
Dose: IV, 0.5–2 mg q 3–4 hr; IM, 1–4 mg q 3–4 hr

Onset: IV, 1–5 min, onset IM: 10 min
DOA: IV/IM, 3–4 hr; IM, 10 min; IM, 4–5 hr
Metabolism: liver
Elimination: kidney
Adverse effects: significant psychomimetic effects (sedation, dysphoria), hypertension, hypotension, nausea/vomiting, palpitations
Drug interactions: synergistic with opioid agonists; additive with phenothiazines, droperidol, barbiturates, and tranquilizers

Calcium Chloride

Effect: essential for cell membrane integrity, enzyme function, muscular excitation-contraction coupling
Uses: positive inotrope, electrolyte replacement
Dose: IV, 500–1000 mg (2–10 mg/kg)
Onset: rapid
DOA: variable
Metabolism/elimination: GI, renal
Adverse effects: hypertension, hypotension, arrhythmias, cardiac arrest, increased risk of ventricular fibrillation
Drug interactions: increased dysrhythmias in digitalized patients, calcium channel blocker antagonism

Calcium Gluconate

Effect: see calcium chloride
Use: see calcium chloride
Dose: IV/p.o., 500–2000 mg (1 g = 4.5 mEqCa^{2+})
Onset: IV, < 30 sec
DOA: IV, 10–20 min
Metabolism/elimination: GI, renal
Adverse effects: see calcium chloride
Drug interactions: see calcium chloride

Captopril (Capoten)

Effects: angiotensin-converting enzyme (ACE) inhibition
Uses: antihypertensive, CHF
Dose: p.o., 25–150 mg q q.v. 8–12 hr
Onset: 15–30 min
DOA: 8–12 hr

Metabolism: liver

Elimination: renal

Adverse effects: hypotension, tachycardia, renal failure, neutropenia, agranulocytosis

Drug interactions: additive with other hypotensive agents, potentiates hypotensive effects of anesthetics, antagonized by nonsteroidal antiinflammatory drugs

Chloroprocaine Hydrochloride (Nesacaine)

Effects: neural blockade (ester)

Uses: infiltration and regional anesthesia (epidural and not IV regional or spinal)

Dose: maximum dose, 800 mg (11 mg/kg); with epinephrine (1:200,000), 1000 mg (14 mg/kg)

Onset: infiltration, 2–5 min; epidural: 3–10 min

DOA: 30–45 min

Elimination: plasma cholinesterase

Adverse effects: systemic effects as with other IV local anesthetics; intrathecal injection of drug with bisulfite may produce neurotoxicity

Cimetidine (Tagamet)

Effects: competitive histamine H_2 receptor antagonist blocking the effects of pentagastrin, acetylcholine, and histamine on gastric acid secretion

Uses: acid pulmonary aspiration prophylaxis, treatment of peptic ulcer disease and hypersecretory states

Dose: p.o./IV, 300 mg q 6–8 hr

Onset: IV/p.o., <45 min

DOA: IV, 4–4.5 hr; p.o., 6–8 hr

Metabolism: liver

Elimination: kidney (75%)

Adverse effects: bradycardia, hypotension, arrhythmias, seizures, confusion, diarrhea, agranulocytosis, hepatic enzyme inhibitions, aplastic anemia, thrombocytopenia

Drug interactions: metabolism of many drugs is inhibited including benzodiazepines, calcium channel blockers, some β-blockers, tricyclic antidepressants, coumarin anticoagulants; decreases serum concentration of digoxin; may increase effects of succinylcholine; absorption may be decreased by antacids, anticholinergics, and metoclopromide

Clonidine (Catapres)

Effect: inhibition of central sympathetic outflow by activation of medullary vasomotor α_2-adrenergic receptors; decreases heart rate, cardiac output, and blood pressure

Uses: antihypertensive, anesthesia supplementation, epidural/spinal anesthesia, sedation, antisialagogue

Dose: p.o., 0.2–0.4 mg; epidural, 150–800 μg (2–10 μg/kg)

Onset: p.o., 30–60 min; epidural, <15 min

DOA: p.o., 8 hr; epidural: 3–4 hr

Metabolism: liver

Elimination: kidney (80%), liver (20%)

Adverse effects: hypotension, use cautiously in elderly, hypovolemic patients and children; can cause CHF, AV block, depression, anxiety, nausea/vomiting, angioneurotic edema

Drug interactions: potentiates opioids, alcohol, barbiturates, sedatives; decreases MAC of volatile anesthetics; effects of clonidine reduced by tricyclic antidepressants

Cocaine HCl

Effects: topical anesthetic that stabilizes neuronal membranes, preventing neuronal impulses; block of catecholamine uptake in adrenergic nerve endings causes vasoconstriction

Uses: topical anesthesia and mucous membrane vasoconstriction

Dose: topical, 1–3 mg/kg

Onset: topical, <1 min

DOA: topical, 30–120 min

Elimination: plasma cholinesterase, hepatic

Adverse effects: hypertension, tachyarrhythmias, VF, tachypnea, euphoria, seizures, sloughing of corneal epithelium

Drug interactions: potentiation of sympathomimetic arrhythmogenic effects

Cyclosporine (Sandimmune)

Use: immunosuppression for organ transplantation, treatment for severe autoimmune disease resistant to corticosteroids

Dantrolene Sodium (Dantrium)

Effects: inhibition of calcium release from the muscle sarcoplasmic reticulum

Uses: treat/prevent malignant hyperpyrexia (MH), upper motor neuron disease spasticity

Dose: MH treatment: IV 1–2 mg/kg q 5–10 min up to 10 mg/kg

Onset: p.o., 1–2 hr; IV, <5 min

DOA: p.o., 8–9 hr; IV, 3 hr

Metabolism: liver

Elimination: kidney

Adverse effects: muscle weakness, drowsiness, sedation, GI upset

Drug interactions: additive with muscle relaxants; hyperkalemia and cardiovascular collapse with calcium channel blockers

Desmopressin Acetate (DDAVP, Stimate)

Effects: increases renal tubule and collecting duct permeability to water; release of von Willebrand's factor

Uses: diabetes insipidus (DI), hemostasis after cardiopulmonary bypass, hemophilia A

Doses: DI, 0.1–0.4 ml qd intranasal; hemostasis, 0.3 μg/kg IV over 30 min

Onset: IV, 15–30 min

Duration: IV, 6–20 hr

Elimination: renal

Adverse effects: water intoxication, hyponatremia, hypertension

Drug interactions: antidiuretic effect potentiated by chlorpropamide, clofibrate, and carbamazepine

Dexamethasone (Decadron, Hexadrol)

Effects: prednisolone derivative with potent antiinflammatory effect; 0.75 mg equal to 20 mg cortisol

Uses: treatment of bronchial asthma, cerebral edema, allergic reactions, aspiration pneumonia, prevention of transplanted organ rejection, adrenocortical replacement

Dose: dexamethasone phosphate IV/IM, 0.5–25 mg/day; dexamethasone p.o.: 0.75–9 mg/day

Onset: IV/IM, minutes

DOA: IV/IM, 36–54 hr

Metabolism: liver

Elimination: kidney, liver (15%)

Adverse effects: arrhythmias, hypertension, seizures, corticosteroid psychosis, increased intraocular pressure, subcapsular cataracts, increased insulin requirement, osteoporosis, increased susceptibility to infection

Drug interactions: enhances potassium wasting of potassium-wasting diuretics; clearance enhanced by phenobarbital, phenytoin, ephedrine, rifampin

Diazepam (Valium)

Effects: benzodiazepine that acts on the limbic system, thalamus, and hypothalamus producing calming effects; increases the availability of the glycine-inhibitory neurotransmitter causing antianxiety and skeletal muscle-relaxing effects

Uses: premedication, anxiolysis, amnesia, sedative/hypnotic, skeletal muscle relaxant, anticonvulsant

Dose: p.o., 0.05–0.15 mg/kg; IV (induction), 0.1–0.5 mg/kg; (anticonvulsant) 5–10mg

Onset: p.o., 15 min–1 hr; IV, <2 min

DOA: p.o., 2–6 hr; IV, 15 min–1 hr

Metabolism: liver (active metabolites)

Elimination: kidney (70%)

Adverse effects: extended sedation through active metabolites, painful IV injection, hypotension, respiratory depression, bradycardia

Drug interactions: depressant effects potentiated by opioids, alcohol, and CNS depressants; reduced requirements for volatile anesthetics; elimination decreased by cimetidine; antagonized by flumazanil

Digoxin (Lanoxin)

Effects: inhibition of Na^+/K^+ ATPase ion transport system, decreased SA node activity and prolonged AV conduction

Uses: treatment for heart failure and supraventricular arrhythmias; increased inotropy

Dose: bolus IV, 0.25–0.5 mg over 5 min (8–12 μg/kg),

Maintenance: IV/p.o., 1/3 of initial bolus (0.125–0.25 mg in 4–8 hr)

Onset: IV, 5–30 min; p.o., 30 min–2 hr

DOA: IV/p.o., 3–4 days
Metabolism: minimal
Elimination: kidney
Adverse effects: arrhythmias, AV block, headache, psychosis, nausea/vomiting; toxicity increased in hypokalemia, hypomagnesemia, hypercalcemia; low therapeutic index
Drug interactions: increased serum levels with calcium channel blockers, esmolol, quinidine, amiodarone, flecainide, captopril, benzodiazepines, anticholinergics, erythromycin, aminoglycosides; arrhythmias with succinylcholine

Diltiazem (Cardizem)

Effects: calcium channel blocker causing slowed SA and AV node conduction, coronary and peripheral artery dilation, reduced myocardial contractility
Uses: antiarrhythmic (Afib/flutter, paroxysmal atrial tachycardia (PAT)), coronary artery spasm, chronic angina
Dose: IV, 0.15–0.25 mg/kg; infusion, 5–15 mg/hr
Onset: 1–3 hr;
DOA: $T_{1/2\,E} = 4$ hr
Metabolism: liver
Elimination: kidney
Adverse effects: bradycardia, heart block, arrhythmias in patients with WPW
Drug interactions: impaired contractility with β-blocking agents, potentiation of cardiac depression by volatile anesthetics, potentiates theophylline, increased biovailability with cimetidine and ranitidine

Diphenhydramine HCl (Benadryl)

Effects: histamine (H_1) receptor antagonism, anticholinergic effect, CNS depression
Uses: allergic reactions, drug-induced extrapyramidal reactions, antiemetic, sedative, antisialagogue, antitussive
Dose: IV/IM/p.o., 25–50 mg
Onset: IV, few minutes; p.o.:< 15 min
DOA: IV/p.o.,< 7 hr
Metabolism: liver
Elimination: kidney

Adverse effects: hypotension, tachycardia, dizziness, wheezing, seizures

Drug interactions: additive effect with other CNS depressants, potentiated anticholinergic effect with MAO inhibitors

Dobutamine HCl (Dobutrex)

Effects: β_1-adrenergic agonist (increases heart rate and contractility)

Uses: heart failure, pharmacologic stress test for coronary artery disease

Dose: 2–30 μg/kg/min

Onset: IV, 2 min

DOA: IV, 10 min

Metabolism: liver, nerve endings

Elimination: kidney, liver

Adverse effects: hypertension, tachycardia, arrhythmias, angina, shortness of breath

Drug interactions: decreased effect with β-blockers, higher cardiac output with nitroprusside, potentiated by bretylium, increased arrhythmias with volatile anesthetics

Dopamine HCl (Intropin)

Effects: dopaminergic, α- and β-adrenergic stimulation

Uses: vasoconstriction, ionotropic support and treatment of oliguria

Dose: IV oliguria (low dose), 2–5 μg/kg/min; IV hypotension (high dose), 5–30 μg/kg/min

Onset: IV, 5 min

DOA: IV, 10 min

Metabolism: liver, kidney, nerve endings

Elimination: kidney

Adverse effects: arrhythmias, angina, AV block, hyper/hypotension, nausea/vomiting

Drug interactions: arrhythmias with volatile anesthetics, seizures with phenytoin, bradycardia, severe hypotension

Doxacuricum Chloride (Nuromax)

Effects: competitive binder of cholinergic receptors at motor endplate leading to acetylcholine antagonism (nondepolarizing blockade), minimal cardiovascular side effects

Uses: muscle relaxation (nondepolarizing)
Dose: IV, 0.05 mg/kg
Onset: IV, 5–7 min
DOA: IV, 40–240 min
Metabolism: minimal
Elimination: renal, bile
Adverse effects: contains benzyl alcohol which could cause neurologic complications in neonates, significant prolongation in hepatic/renal failure
Drug interactions: potentiation by volatile anesthetics, hypokalemia, aminoglycosides, lithium, magnesium, local anesthetics, anticonvulsants, procainamide, quinidine

Doxapram HCl (Dopram)

Effects: respiratory stimulation via the peripheral carotid chemoreceptors; with higher doses, medulla respiratory receptors are stimulated
Use: stimulation of respiration
Dose: slow IV, 0.5–1.5 mg/kg to maximum of 2 mg/kg
Onset: IV, 20–40 sec
DOA: IV, 5–12 min
Elimination: hepatic
Adverse effects: hypertension, tachy/bradycardia, laryngospasm, bronchospasm, seizures, clonus, nausea/vomiting, anemia, leukopenia
Drug interactions: additive pressor with sympathomimetics and MAO inhibitors, increased arrhythmias with volatile anesthetics, precipitation with alkaline solutions

Droperidol (Inapsine)

Effects: interferes with CNS transmission at dopamine, GABA, serotonin, and norepinephrine synaptic sites; has some α_1-adrenergic antagonist action
Uses: antiemetic, anxiolytic, sedative
Dose: IV antiemetic, 0.625–2.5 mg; IV/IM premedicant, 2.5–10 mg
Onset: IV/IM, 5–8 min
DOA: IV/IM, 3–6 hr
Metabolism: liver

Elimination: kidney, liver

Adverse effects: hypotension, tachycardia, extrapyramidal symptoms, hyperactivity, laryngospasm, sedation, oculogyric crisis

Drug interactions: potentiation of CNS depressants and vasodilators, antagonism of epinephrine effects

Edrophonium Chloride (Enlon, Tensilon, Reversol)

Effects: binds acetylcholinesterase, inhibiting the hydrolysis of acetylcholine at the neuromuscular junction; faster onset of action with fewer muscarinic side effects than other relaxant reversal drugs

Uses: muscle relaxant reversal, antidysrhythmic, diagnostic assessment for myasthenia gravis

Dose: IV, 0.5–1.0 mg/kg

Onset: IV, 1–5 min

DOA: IV, 1.0 hr

Metabolism/elimination: liver/kidney

Adverse effects: bradycardia, salivation, bronchospasm, tachycardia, AV block, hypotension, seizures, nausea, increased peristalsis

Drug interactions: prolonged phase 1 block of succinylcholine; reduced effect with aminoglycosides, corticosteroids, magnesium

Ephedrine Sulfate

Effects: sympathomimetic with direct and indirect α and β actions; increases cardiac output, blood pressure, and heart rate

Uses: vasopressor and bronchodilator

Dose: IV, 5–10 mg; IM, 25–50 mg

Onset: IV, rapid

DOA: IV/IM, 10–60 min

Metabolism: liver

Elimination: kidney

Adverse effects: hypertension, tachycardia, arrhythmias, pulmonary edema

Drug interactions: arrhythmias with volatile anesthetics, potentiated by MAO inhibitors and tricyclic antidepressants

Epinephrine HCl (Adrenaline, Epinephrine, Vaponefrin, Micronefrin)

Effects: Endogenous catecholamine with α- and β-adrenergic effects

Uses: resuscitation, inotrope, bronchodilator, prolongs effect of local anesthetics, treatment of allergic reactions

Dose:

Cardiac arrest, 0.5–1 mg IV bolus

Anaphylaxis/asthma, 0.1–0.5 mg s.c./IM

Bronchodilation (racemic epinephrine): 1:3 to 1:6 dilution in NS solution inhaled

Inotropic support: 10–100 μg IV bolus; infusion 0.01–0.02 μg/kg/min

Onset: IV, rapid; s.c./IM, 3–5 min; inhaled, 1–5 min

DOA: IV, 10 min; IM, 10–60 min; inhaled, 2–3 hr

Metabolism: liver/nerve endings

Elimination: kidney (90%), liver (10%)

Adverse effects: hypertension, tachycardia, arrhythmias, angina, pulmonary edema, anxiety, cerebrovascular hemorrhage, hyperglycemia

Drug interactions: ventricular arrhythmias with volatile anesthetics; enhanced effect with tricyclic antidepressants, bretylium, MAO inhibitors, and antihistamines

Ergonovine Maleate (Ergotrate)

Effects: contraction of uterine and vascular smooth muscle

Uses: postpartum uterine atony and bleeding, uterine involution

Dose: IV/IM, 0.2 mg; p.o., 0.2–0.4 mg q 6–12 hr $\times$ 2 days

Onset: IV, rapid; IM, 2–5 min; p.o., 5–15 min

DOA: IV, 45 min; IM, 3 hr; p.o., 3 hr

Metabolism: hepatic

Elimination: hepatic

Adverse effects: tachycardia, hypertension, seizures, cerebrovascular accidents, nausea/vomiting, coronary spasm

Drug interactions: vasoconstrictive effects potentiated by sympathomimetics

Esmolol (Brevibloc)

Effects: cardioselective β-blockade with rapid onset and short DOA

Uses: PSVT, hypertension

Dose: bolus IV, 0.25–1 mg/kg; infusion: 50–500 μg/kg/min

Onset: 1–2 min

DOA: 10 min

Metabolism: hydrolysis by RBC esterases

Adverse effects: hypotension, bradycardia, bronchospasm, urinary retention

Drug interactions: potentiated myocardial depression of some anesthetic drugs, incompatible with sodium bicarbonate, negative ionotropic effect of ketamine unmasked, possible enhancement of muscle relaxers

Etomidate (Amidate)

Effects: nonbarbiturate nonanalgesic hypnotic

Uses: induction agent

Dose: IV, 0.3–0.4 mg/kg (0.2–0.3 mg/kg in ill patients)

Onset: one circulation time (30–60 sec)

DOA: 7–14 min

Metabolism: liver, plasma esterases

Adverse effects: hypotension, hypertension, arrhythmias, laryngospasm, myoclonus, adrenocortical suppression, thrombophlebitis

Drug interactions: potentiation with sedatives and narcotics

Famotidine (Pepcid)

Effects: competitive inhibition of histamine H_2 receptors

Uses: acid pulmonary aspiration prophylaxis, peptic ulcer disease, longest-acting H_2 blocker

Dose: IV, 20 mg bid; p.o., 20 mg bid or 40 mg at bedtime

Onset: IV: <30 min; p.o., 1 hr

DOA: IV/p.o., 10–12 hr

Elimination: renal

Adverse effects: hypotension, arrhythmias, bronchospasm, tinnitus, depression, nausea/vomiting, arthralgia, myalgia, thrombocytopenia

Drug interactions: decreased bioavailability with antacids

Fentanyl (Sublimaze)

Effects: potent opioid agonist (100 μg equal to 10 mg morphine)

Uses: analgesia, anesthesia; transdermal used only in patients with chronic pain

Dose: Sedation (IV): 1–2 μg/kg
      Induction(IV): 5–8 μg/kg
      Cardiac surgery: 50–100 μg/kg
      Epidural: bolus, 50–100 μg; infusion: 10–80 μg/hr
      Transdermal: 25–100 μg/hr

Onset: IV, within 30 sec; epidural, 4–10 min; transdermal: 12–18 hr

DOA: IV, 30–60 min; epidural, 4–8 hr; transdermal: 3 days

Metabolism: liver

Elimination: kidney

Adverse effects: hypotension, bradycardia, apnea, seizure, nausea/vomiting, muscle rigidity, biliary tract spasm

Drug interactions: depressant effects potentiated by narcotics, sedatives, nitrous oxide, volatile anesthetics; analgesia enhanced by α_2-agonists; ventilation depression enhanced by amphetamines, MAO inhibitors, phenothiazines, and tricyclic antidepressants

Flumazenil (Romazicon)

Effects: competitive inhibition of activity at the benzodiazepine recognition site on the GABA receptor in the central nervous system

Uses: reversal of benzodiazepine receptor agonists

Dose: bolus IV, 0.2–1 mg (4–20 μg/kg) at 0.2 mg/min (max 3 mg/hr)

Onset: 1–2 min

DOA: 45–90 min

Elimination: hepatic

Adverse effects: arrhythmias, tachycardia, bradycardia, hypertension, angina, seizures, agitation, nausea/vomiting, resedation when reversing long-acting benzodiazepines

Drug interactions: seizures in patients with prior seizure activity, tricyclic antidepressant poisoning, major hypnotic drug withdrawal

Furosemide (Lasix)

Effects: diuretic inhibiting reabsorption of sodium and chloride ions in the medullary part of loop of Henle

Uses: diuretic used to treat fluid overload, hypertension, pulmonary edema, increased intracranial pressure, CHF, edema

Dose: 10–40 mg IV; 20–200 mg/day p.o

Onset: IV, 2–15 min; p.o., 30–60 min

DOA: IV, 2 hr; p.o., 6–8 hr

Metabolism: minimal

Elimination: renal (some liver)

Adverse effects: orthostatic hypotension, tinnitus, hearing loss, paresthesias, urinary bladder spasm, nausea/vomiting, pancreatitis, diarrhea, aplastic anemia, thrombocytopenia, neutropenia, hyperglycemia, hypovolemia, hypokalemia, hyperuricemia

Drug interactions: increased renal toxicity with aminoglycosides, ethacrynic acid; reduces clearance of salicylates and lithium; potentiates adrenergic blocking drugs; decreased effects with indomethacin and NSAIDs

Glycopyrrolate (Robinul)

Effects: quaternary ammonium anticholinergic with high polarity causing minimal passage through the blood-brain barrier; reversibly binds with muscarinic cholinergic receptors; fewer CNS effects and tachycardia than atropine

Uses: antisialagogue, bradycardia, anticholinergic, blocks muscarinic effects of anticholinesterases

Dose: IV, 0.1–0.4 mg; IM, 0.1–0.3 mg

Onset: IV, less than 60 sec; IM: 15–30 min

DOA: IV: 2–4 hr; IM: 4–6 hr

Metabolism: minimal

Elimination: renal

Adverse effects: tachycardia (high doses), bradycardia (low doses), headache, confusion, urine retention, nausea/vomiting, increased intraocular pressure

Drug interactions: minimal

Heparin Sodium (Lipo-Hepin, Liquaemin sodium, Panheprin)

Effects: in combination with antithrombin III, inhibits thrombosis by inactivating active factors IX, X, XI, and XII and inhibiting the conversion of prothrombin to thrombin

Uses: anticoagulant

Dose: (cardiopulmonary bypass) IV, 350–450 units/kg, titrated against activated clotting time (ACT); s.c., 8,000–10,000 units q 8 hr (phlebitis)

Onset: IV, seconds; s.c., 20 min–1 hr

DOA: IV, 2–6 hr; s.c., 12–16 hr

Metabolism: liver

Elimination: renal

Adverse effects: hemorrhage, thrombocytopenia, elevated liver function tests, osteoporosis, priapism

Drug interactions: increased plasma diazepam levels, nitroglycerin may produce antagonism of effects, anticoagulation properties interfered with by digitalis and antihistamines

Hetastarch (Hespan)

Uses: plasma volume expansion

Adverse effects: pulmonary edema, urticaria, anaphylactoid reactions, coagulopathy with large volumes

Hydralazine (Apresoline)

Effects: direct relaxant effect on arteriolar smooth muscle causing a decrease in systemic vascular resistance

Uses: systemic arterial hypertension, CHF

Dose: IV, 2.5–5 mg

Onset: 5–15 min

DOA: 2–4 hr

Metabolism: liver

Elimination: kidney

Adverse effects: tachycardia, angina, hypotension, dyspnea, peripheral neuritis, SLE-like syndrome, urticaria, eosinophilia, splenomegaly, agranulocytosis

Drug interactions: enhanced defluorination of enflurane, enhanced hypotensive effects of other antihypertensives, reduced pressor response to epinephrine

Hydrocortisone (Solu-Cortef)

Uses: treatment of allergic reactions, antiinflammatory, steroid replacement, organ transplantation

Dose: IV/IM, 100 mg (1–2 mg/kg) q 2–10 hr (stress dose), p.o., 5–30 mg bid to qid (replacement dose)

Hydroxyzine (Vistaril, Atarax)

Effects: antagonism of histamine action on H_1 receptors, CNS depression, antiemetic effect
Uses: sedation, nausea/vomiting, anxiety, allergies
Dose: IM, 25–100 mg q 4–6 hr; p.o., 25–100 mg q 6–8 h

Hydromorphone HCl (Dilaudid, Dilaudid HP)

Effects: opiate agonist; 7 times more potent than morphine (1.5 mg equal to 10 mg morphine)
Uses: analgesia, anesthesia, premedication
Dose: IV, 0.5–2 mg (0.007–0.01 mg/kg); IM, 0.01–0.02 mg/kg; p.o., 2–4 mg q 4–6 hr
Onset: IV, rapid; p.o., 15–30 min
DOA: IV, 2–4 hr; p.o., 4–6 hr
Metabolism: liver
Elimination: liver, kidney
Adverse effects: hypotension, hypertension, bradycardia, chest wall rigidity, bronchospasm, syncope, dysphoria, biliary tract spasm, nausea/vomiting, pruritus
Drug interactions: CNS and circulatory depressant effects potentiated by sedatives, phenothiazines, tricyclic antidepressants and MAO inhibitors; decreases effects of diuretics in CHF

Isoproterenol (Isuprel)

Effects: synthetic sympathomimetic amine acting almost exclusively on β_1 and β_2-adrenergic receptors
Uses: chronotrope, inotrope, bronchodilator, treatment of bradycardia, heart block, and cardiogenic shock
Dose: bolus IV, 10–60 μg; infusion IV, 0.02–0.15 μg/kg/min
Onset: IV, rapid
DOA: IV, 1–5 min
Metabolism: liver, nerve endings
Elimination: liver, kidney
Adverse effects: arrhythmias, angina, hyper/hypotension, pulmonary edema, CNS excitement, nausea/vomiting
Drug interactions: arrhythmias with volatile agents and sympathomimetics, antagonized by β-blocking drugs

Ketamine (Ketalar, Ketaject)

Effects: a phencyclidine derivative producing rapid-acting dissociative anesthesia useful in hypovolemic patients because of sympathetic stimulating effects

Uses: anesthesia induction, anesthesia, sedation with local anesthesia

Dose: IV, 1–3 mg/kg (induction); IM, 5–10 mg/kg

Onset: IV, 30–60 sec; IM, 3–4 min

DOA: IV, 10–15 min; IM, 12–25 min

Metabolism: liver

Elimination: kidney, liver

Adverse effects: hypertension, tachycardia, increased intracranial and intraocular pressure, hypotension, arrhythmias, apnea, laryngospasm, emergence delirium, hypersalivation, nausea/vomiting, nystagmus

Drug interactions: hemodynamic depression with α-blockers, β-blockers, calcium channel blockers, benzodiazepines, opioids, and inhalation anesthetics; enhancement of neuromuscular blocking drugs; reduction of seizure threshold with aminophylline

Ketorolac Tromethamine (Toradol)

Effects: NSAID with analgesic, antiinflammatory, antipyretic activity; inhibitor of prostaglandin synthesis and platelet aggregation causing prolongation of bleeding time; analgesic potency of 30 mg is equivalent to 9 mg morphine

Uses: analgesic

Dose: IM, 15–60 mg; p.o., 10 mg q 4–6 hr

Onset: IM, less than 10 min; p.o., 1 hr

DOA: IM/p.o., 3–7 hr

Elimination: hepatic, renal

Adverse effects: vasodilation, angina, dyspnea, asthma, dizziness, headache, GI ulceration, bleeding, nausea/vomiting, GI pain, renal failure in susceptible patients

Drug interactions: potentiated by concomitant salicylates, enhanced toxicity of methotrexate and lithium

Labetalol (Normodyne, Trandate)

Effects: Adrenergic receptor-blocking agent with predominant β- and mild α-adrenergic receptor blocking action; ratios of

α- to β-blockade are 1:3 and 1:7 after oral and IV use, respectively

Uses: antihypertensive, β- and α-adrenergic blockade

Dose: IV bolus, 2.5–5 mg; IV infusion, 0.2–2 mg/kg/hr

Onset: 2–5 min

DOA: 40–90 min

Metabolism: liver

Elimination: kidney, liver

Adverse effects: hypotension, bradycardia, CHF, ventricular arrhythmias, bronchospasm, elevated liver function tests, paresthesia, diarrhea, positive antinuclear antibody (ANA) titers

Drug interactions: increased bioavailability with cimetidine, hypotensive effect potentiated by volatile anesthetics

Lidocaine HCl (Xylocaine)

Effects: amide-derivative local anesthetic that inhibits initiation and conduction of nerve impulses by inhibiting sodium flux across the neuronal membrane, suppresses automaticity and shortens the refractory period and action potential duration of the His-Purkinje system

Uses: regional anesthesia, antidysrhythmic for ventricular arrhythmias, attenuation of pressor response to intubation

Dose: for arrhythmias, IV bolus, 1 mg/kg slowly, then 0.5 mg/kg in 5-min (decrease 25–50% in CHF); IV infusion, 10–50 μg/kg/min

Onset: IV, 45–90 sec

DOA: IV, 10–20 min

Metabolism: liver

Elimination: liver, pulmonary

Adverse effects: hypotension, bradycardia, arrhythmias, heart block, respiratory arrest, tinnitus, seizures, angioneurotic edema, circumoral paresthesias

Drug interactions: potentiation of effect of succinylcholine and d-tubocurarine, reduced clearance with β-blocking agents and cimetidine, DOA prolonged in local and regional anesthesia by use of vasoconstrictor agents such as epinephrine, cardiac effects may be additive or antagonistic with other antiarrhythmics

Lorazepam (Ativan)

Effects: dose-related sedation and anxiolysis, amnesia, facilitates GABA effects in the CNS

Uses: preoperative sedation, amnesia, acute alcohol withdrawal treatment, nausea/vomiting induced by chemotherapy, long-acting amnesia (10–20 hr)

Dose: IV/IM, 1–4 mg (0.05 mg/kg); p.o., 0.05 mg/kg

Onset: IV, 5–20 min; IM, 0.5–2 hr; p.o., 1–2 hr

DOA: IV, 4–6 hr; IM, 8 hr; p.o., 10–20 hr

Metabolism: liver

Elimination: kidney

Adverse effects: hypo/hypertension, tachy/bradycardia, respiratory depression, agitation, psychosis, visual disturbance, urticaria

Drug interactions: potentiation of CNS effects by other CNS depressants, cimetidine, MAO inhibitors, volatile anesthetics; antagonized by flumazenil; decreased MAC for volatile anesthetics

Magnesium Sulfate

Effects: decreased acetylcholine release, reduced amplitude of motor endplate potential, decreased sensitivity of motor endplate to acetylcholine, vasodilation, prolonged cardiac conduction time

Uses: toxemia, preeclampsia, hypomagnesemia, tocolytic therapy

Dose: IV, Toxemia, 1–4 g then 1–2 g/hr; hypomagnesemia, 10–15 mg/kg, then 1 g/hr

Onset: IV, rapid

DOA: IV, 30 min

Elimination: renal

Adverse effects: hypotension, circulatory collapse, flaccid paralysis, heart block, decreased reflexes, hypocalcemia

Drug interactions: muscle relaxant potentiation; potentiation of CNS effects of volatile anesthetics, sedatives, narcotics; CNS depression and neuromuscular effects antagonized by calcium

Mannitol (Osmitrol)

Effects: osmotic diuretic that inhibits tubular reabsorption of water and electrolytes in patients susceptible to renal failure

Uses: diuretic, "renal protection," to help reduce increased intracranial and intraocular pressure

Dose: IV (oliguria), 0.25–1 g/kg; IV (intracranial and/or intraocular hypertension), 0.5–2 g/kg

Onset: diuresis, 15–60 min; increased ICP, <15 min; increased IOP, 30–60 min

DOA: diuresis, 3–8 hr; increased ICP, 4–6 hr; increased IOP, 3–8 hr

Metabolism: minimal

Elimination: kidney

Adverse effects: hyper/hypotension, pulmonary edema, tachycardia, seizures, nausea/vomiting, electrolyte imbalances, hypervolemia

Drug interactions: urinary lithium excretion increased

Meperidine (Pethidine, Demerol)

Effects: synthetic opioid with more rapid onset and shorter DOA than morphine, 100 mg equivalent to 10 mg morphine

Uses: analgesia, premedication, antishivering

Dose: IV, 0.2–0.5 mg/kg; IM, 1 mg/kg

Onset: IV, 1–5 min; IM, 5–10 min

DOA: 3–5 hr

Metabolism: liver

Elimination: kidney

Adverse effects: tachycardia, hypotension, respiratory arrest, laryngospasm, dysphoria, seizures, biliary tract spasm, chest wall rigidity

Drug interactions: potential fatal reaction with MAO inhibitors, potentiates CNS-depressant drugs, analgesia enhanced by α-agonists, aggravates adverse effects of isoniazid, chemically incompatible with barbiturates

Mephentermine (Wyamine)

Effects: synthetic noncatecholamine α- and β-receptor sympathetic agonist

Uses: inotrope, vasoconstriction
Dose: IV/IM, 15–45 mg (0.4 mg/kg)

Mepivacaine HCl (Carbocaine, Polocaine)

Effects: tertiary amine, local anesthetic that inhibits initiation and transmission of neuronal impulses; similar to lidocaine with slightly longer DOA
Uses: regional, local anesthesia
Dose: infiltration, 50–400 mg; nerve block, 300–400 mg; epidural, 150–400 mg (5–6 mg/kg); epidural with epi, 500 mg maximum
Onset: infiltration, 3–5 min; epidural, 5–15 min
DOA: infiltration, 45 min–1.5 hr; epidural, 3–5 hr
Elimination: liver
Adverse effects: hypotension, bradycardia, cardiac arrest, respiratory arrest, seizure, tinnitus
Drug interactions: cimetidine and β-blockers reduce clearance

Metaproterenol (Alupent, Orciprenaline)

Effects: β-adrenergic stimulation (β_2 mostly) causing bronchodilation
Use: bronchospasm
Dose: aerosol, 2–3 puffs (0.65 mg/puff) g 3–4 hr; inhaled, 0.2–0.3 ml of 5% solution in 2.5 ml NS q 4 hr; p.o., 20 mg q 6–8 hr

Methadone HCl (Dolophine, Westadone)

Effects: synthetic narcotic analgesic with actions similar to those of morphine
Uses: analgesia, premedication, detoxification of narcotic addiction
Dose: analgesia IV/IM/p.o., 2.5–10 mg q 3–4 hr
Onset: IV, minutes; IM/p.o., 30–60 min
DOA: IV/IM/p.o., 4–6 hr
Metabolism: liver
Elimination: liver, kidney
Adverse effects: hypotension, bradycardia, respiratory depression, dysphoria, biliary tract spasm, urticaria
Drug interactions: antagonized by rifampin, severe reactions

with MAO inhibitors, CNS and cardiovascular depressants are potentiated, enhanced by α_2 agonists

Methohexital Sodium (Brevital)

Effects: oxybarbiturate producing rapid, ultrashort anesthesia, no analgesia or muscle relaxation
Use: induction agent
Dose: IV, 1.5–2.5 mg/kg; IM, 7–10 mg/kg; p.r., 20–30 mg/kg
Onset: IV, rapid, p.r., 5–7 min
DOA: IV, 5–10 min; p.r., 45 min
Metabolism: liver
Elimination: liver, kidney
Adverse effects: cardiovascular depression, apnea, laryngospasm, arrhythmias, hiccups, muscle tremors, pain at injection site
Drug interactions: potentiation of CNS and circulatory depressants; decreased effects of digoxin, β-blockers, corticosteroids, quinidine and theophylline; prolonged by MAO inhibitors; incompatible with lactated Ringer's, atropine sulfate, succinylcholine, metocurine iodide

Methoxamine HCl (Vasoxyl)

Effects: α_1 receptor agonist causing prompt and prolonged rise in blood pressure with increases in peripheral vascular resistance
Uses: vasoconstrictor, paroxysmal atrial tachycardia
Dose: IV, 1–5 mg (slowly); IM, 5–15 mg

Methyldopa (Aldomet, Methyldopate)

Effects: acts on the CNS to lower blood pressure; in the CNS, it is converted to α-methylnorepinephrine, which acts on α_2-receptors to decrease sympathetic output
Use: hypertension
Dose: IV/p.o., 250–500 mg bid or tid (20–40 mg/kg/day)
Onset: IV, 1–2 hr; p.o., 3–6 hr
DOA: IV, 10–16 hr; p.o., 12–24 hr
Metabolism: liver
Elimination: kidney
Adverse effects: bradycardia, hypotension, sedation, Bell's palsy,

nausea/vomiting, jaundice, thrombocytopenia, positive Coomb's test

Drug interaction: reduced MAC for volatile anesthetics, paradoxical hypertension when given with propranolol, Coomb's positive test for hemolytic anemia

Methylene Blue (Methylthionine Chloride, Urolene Blue)

Effects: oxidation-reduction action, tissue-staining property

Uses: treatment of drug-induced methemoglobinemia, urinary aseptic, body tissue dye

Dose: IV, 1–2 mg/kg; p.o., 65–130 mg tid

Methylergonovine Maleate (Methergine)

Effects: semisynthetic ergot alkaloid with direct action on the smooth muscle of the uterus to increase the amplitude, rate, and tone of uterine contractions

Uses: postpartum hemorrhage and uterine atony

Dose: IV/IM, 0.2 mg (over 60 sec IV); p.o., 0.2–0.4 mg q 4–6 hr

Methylprednisolone (Solu-Medrol)

Effects: prednisolone derivative with antiinflammatory potency (4 mg is equal to 5 mg prednisolone) with less tendency toward salt and water retention than with other steroids

Dose: (non-life-threatening conditions) IV/IM 10–250 mg q 4–24 hr; (life-threatening conditions) IV, 100–250 mg q 2–6 hr

Uses: allergic reactions, steroid replacement, inflammation, organ transplantation

Onset: IV, rapid

DOA: IV, 12–36 hr

Metabolism: liver microsomes

Elimination: kidney

Adverse effects: arrhythmias, hypertension, seizures, psychosis, increased intracranial pressure, impaired wound healing, osteoporosis, aseptic necrosis

Drug interactions: clearance increased by phenytoin, phenobarbital, ephedrine, and rifampin; enhanced effect in hypothyroid and cirrhotic patients; increased potassium wasting with potassium-wasting diuretics

Metoclopramide (Reglan)

Effects: stimulation of upper GI tract motility and increased lower esophageal sphincter tone, inhibition of vomiting mediated by the chemoreceptor trigger zone

Uses: stimulate gastric emptying, antiemetic, gastric reflux, diabetic gastroparesis, aspiration prophylaxis

Dose: IV/IM/p.o., 5–20 mg

Onset: IV, 1–3 min; IM, 10–15 min; p.o., 30–60 min

DOA: IV/IM/p.o., 1–2 hr

Metabolism: liver

Elimination: kidney

Adverse effects: hyper/hypotension, arrhythmias, extrapyramidal reactions, anxiety, nausea, diarrhea, hypoglycemia

Drug interactions: sedative effects enhanced by other CNS depressants, GI motility effects antagonized by anticholinergics and narcotics

Metocurine Iodide (Metubine)

Effects: nondepolarizing neuromuscular blockade of the myoneural junction, hemodynamic stability with small doses

Use: nondepolarizing muscle relaxant

Dose: IV (intubation), 0.4 mg/kg

Onset: IV, 4–6 min

DOA: IV, 40–80 min

Metabolism: minimal

Elimination: kidney, liver (slight)

Adverse effects: mild histamine release, autonomic ganglion blockade

Drug interactions: potentiated by volatile anesthetics, aminoglycoside antibiotics, local anesthetics and numerous other drugs; decreased effect with phenytoin

Metoprolol Tartrate (Lopressor, Toprol XL)

Effects: cardioselective β-blockade, slows AV conduction

Uses: hypertension, supraventricular and ventricular arrhythmias, acute myocardial infarction

Dose: IV, 1–5 mg (1–2 mg for hypertension); p.o., 50–100 mg qid or bid

Onset: IV, rapid; p.o., within 15 min

DOA: IV/p.o., 5–8 hr

Metabolism: liver

Elimination: kidney

Adverse effects: hypotension, bronchospasm, depression, nausea/vomiting, thrombocytopenia purpura, rebound hypertension with abrupt withdrawal, may produce significant first-, second-, or third-degree heart block

Drug interactions: potentiation of muscle relaxants, hypotensive effects potentiated by volatile anesthetics, causes prolonged hyperkalemia after succinylcholine, increases serum levels of digoxin and morphine

Midazolam HCl (Versed)

Effects: short-acting benzodiazepine that facilitates the effects of GABA in the CNS, 2–3 times more potent than diazepam

Uses: sedation, premedication, amnesia, induction of anesthesia, anesthetic supplements

Dose:

Induction IV, 0.2–0.3 mg/kg (healthy patients)

Induction IV, 0.1–0.2 mg/kg (ill patients)

Sedation IM, 0.04–0.08 mg/kg

Sedation IV, 0.02–0.05 mg/kg

Sedation p.o., 0.2–0.5 mg/kg

Sedation IN, 0.2–0.8 mg/kg

Onset: IV, 1–3 min

DOA: IV, 12–60 min

Metabolism: liver

Elimination: kidney

Adverse effects: tachycardia, hypotension, bronchospasm, apnea especially in combination with narcotics, agitation, pruritus

Drug interactions: circulatory and CNS effects potentiated by other CNS depressants, MAC of volatile anesthetics decreased, effects antagonized by flumezanil

Mivacurium Chloride (Mivacron)

Effects: Short-acting nondepolarizing neuromuscular blocking agent, metabolized by plasma cholinesterase, has minimal cumulative effect

Uses: nondepolarizing muscle relaxant

Doses: IV, (intubation), 0.15 mg/kg
Onset: IV, 2–4 min
DOA: IV, 8–15 min
Metabolism/elimination: plasma cholinesterase
Adverse effects: hypotension, tachy/bradycardia, vasodilation, bronchospasm, urticaria, rash, histamine release
Drug interactions: resistance or reversal of effects with administration of theophylline; potentiated by succinylcholine, volatile anesthetics, aminoglycosides, antibiotics, local anesthetics, magnesium, lithium, ganglionic-blocking agents

Morphine Sulfate (Astramorph, Duramorph, Morphine, MS Contin)

Effects: CNS effects causing analgesia, drowsiness, euphoria, respiratory depression (dose-related); vascular effects causing decreased peripheral vascular resistance via arteriolar and venous dilation; adverse effects on GI tract contractions; activation of the chemoreceptor trigger zone causing nausea, histamine release
Uses: analgesia, premedication, anesthesia, pain and dyspnea of myocardial ischemia
Dose: premedication/analgesia, IV, 0.05–0.1 mg/kg; IM/s.c., 0.1 mg/kg
Onset: IV, rapid; IM, 1–5 min
DOA: IV/IM/s.c., 3–5 hr
Metabolism: liver
Elimination: kidney
Adverse effects: respiratory depression, bronchospasm, bradycardia, hypotension, chest wall rigidity, dysphoria, nausea/vomiting, pruritus, histamine release, increased biliary pressure
Drug interactions: depressant effects potentiated by other CNS depressant drugs, analgesia enhanced by α_2 agonists, decreased effects of diuretics in patients with CHF

Nadolol (Corgard)

Effects: nonselective β-adrenergic blocker
Uses: hypertension, angina
Dose: p.o., 40–320 mg/day

Nalbuphine HCl (Nubain)

Effects: κ receptor agonist, moderately potent μ-receptor antagonist; less sedating than butorphanol, initial respiratory depression similar to that with morphine but a ceiling effect with larger doses, mixed narcotic agonist/antagonist

Uses: anesthesia, analgesia

Dose: IV/IM/s.c., 10 mg

Onset: IV, 2–3 min; IM/s.c., within 15 min

DOA: IV/IM/s.c., 3–5 hr

Adverse effects: hyper/hypotension, tachy/bradycardia, dyspnea, asthma, euphoria, dysphoria, sedation, urticaria, bitter taste, withdrawal symptoms in narcotic-dependent patients

Drug interactions: potentiated depression by other narcotics and CNS depressants

Naloxone HCl (Narcan)

Effects: pure opioid antagonism with no agonist activity; reverses opiate-induced respiratory depression, sedation, hypotension, and analgesia

Uses: reversal of narcotic effects

Dose: IM/s.c., 0.1–1.0 mg; IV, 20–100 μg (0.3–0.6 μg/kg/min titrated to effect up to 10 μg/kg)

Onset: IV, 1–2 min; IM/s.c., 2–5 min

DOA: IV/IM/s.c., 1–4 hr

Metabolism: liver

Elimination: kidney

Adverse effects: hyper/hypotension, tachycardia, pulmonary edema, seizures, nausea/vomiting, cardiac arrhythmias in patients with cardiac disease, narcotic effect may outlast naloxone effects

Drug interactions: reversal of narcotic effects, can cause acute abstinence syndrome

Neostigmine (Prostigmine)

Effects: inhibition of acetylcholine hydrolysis by competitively attaching to the ester site of acetylcholinesterase

Uses: reversal of neuromuscular blockade; treatment of myasthenia gravis, postoperative ileus, and urinary retention

Dose: IV (reversal), 40–70 μg/kg (given with atropine 0.015 mg/kg or glycopyrrolate 0.01 mg/kg); myasthenia gravis, IM/IV (slow) 0.5–2 mg; p.o., 15–375 mg (divided in tid doses)

Onset: IV, 1–5 min; IM, within 20 min; p.o., 45–75 min

DOA: IV, 40–60 min; IM/p.o., 2–4 hr

Metabolism: liver

Elimination: kidney

Adverse effects: bradycardia, AV block, nodal rhythm, hypotension, increased oral and respiratory secretions, bronchospasm, respiratory depression, seizures, increased peristalsis, urinary frequency, rash

Drug interactions: may prolong the phase 1 block of succinylcholine, reduced neuromuscular blockade antagonism in the presence of aminoglycoside antibiotics

Nifedipine (Procardia, Adalat)

Effects: calcium channel blockade, inhibiting the influx of calcium ions across the cell membranes of smooth muscle and cardiac muscle, has greater arterial vasodilatory properties than verapamil, improves myocardial oxygen supply and demand

Uses: hypertension, angina

Dose: p.o., 10–60 mg tid; (unlabeled use), 10 mg s.l. (via punctured capsule)

Onset: p.o., 15–20 min

DOA: p.o., 4–12 hr

Metabolism: liver

Elimination: liver, kidney

Adverse effects: hypotension, bronchospasm, dyspnea, dizziness, diarrhea, joint inflammation

Drug interactions: potentiates effects of muscle relaxants, additive cardiovascular depression with other myocardial depressants, sinus bradycardia when given with concurrent β-blocking drugs, severe hypotension and bradycardia with bupivacaine, when given with IV verapamil and dantrolene may cause cardiovascular collapse

Nimodipine (Nimotop)

Effects: calcium channel blocker
Use: prevention of cerebral arterial spasm (in cases of subarachnoid hemorrhage)
Dose: p.o., 60 mg q 4 hr

Nitroglycerin (Nitrol, Tridil, Nitrostat, Nitrocine, Nitro-bid, Transderm-nitro, Nitrodisc and Ointment)

Effects: an organic nitrate that has a vasodilatory effect primarily on venous capacitance vessels, also causes redistribution of blood to areas of the subendocardium that are ischemic
Uses: myocardial ischemia, CHF, hypertension, pulmonary hypertension
Dose: bolus IV, 50–100 μg; infusion IV, 0.25–2.0 μg/kg/min; s.l., 0.15–0.6 mg q 5 min $\times$3 doses (if needed); ointment, 1/2–2 inches q 8 hr
Onset: IV, 30–60 sec; s.l., 1–3 min; t.d., 40–60 min
DOA: IV, 3–5 min; s.l., 30–60 min; t.d., 18–24 hr
Metabolism: liver
Elimination: liver, kidney
Adverse effects: tachycardia, hypotension, paradoxical bradycardia, angina, headache, abdominal pain, nausea/vomiting, contact dermatitis, methemoglobinemia (in high doses)
Drug interactions: increases bioavailability of dihydroergotamine; hypotensive effects potentiated by antihypertensives, alcohol, phenothiazines, calcium channel blockers, β-adrenergic blockers

Nitroprusside, Sodium (Nipride, Nitropress)

Effects: relaxation of vascular smooth muscle, causing dilation of peripheral arteries and veins with comparatively less effect on veins than nitroglycerin
Uses: hypertension, controlled hypotension, CHF, pulmonary hypertension
Dose: bolus IV, 10–50 μg; infusion IV, begin at 0.1–0.5 μg/kg/min (toxicity more likely with more than 1 mg/kg over 2.5 hr or 0.5 mg/kg/hr over 24 hr)
Onset: IV, 15–30 sec
DOA: IV, 2–5 min

Metabolism: RBC and tissues to convert nitroprusside to cyanmethemoglobin followed by liver metabolism to thiocyanate

Elimination: kidneys

Adverse effects: accumulation of cyanide in liver dysfunction; accumulation of thiocyanate in renal dysfunction; avoid in tobacco amblyopia, hypothyroidism, Leber's hereditary optic atrophy, vitamin B_{12} deficiency; can cause reflex tachycardia and excessive hypotension; unstable when exposed to light; cyanide toxicity should be considered when increasing doses are required, mixed venous O_2 is increased, or metabolic acidosis occurs

Drug interactions: incompatible with other drugs in the same solution, treatment of cyanide toxicity includes sodium nitrate to convert hemoglobin to methemoglobin and infusion of sodium thiosulfate to convert the cyanide to thiocyanate

Norepinephrine Bitartrate (Levophed, Levarterenol)

Effects: potent peripheral vasoconstriction of arteries and veins (α-adrenergic action), ionotropic stimulation of the heart (β-adrenergic action)

Uses: vasoconstriction, inotropy

Dose: infusion IV, 0.1–0.4 μg/kg/min

Onset: infusion IV, within 1 min

DOA: IV, 2–10 min

Metabolism: liver, nerve endings

Elimination: kidney

Adverse effects: hypertension, bradycardia, tachyarrhythmias, CHF, headache

Drug interactions: increased arrhythmias with volatile anesthetics or bretylium; enhanced pressor effect in patients on MAO inhibitors, tricyclic antidepressants, and guanethidine

Ondansetron (Zofran)

Effects: selective serotonin (5-HT$_3$) receptor antagonism, which may prevent serotonin stimulation of vagal afferents; effective without significant sedation

Uses: antiemetic (used against chemotherapy-induced emesis and against vomiting in the perioperative period)

Doses: IV, 4–8 mg (0.15 mg/kg $\times$3 doses); p.o., 4 mg

Elimination: $T_{1/2} = 4$ hr

Metabolism: liver (cytochrome P-450 enzymes)

Elimination: kidney

Adverse effects: diarrhea, headache, constipation, elevated liver enzymes, potentiated in liver disease, rash, bronchospasm, extrapyramidal reactions

Drug interactions: inducers or inhibitors of the cytochrome P-450 enzymes will change the clearance of ondansetron

Oxytocin (Pitocin, Syntocinon)

Effects: natural nonapeptide hormone that stimulates uterine smooth muscle contractions raising their force and frequency and the tone of uterine musculature

Uses: control of postpartum hemorrhage, induction of labor, improvement of uterine contractions

Dose: bolus IV, 0.5–1.0 unit slowly (10–40 U may be placed in 1 liter of IV fluid and given slowly); infusion IV, 10–30 mU/min

Pancuronium Bromide (Pavulon)

Effects: a synthetic bisquarternary amino corticosteroid with long-acting nondepolarizing neuromuscular blockade

Uses: nondepolarizing muscle relaxant

Doses: IV, 0.1 mg/kg (intubation)

Onset: 3–6 min

DOA: 40–90 min

Metabolism: liver (partial)

Elimination: kidney (mostly), liver

Adverse effects: tachycardia, hypertension, apnea, bronchospasm, salivation, anaphylactoid reactions, prolonged neuromuscular block especially in patients with renal or hepatic disease

Drug interactions: potentiated by volatile anesthetics, aminoglycosides, magnesium, local anesthetics, procainamide, quinidine, hypokalemia; patients taking tricyclic antidepressants anesthetized with halothane may develop cardiac dysrhythmias if given pancuronium

Pentobarbital (Nembutal)

Effects: CNS depression, anticonvulsant

Uses: sedation, preoperative medication, acute convulsive episodes

Doses: IV, 50–100 mg, incrementally to a total of 500 mg; IM/
p.o., 100–200 mg/kg (1–2 mg/kg)
Onset: IV, 1 min; IM, 10–30 min; p.o., 30–60 min
DOA: IV, 15 min; IM, 2–3 hr; p.o., 3–4 hr
Metabolism: liver
Elimination: kidney (mostly), liver
Adverse effects: hypotension, hiccups, laryngospasm, porphyria,
respiratory depression
Drug interactions: may antagonize oral anticoagulants

Pentazocine (Talwin)

Effects: κ receptor agonist, mixed agonist/antagonist opioid ef-
fects
Uses: analgesia, opioid agonist/antagonist
Dose: IV/IM or s.c., 20–40 mg
DOA: 3–4 hr
Adverse effects: can cause dysphoria in high doses, withdrawal
symptoms in opioid-dependent patients, hypertension

Phenoxybenzamine (Dibenzyline)

Effects: noncompetitive α-adrenergic antagonism
Uses: vasospasm, hypertension induced by catecholamine ex-
cess, malignant hyperreflexia
Doses: p.o., 10–200 mg/day

Phentolamine (Regitine)

Effects: competitive α-adrenergic antagonism producing vasodilation
Uses: vasospasm, arterial dilation, hypertension from excess catecholamines, pulmonary hypertension, counteract α-agonist
effect
Dose: antihypertensive IV/IM, 2–5 mg; infusion IV, 0.1–1 mg/
min
Onset:IV, 1–2 min; IM, 5–20 min
DOA: IV, 10–15 min; IM, 30–45 min
Metabolism/elimination: liver
Adverse effects: hypotension, reflex tachycardia, myocardial infarction, cerebrovascular spasm, flushing, nausea/vomiting,
diarrhea
Drug interactions: paradoxical fall in blood pressure with epinephrine, ephedrine, dobutamine, and isoproterenol

Phenylephrine HCl (Neo-synephrine)

Effects: α-adrenergic receptor agonism with minimal β-adrenergic activity

Uses: vasoconstriction, hypotension, supraventricular tachyarrhythmias, nasal congestion

Dose: bolus IV, 50–100 μg; infusion IV, 0.10–0.75 μg/kg/min

Onset: IV, within seconds

DOA: IV, 15–20 min

Metabolism: liver, intestine

Adverse effects: reflex bradycardia, arrhythmias, hypertension, headache, uterine contraction, uterine vasoconstriction, extravasation may cause sloughing

Drug interactions: pressor effects enhanced by other sympathomimetics, bretylium, guanethidine, MAO inhibitors, oxytocics; increased arrhythmias with volatile anesthetics

Phenytoin Sodium (Diphenylhydantoin, Dilantin)

Effects: anticonvulsant primarily acting in the motor cortex; it stabilizes neuronal cell membranes by preventing influx or enhancing efflux of sodium ions; it is also a class 1B antiarrhythmic agent decreasing automaticity, action potential duration, velocity of conduction, and effective refractory period of cardiac fibers

Uses: anticonvulsant, lidocaine-resistant ventricular arrhythmias, digitalis toxic arrhythmias, congenital prolonged QT syndrome, trigeminal neuralgia

Dose: anticonvulsant loading IV/p.o., 10–15 mg/kg in 3 divided doses given < 50 mg/min IV with ECG monitoring; maintenance IV/p.o., 100 mg tid; arrhythmias IV, 100 mg (at <50 mg/min) q 10–15 min to maximum 10–15 mg/kg; arrhythmias p.o., 200–400 mg qd

Physostigmine Salicylate (Eserine, Antilirium)

Effects: tertiary amine anticholinesterase agent that increases acetylcholine concentrations, it can crosses the blood-brain barrier

Uses: reversal of anticholinergic effects in the CNS including central anticholinergic syndrome; also reverses peripheral anticholinergic effects associated with drugs such as atropine, scopolamine, and tricyclic antidepressants; nonspecific reversal of the sedative effect of benzodiazepines, phenothiazines, and opioid-induced ventilatory depression

Doses: IV/IM, 0.5–1 mg q 10–30 min for total of 2 doses

Onset: IV/IM, 3–8 min

DOA: IV/IM, 30 min–5 hr

Metabolism: plasma esterases

Elimination: kidney

Adverse effects: bradycardia, seizures, bronchospasm, vomiting, dyspnea, salivation, miosis, tremors, hallucinations, cholinergic crisis

Drug interactions: as above

Pipecuronium Bromide (Arduan)

Effects: long-acting neuromuscular blocking agent that competes for cholinergic receptors at the motor endplate

Uses: neuromuscular blockade

Doses: IV, 0.07–0.085 mg/kg

Onset: IV, 2.5–3 min

DOA: IV, 45–120 min

Metabolism: 75% excreted unchanged

Elimination: kidney

Adverse effects: hyper/hypotension, bradycardia, myocardial infarction, apnea, anuria, rash, hyperkalemia, increased creatinine

Drug interactions: recurrent paralysis with quinidine, decreased effect with theophylline, potentiated by the muscle relaxant activities of other agents

Potassium Chloride

Effects: major intracellular cation with concentration inside the cell up to 40 times that outside the cell

Uses: treatment of hypokalemia, digitalis toxicity, arrhythmias, electrolyte replacement

Doses: IV, 10–20 mEq/hr (concentration in IV fluid not to exceed 40 mEq/liter)

Onset: IV, immediate

DOA: IV, variable

Adverse effects: cardiac arrest, arrhythmias, coma, nausea/vomiting, abdominal pain, ulceration of the esophagus and/or small intestine (oral administration)

Drug interactions: potential life-threatening hyperkalemia with ACE inhibitors, potassium-sparing diuretics; GI toxicity enhanced by anticholinergic drugs

Prilocaine HCl (Citanest)

Effects: amide local anesthetic that prevents initiation of transmission of impulses across the neuronal membrane

Use: regional anesthesia

Dose: IV regional block, 200–300 mg; brachial plexus block, 300–600 mg; epidural, 200–300 mg

Onset: infiltration, 1–2 min; epidural, 5–15 min (can be tripled by adding epinephrine)

DOA: infiltration, 0.5–1.5 hr; epidural, 1–3 hr, prolonged with epinephrine

Metabolism/elimination: liver, lungs

Adverse effects: methemoglobinemia (treated with methylene blue 1–2 mg/kg), hypotension, arrhythmias, cardiovascular collapse, respiratory paralysis, seizures, urticaria, anaphylactoid reactions

Drug interactions: reduced clearance with β-blockers and cimetidine, DOA prolonged with addition of epinephrine

Procainamide HCl (Procan SR, Pronestyl)

Effects: class 1A antiarrhythmic (membrane stabilizer); increases the effective refractory period and reduces impulse conduction velocity in the atria, His-Purkinje fibers, and ventricular muscle; fast sodium channel blockade

Uses: lidocaine-resistant ventricular arrhythmias, premature ventricular contraction (PVC), arrhythmias in malignant hyperpyrexia, atrial fibrillation or PSVT

Dose: loading dose IV, 100 mg (7–10 mg/kg); infusion IV, 100 mg q 5 min to maximum 1 g; maintenance infusion, 2–6 mg/min

Onset: IV, immediate

DOA: IV, 2.5–5 hr (depending on fast vs slow acetylator)

Metabolism: liver (acetylation)

Elimination: kidney

Adverse effects: hypotension, heart block, prolonged QT interval, cardiac arrhythmias, seizures, diarrhea, thrombocytopenia, neutropenia, anemia, agranulocytosis, angioneurotic edema

Drug interactions: hypotension potentiated with other antiarrhythmics, ventricular asystole with digitalis toxic heart block,
potentiation of muscle relaxants, increased serum levels with
either cimetidine or ranitidine

Procaine HCI (Novocaine)

Effects: benzoic acid, ester local anesthetic with vasodilator ac-
tivity, has a rapid onset of action and short duration
Use: regional anesthesia
Dose: infiltration/epidural, less than 500 mg; spinal, 50–200 mg
Elimination: plasma pseudocholinesterase

Prochlorperazine (Compazine)

Effects: a piperazine phenothiazine with central antidopaminergic actions
Uses: antiemetic, antipsychotic
Dose: antiemetic p.o., 5–10 mg; IV/IM, 5–10 mg; rectal, 25 mg
bid

Promethazine HCI (Phenergan)

Effects: a histamine H_2 receptor antagonist with sedative, anti-
emetic and anticholinergic effects
Uses: antiemetic, premedication, sedation, allergies
Dose: IV/deep IM/p.o./rectal, 12.5–50 mg

Propofol (Diprivan)

Effects: diisopropylphenol, a hypnotic agent given IV that in-
duces a rapid onset of anesthesia with extensive redistribution and rapid elimination, it is associated with some slight
excitatory activity such as myoclonus, more rapid recovery
with less nausea/vomiting than with thiopental
Uses: induction and/or maintenance of anesthesia, sedation
Dose: IV bolus, 1.5–3 mg/kg (in sick patients; 1–2 mg/kg); infusion, 0.1–0.2 mg/kg/min
Onset: IV, one circulation time
DOA: IV, 2–5 min
Metabolism/elimination: hepatic, extrahepatic
Adverse effects: pain on injection, hypotension, tachy/bradycar-
dia, apnea, hiccups, broncho/laryngospasm, euphoria, clo-
nic, myoclonic movement, erythema, pruritus; must be used

within 6 hr after vial is opened to prevent bacterial growth in the solution

Drug interactions: potentiates CNS and circulatory depressant effects of volatile anesthetics, narcotics, and hypnotics

Propranolol HCl (Inderal)

Effects: nonselective β-adrenergic receptor antagonist with no intrinsic sympathomimetic activity

Uses: antiarrhythmic for both supraventricular and ventricular arrhythmias; antihypertensive; antianginal; used in the treatment of myocardial infarction; thyrotoxicosis, tremors, pheochromocytoma; used in migraine prophylaxis

Dose: IV, 0.5–1 mg

Onset: IV, within 2 min

DOA: IV, 1–6 hr

Metabolism: liver

Elimination: kidney, liver

Adverse effects: CHF, AV dissociation, bronchospasm, bradycardia, drowsiness, hypoglycemia

Drug interaction: myocardial depression of inhaled and injected anesthetics is potentiated; additive effects with calcium channel blockers and catecholamine-depleting drugs; theophylline and lidocaine clearance is decreased; potentiates digoxin, succinylcholine, d-tubocurarine and vasoconstrictive effects of epinephrine

Prostaglandin E$_1$, Alprostadil (Prostin VR)

Effects: vasodilation and decreased blood pressure, relaxes smooth muscle of the ductus arteriosus

Uses: maintain patency of the ductus arteriosus, treatment of pulmonary hypertension and right heart failure

Dose IV: 0.05–0.4 μg/kg/min

Protamine Sulfate

Effects: combines with heparin to form a stable complex with no anticoagulant activity

Uses: reversal of heparin effects

Dose: slow IV, 1 mg per 90 U of lung heparin or 1 mg per 115 U of intestinal heparin

Onset: IV, within 1 min

DOA: IV, 2 hr

Metabolism/elimination: liver

Adverse effects: hyper/hypotension, bradycardia, pulmonary hypertension, bronchospasm, myocardial depression, thrombocytopenia, anaphylaxis with hypotension especially if given too rapidly

Drug interactions: potentiates vasodilators, incompatible with solutions of penicillin and cephalosporin

Pyridostigmine Bromide (Mestinon, Regonol)

Effects: anticholinesterase agent with slower onset and longer DOA than neostigmine, no significant crossing of blood-brain barrier

Uses: muscle relaxant reversal, treatment of myasthenia gravis

Dose: IV (for reversal), 0.15–0.25 mg/kg given with atropine 15 μg/kg; p.o. (for myasthenia), 60–1500 mg/day

Onset: IV, 2–5 min; p.o., 20–30 min

DOA: IV, 1–3 hr; p.o., 3–6 hr

Metabolism: cholinesterases in liver and tissue

Elimination: kidney (75%), liver

Adverse effects: bradycardia, AV block, increased bronchial secretions, bronchospasm, abdominal cramps, increased peristalsis, increased salivation, muscle cramps, fasciculations, miosis, diaphoresis

Drug interactions: may prolong the phase 1 block of succinylcholine, effectiveness in antagonism of neuromuscular blockade is decreased by aminoglycoside antibiotics

Quinidine Gluconate (Quinaglute)

Effects: class IA antiarrhythmic; depressing myocardial excitability, conduction velocity and contractility

Uses: atrial and ventricular arrhythmias

Dose: IV, 300–750 mg at no more than 16 mg/min (monitor ECG)

Ranitidine (Zantac)

Effects: a histamine H_2 receptor antagonist that blocks induced secretion of hydrogen ions by gastric parietal cells, produces suppression of histamine-induced peripheral vasodilation and inotropic effects, minimal crossing of blood-brain barrier

Uses: treatment of gastroesophageal reflux, prophylaxis against acid pulmonary aspiration, treatment of duodenal ulcer

Dose: IV/IM, 50 mg q 6–8 hr (IV dose given over 5–15 min); p.o., 150 mg bid

Onset: IV, within 15 min; p.o., within 30 min

DOA: IV, 6–8 hr; p.o., 8–12 hr

Metabolism: liver

Elimination: kidney

Adverse effects: tachy/bradycardia, PVCs with rapid IV injection, bronchospasm, headache, depression, hepatitis, diarrhea, thrombocytopenia, erythema multiforme

Drug interactions: may interfere with warfarin clearance, absorption decreased by antacids, may decrease diazepam absorption

Ritodrine HCl (Yutopar)

Use: tocolytic (uterine relaxation)

Rocuronium Bromide (Zemuron)

Effects: rapid onset, medium duration, neuromuscular blocking agent

Use: nondepolarizing muscle relaxant

Dose: bolus IV, 0.45–0.6 mg/kg (intubation); infusion IV, 0.01–0.012 mg/kg/min

Onset: 60–78 sec

DOA: 22–31 min

Metabolism/elimination: liver

Adverse effects: prolonged neuromuscular block in hepatic failure, arrhythmias, ECG abnormalities, tachycardia, nausea/vomiting, asthma, rash, localized edema, pruritus, local irritation with extravasation

Drug interactions: slightly prolonged DOA with isoflurane and enflurane, shorter DOA in patient on anticonvulsant drugs, possible prolonged DOA with antibiotics, possible enhanced neuromuscular blockade with magnesium sulfate

Scopolamine Hydrobromide

Effects: antagonizes the action of acetylcholine at postganglionic nerve endings with more sedative effect than atropine, crosses the blood-brain barrier, less tachycardia than with atropine

Uses: amnestic, premedication, sedation, antisialagogue, antiemetic

Dose: IV/IM/s.l., 0.20–0.6 mg; p.o., 0.4–0.8 mg; patch, behind ear night before or after surgery for treatment of nausea or motion sickness, 1.5mg

Sodium Citrate (Shohl's Solution, Bicitra)

Effects: nonparticulate buffer used to neutralize gastric acid
Uses: aspiration prophylaxis, antacid, systemic alkalinization
Dose: p.o., 15–30 ml diluted with 15–30 ml water
Onset: p.o., rapid
DOA: p.o., 2 hr
Metabolism/elimination: liver
Adverse effects: seizures, nausea/vomiting, alkalosis
Drug interactions: alkalosis more pronounced in hypocalcemia

Sodium Nitrite

Effects: forms methemoglobin (metHb), which can bind with cyanide
Use: cyanide poisoning
Dose: IV, 300 mg in 10 ml at 2.5–5 ml/min

Succinylcholine Chloride (Anectine, Quelicin, Sucostrin)

Effects: extremely short-acting depolarizing skeletal muscle relaxant, combines with the cholinergic receptors of the motor endplate producing depolarization
Uses: neuromuscular blockade
Dose: IV, 1 mg/kg; if pretreatment with a small dose of nondepolarizing muscle relaxant is used, give 1.5–2 mg/kg
Onset: IV, 30–60 sec
DOA: IV, 3–5 min
Metabolism: blood pseudocholinesterase
Elimination: kidney

Adverse effects: arrhythmias, bradycardia, myoglobinuria, transient muscarinic and nicotinic stimulation, increases in intraocular and intragastric pressures, prolonged blockade with pseudocholinesterase deficiency, phase II block with large doses, hyperkalemia with accentuated potassium release in certain clinical states: burns, paralysis, massive tissue trauma, Guillain-Barré syndrome, muscular dystrophy

Drug interactions: prolonged block in patients receiving β-adrenergic blockers, lidocaine, magnesium, anticholinesterases, trimethaphan, volatile anesthetics, procainamide, phenelzine; precipitation with sodium thiopental and incompatible with alkaline solutions

Sufentanil Citrate (Sufenta)

Effects: an analogue of fentanyl with 5–7 times more analgesic potency with similar cardiovascular effects

Uses: induction of general anesthesia, analgesia, anesthesia

Dose: induction IV, 0.5–1.5 μg/kg with barbiturate or benzodiazepines; infusion IV, 0.1–1 μg/kg/hr; sedation IV, 5–10 μg q 10–30 min; cardiac surgery IV, 8–30 μg/kg; epidural bolus, 5–20 μg; epidural infusion, 2–10 μg/hr

Onset: IV, immediate; epidural, 4–10 min

DOA: IV, 20–45 min; epidural, 4–8 hr

Metabolism: liver, small intestine

Elimination: kidney

Adverse effects: dose-related muscle rigidity and bradycardia, hypotension, apnea, euphoria, dysphoria, nausea/vomiting, biliary tract spasm, delayed gastric emptying

Drug interactions: circulatory and ventilatory depression potentiated by other narcotics, sedatives, volatile anesthetics and nitrous oxide; ventilatory depression enhanced by MAO inhibitors, phenothiazines, and tricyclic antidepressants; bradycardia with vecuronium

Terbutaline Sulfate (Brethaire, Bricanyl)

Effects: β_2-adrenergic receptor agonist with some β_1 effects

Uses: bronchodilation, premature labor (tocolytic)

Dose:

Bronchodilation, s.c., 0.25 mg

Bronchodilation, inhalation, 2 puffs q 4–6 hr

Bronchodilation, p.o., 2.5–5 mg tid
To inhibit premature labor, IV, 10–80 μg/min
To inhibit premature labor, p.o., 2.5 mg q 4–6 hr

Tetracaine (Pontocaine)

Effects: potent long-acting local anesthetic with prolonged DOA compared with procaine or chloroprocaine because of slower rate of hydrolysis by plasma cholinesterase
Uses: topical and regional anesthesia
Dose: spinal, 5–20 mg; topical (2% solution), 1-sec application (average 1-sec spray contains 200 mg)
Onset: spinal, < 10 min
DOA: spinal, 1.25–3.0 hr
Metabolism/elimination: plasma cholinesterase
Adverse effects: hypotension, peripheral vasodilation, bradycardia, heart block, respiratory paralysis, seizures, angioneurotic edema
Drug interactions: duration of regional anesthesia prolonged by vasoconstrictor agents such as epinephrine, prolongs effects of succinylcholine, toxicity is enhanced by cimetidine and anticholinesterase

Thiopental Sodium (Pentothal, Thiopentone)

Effects: ultra-short-acting barbiturate with CNS depressant effects producing hypnosis and anesthesia, but no analgesia
Uses: induction of anesthesia, sedation, anticonvulsant, reduction of increased intracranial pressure
Dose: IV, 3–5 mg/kg (in healthy patients), 2–3 mg/kg (in sick patients); rectal, 25 mg/kg
Onset: IV, one circulation time rectal, 5–8 min
DOA: IV, 5–15 min;
Metabolism: liver
Elimination: kidney
Adverse effects: respiratory and circulatory depression, apnea, broncho/laryngospasm, delirium on emergence, nausea/vomiting, thrombophlebitis (high pH), pruritus, anaphylactic reactions
Drug interactions: potentiates the CNS and circulatory depressant effects of other hypnotics, narcotics, volatile anesthetics, and alcohol; decreased effects of oral anticoagulants, β-block-

ers, digoxin, corticosteroids, theophylline; effects prolonged by MAO inhibitors and chloramphenicol; incompatible with solutions at an acid pH (e.g., d-tubocurarine, succinylcholine)

Trimethaphan Camsylate (Arfonad)

Effects: nicotinic ganglionic receptor blockade; rapid, extremely brief onset, therefore is given as a continuous IV infusion; dilates capacitance vessels

Uses: hypertension, vasodilation, controlled hypotension

Dose: infusion, 0.3–6 mg/min

Onset: rapid

DOA: 10–30 min

Metabolism: plasma cholinesterase

Adverse effects: mydriasis, histamine release

d-Tubocurarine Chloride

Effect: an intermediate, nondepolarizing neuromuscular blocking agent that competes for motor endplate cholinergic receptors, releases histamine, has autonomic ganglion blockade

Uses: nondepolarizing muscle relaxant, defasciculating agent prior to succinylcholine

Dose: IV, 0.3–0.6 mg/kg (intubation); infusion, 2 μg/kg/min

Onset: IV, 2–4 min

DOA: IV, 30–90 min

Metabolism: minimal

Elimination: liver (40%), kidney (60%)

Adverse effects: significant histamine release, autonomic ganglion blockade producing hypotension, duration increased in renal failure, bradycardia, apnea, rash

Drug interactions: effects potentiated by inhalation anesthetics, aminoglycoside antibiotics, local anesthetics, diuretics, magnesium, lithium; resistance to effects in the presence of phenytoin; reduces MAC requirement for inhalation anesthetics

Vasopressin (Pitressin, Antidiuretic Hormone)

Effects: a synthetic analogue of arginine vasopressin or antidiuretic hormone (ADH) which increases the reabsorption of water by the renal tubules, contracts smooth muscle of the GI tract and vascular bed

Uses: diagnosis and treatment of diabetes insipidus; treatment of GI hemorrhage and hemophilia; control of postoperative ileus

Dose: diabetes insipidus, s.c./IM, 5–10 units bid or tid; GI hemorrhage, infusion 0.2–0.4 units/min to maximum of 0.9 units/min

Vecuronium Bromide (Norcuron)

Effects: nondepolarizing muscle relaxant of intermediate duration, a monoquaternary analogue of pancuronium that competes for cholinergic receptors at the motor endplate, minimal cardiovascular effects, minimal histamine release

Uses: nondepolarizing muscle relaxant

Dose: IV, 0.08–0.12 mg/kg (intubating); infusion IV, 1–2 μg/kg/min

Onset: IV, 2.5–3 min

DOA: IV, 45 min

Metabolism: liver

Elimination: liver, kidney

Adverse effects: duration increased 40–60% in hepatic/renal disease

Drug interactions: potentiated by inhalation anesthetics, succinylcholine, aminoglycoside antibiotics, diuretics, local anesthetics, magnesium, lithium; reversal of effects with theophylline

Verapamil HCl (Calan, Isoptin)

Effects: calcium channel blockade, decreases AV nodal conduction, reduces ventricular rate in atrial flutter or fibrillation; interrupts reentry at the AV node and restores normal sinus rhythm in patients with PSVT

Uses: Treatment of PSVT (not WPW), hypertension, angina, treatment of atrial fibrillation/flutter with rapid ventricular response

Doses: arrhythmias, IV, 1.25–5.0 mg (may repeat in 30 min); angina, p.o., 40–120 mg tid; antihypertensive, p.o., 40–80 mg tid

Onset: IV, 2–5 min; p.o., 30 min

DOA: IV, 30–60 min; p.o., 3–7 hr
Metabolism: liver
Elimination: liver, kidney
Adverse effects: significant hypotension can occur because of negative inotropic effects (may be treatable with IV calcium), brady/tachycardia, broncho/laryngospasm, seizures, urticaria
Drug interactions: potentiates all classes of muscle relaxants; cardiovascular depression enhanced by inhalation anesthetics and antihypertensives; with β blockers, can cause CHF, severe AV conduction anomalies and sinus bradycardia; severe hypotension and bradycardia with bupivacaine; cardiovascular collapse with IV dantrolene; decreases lithium effects; decreased clearance with cimetidine; incompatible with bicarbonate and nafcillin

Warfarin (Coumadin, Panwarfin, Athrombin-k)

Effects: interferes with vitamin K utilization by the liver causing inhibition of synthesis of factors II, VII, IX and X
Uses: anticoagulation
Dose: p.o., 2–15 mg q d based on prothrombin time

Index

Page numbers followed by "t" denote tables, those followed by "f" denote figures.

relation of amount to duration
of, 102
toxicity of, 92
Buprenorphine (Buprenex), 544
pharmacology of, 42
transmucosal bioavailability of,
492
Burns
airway management of, 380
altered pharmacokinetics/phar-
macodynamics with,
386–387
assessment of, 379
carbon monoxide poisoning
potential with, 385–386
classification of, 379–380
fluid resuscitation in, 384
hypothermia potential with,
384–305
infection potential with, 385
monitoring and vascular access
in, 386
outcome of, 379
pathophysiology of, 380–383
skin, postoperative, 481
third degree, anesthetic technique for, 405
Busulfan
interstitial pulmonary fibrosis
with, 235
pulmonary pathophysiology
with, 228t
Butorphanol (Stadol), 544–545
in obstetrics, 450
pharmacology of, 42

Calcitonin, increased levels, 382
Calcium
abnormal levels of, 54–56
body distribution of, 54–56
functions of, 54
for hypocalcemia, 289
rapid replacement in trauma
victims, 391–392
regulation of, 286–287

Calcium channel blockers
before cardiac surgery, 329
in perioperative period, 18
for postoperative hypertension,
475
Calcium chloride, 545
Calcium gluconate, 545
Calcium salts, 49
CaO_2. *See* Arterial blood oxygen
content
Capnography, 21, 246
setup for awake patient, 247f
Capnometer, 160
Capsaicin, topical, 504
Captopril (Capoten), 545–546
for postoperative hypertension,
475
Carbachol, 166
Carbamazepine, 513
Carbon dioxide
absorption of during pneumoperitoneum, 272–273
diminished removal of, 133
end-tidal, with malignant hyperthermia, 139
exhaled, monitoring in pediatric patient, 430–431
increased production of, 132–
133
monitoring, in hypercarbia,
132–133
removal of, 68
retention of, 133
Carbon monoxide
diffusion capacity of lung,
220
poisoning, 227
with burn injury, 381, 383,
385–386
pulse oximetry with, 130
treatment of, 227
Carbonic anhydrase inhibitors,
169
Carboxyhemoglobin, 130
in burn injury, 385